Torres'
Patient Care in Imaging Technology

TENTH EDITION

TerriAnn Ryan, MEd, ARRT (R, M), CRT (R, M, F)

Program Director, Radiologic Technology (Retired)
MercyHealth System
Rockford, Illinois

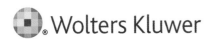 Wolters Kluwer

Philadelphia • Baltimore • New York • London
Buenos Aires • Hong Kong • Sydney • Tokyo

Acquisitions Editor: Nicole Dernoski
Development Editor: Eric McDermott
Editorial Coordinator: Remington Fernando
Editorial Assistant: Kristen Kardoley
Marketing Manager: Kirsten Watrud
Production Project Manager: Kirstin Johnson
Manager, Graphic Arts & Design: Stephen Druding
Manufacturing Coordinator: Beth Welsh/Lisa Bowling
Prepress Vendor: S4Carlisle Publishing Services

Tenth Edition

Library of Congress Cataloging-in-Publication Data

ISBN-13: 978-1-975192-51-8

Cataloging in Publication data available on request from publisher.

QUADM 0523

In loving memory of Leslie Linn

Preface

DEVELOPING SKILLS FOR SAFE, PERCEPTIVE, AND EFFECTIVE PRACTITIONERS

The tenth edition of *Torres' Patient Care in Imaging Technology* not only provides the knowledge and skills that empower students to become safe, perceptive, and effective in providing excellent patient care but also brings attention to real consequences of failed actions. *Focused on connecting classroom learning to clinical practice*, the text is designed to present key concepts effectively for beginning students as well as more advanced students and practitioners who want to improve their skills in patient care and imaging technology for Continuing Qualifications Requirements (CQR).

UPDATED, ENGAGING, AND EFFECTIVE

Torres' Patient Care in Imaging Technology is engaging with its focused, visually attractive, comprehensive approach. Chapters have been redesigned to follow the curriculum and address elements listed in the American Registry of Radiologic Technologists (ARRT) exam content. Outlining key concepts, current trends, and advances in imaging technology and patient care, this book uses a concise style and logical organization to ensure that crucial topics are addressed effectively and efficiently. The appealing full-color design breaks up the text with illustrations and pedagogic features in a way that enhances learning. Bulleted key concepts in the Summary reinforce critical information.

CULTURAL CONSIDERATIONS AND OTHER REAL-WORLD EXPERIENCE

Torres' Patient Care in Imaging Technology's student-centered approach is designed to move from theory to practice quickly. *Cultural Considerations* boxes bring awareness to the diverse cultural and ethnic backgrounds of patients. This complements the strong pedagogic approach of *Torres' Patient Care in Imaging Technology*, which includes online situational judgment questions, skills checklists, and laboratory activities. The newly added "Medical Ethics and the Law" chapter enforces the learning component regarding consequences of actions that are not effectively carried out and care falls below the standard practice of care.

AN INTEGRATED, EFFICIENT, AND EFFECTIVE LEARNING SYSTEM

Torres' Patient Care in Imaging Technology is designed to help every class become a dynamic learning experience. The concise text enables coverage of key concepts in a limited amount of time, yet it is also integrated with rich pedagogic resources that engage students, present concepts in a relevant way, and provide many ways in which to practice and build important skills. The new edition includes *real-world case studies*, *demonstration videos*, and *laboratory activities* to bring to life situations that will be faced every day on the job.

FROM THE AUTHOR

Forty years ago, the first edition of this book was published. It was first named *Basic Medical Techniques and Patient Care for Radiologic Technologists*. The author, Lillian Torres, and her consultants had no idea of the degree or magnitude of changes that would take place in the profession of radiologic technology. Each edition of this book has made contributions to the education in the field by meeting the changing needs of students and educators and by making improvements in the teaching of patient care. Patient care is the foundation of medical imaging, and although health care may change, high-quality patient care should not.

The tenth edition of this book has been altered to address the needs of the beginning student in the profession. It includes the latest techniques used in imaging and meets the current requirements of the American Society of Radiologic Technologists (ASRT) and the ARRT. Cultural diversity is addressed throughout the text and is expanded upon in the new chapter "Patient Populations." Students studying for their board exams will find that this new edition addresses all components of the ARRT curriculum and the exam for radiologic technology.

HIGHLIGHTS OF THE TENTH EDITION

- The chapters have been completely revamped to address the components of the most current ARRT radiologic technology curriculum.
- A new chapter devoted to medical ethics and the law has been added to adequately address legal considerations and the standard practice of care. More real-life case studies have been added and demonstrate how the radiographer can be held accountable for a "mistake" that resulted in harm to a patient.
- All chapters have been reviewed and updated to include the most current and relevant information.
- The pharmacology and drug administration chapters have been revised to more accurately reflect the ARRT curriculum.
- Some chapters have been deleted completely or combined with other chapters as the field and profession of radiologic technology have changed.

- Chapters are now more in line with the ARRT curriculum.
- All tables and displays have been updated; more color photos have been added and more radiographic images have been included to enhance the information presented.
- Procedures are placed in a step-by-step format for quick and easy reference for student and instructor use.
- Infection control in imaging is stressed and includes the current threats to the health care of patients and all health care workers. Methods of protecting all involved in patient care from nosocomial infections are emphasized.
- More call out and warning boxes have been added to provide students with notice of vital concepts.

It is the hope of the author that the changes in the tenth edition will assist radiologic technology students to be safe and sensitive practitioners in every aspect of patient care.

TerriAnn Ryan, *MEd, ARRT (R, M), CRT (R, M, F)*

Acknowledgments

A large revision like this does not come together without the help of many people working to pull it all together. I would like to extend a special thank you to those people at this time.

To the members of Beloit Health Care, Beloit, WI; Mayo Clinic, Rochester, MN; Alamar Health, Alexandria, MN; SSM Health, Janesville, WI; and Physician's Immediate Care, Machesney Park, IL—Thank you! All of you allowed me to be a patient and an author concurrently. Being a patient at the same time as revising a book gave me a new perspective on patient care. Some of the scenarios and case studies stem from my experiences.

To Heather Shaw, RT (R); Michael Ayers, RT (R); Megan Johnson, RT (R); Vanessa Tellez, RN; Luis Rivera, MD; and Michael Hess—Thank you! You were all perfect models to demonstrate the necessary operations of quality patient care.

For the professional advice from the acquisitions editors, production managers, and editorial coordinators at Wolters Kluwer/Lippincott Williams & Wilkins—Thank you! Remington Fernando, you have my special thanks for always being there to answer my questions or direct them on to someone you knew could help. Eric McDermott has been with me through the entire process when we started in May 2021. You deserve a raise for putting up with me! To Samson Premkumar Charly who headed up the typesetting and whatever magic he and his team worked to change my duplicated or missing information into a finished and polished product—Thank you all!

For my husband Jack—Thank you! Thank you for your understanding throughout a crazy year of my living in "the hole" where my office is. I know I promised working on this would not consume my entire waking hours for the last 16 months. Many times, it did and you were always there, with dinner ready. You mean the world to me.

TerriAnn Ryan

Brief Contents

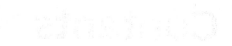

Contents

User's Guide

This User's Guide shows how to put the features of *Torres' Patient Care in Imaging Technology*, 10th Edition, to work.

CHAPTER-OPENING ELEMENTS

Each chapter begins with the following elements to provide orientation to the material.

Objectives provide a quick overview of the content to be covered.

Key Terms are listed and defined at the beginning of each chapter. These help bring extra attention to alert the student of those terms that have significance in the text.

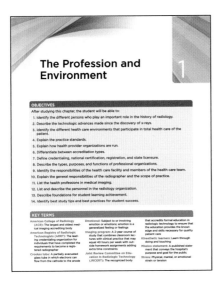

SPECIAL FEATURES

Unique chapter features aid in comprehension and retention of information. These include:

Procedure Boxes with accompanying online videos help master the steps needed to ensure the safety of everyone involved.

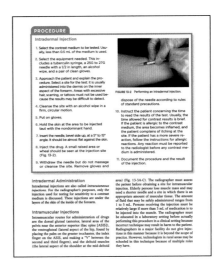

Full-Color Photos and Radiographic Images allow visualization of key techniques and procedures.

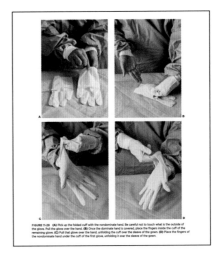

Display Boxes highlight important accreditation, competency, and skills information.

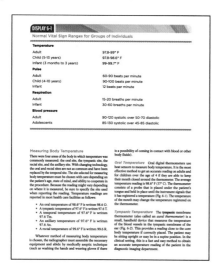

Call Out and Warning Boxes bring attention to important facts and away from common pitfalls.

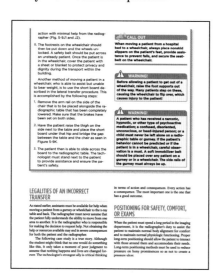

Case Studies with Issues to Consider provide real-life (and, in many cases, true) situations that stimulate thought-provoking discussions that allow students to think through what occurred and determine what could have been done for different outcomes.

Cultural Considerations have been set aside in boxes to bring attention to this important aspect of patient care in every chapter. An entire section is now devoted to cultural awareness in Chapter 4, which brings awareness to the diverse cultural and ethnic backgrounds of patients.

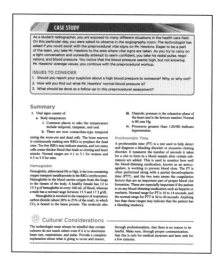

CHAPTER-CLOSING ELEMENTS

Each chapter closes with the following elements, which helps aid in further study.

A **Summary** with bulleted highlights on the important topics. This brief text format brings attention to the most important aspects of the text to aid in the students' retention.

A **Chapter Test** allows assessment of knowledge and retention of critical elements.

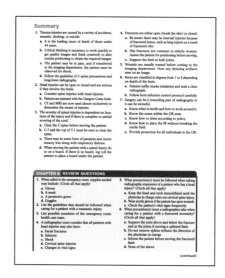

ADDITIONAL LEARNING RESOURCES

This powerful tool also includes a host of resources for instructors and students on the companion website at http://thepoint.lww.com. See the inside front cover for details on how to access these resources.

Student Resources include videos, a question bank, audio glossary, skills checklists, lab activities, and more!

Instructor Resources include PowerPoint slides with lecture material, lesson plans, an image bank, a test generator, and answers to the chapter tests. New with this edition is an instructor guide to the areas within the text that address specific Patient Care content that may be found on the ARRT.

INTRODUCTION TO THE HEALTH CARE ENVIRONMENT AND MEDICAL IMAGING

The Profession and Environment

1

OBJECTIVES

After studying this chapter, the student will be able to:

1. Identify the different persons who play an important role in the history of radiology.

2. Describe the technologic advances made since the discovery of x-rays.

3. Identify the different health care environments that participate in total health care of the patient.

4. Explain the practice standards.

5. Explain how health provider organizations are run.

6. Differentiate between accreditation types.

7. Define credentialing, national certification, registration, and state licensure.

8. Describe the types, purposes, and functions of professional organizations.

9. Identify the responsibilities of the health care facility and members of the health care team.

10. Explain the general responsibilities of the radiographer and the scope of practice.

11. List the health professions in medical imaging.

12. List and describe the personnel in the radiology organization.

13. Describe foundations for student learning achievement.

14. Identify best study tips and best practices for student success.

KEY TERMS

American College of Radiology (ACR): The largest and oldest medical imaging accrediting body

American Registry of Radiologic Technologists (ARRT): The leading credentialing organization for individuals that have completed the requirements to become a registered radiographer

Crookes tube: A partially evacuated glass tube in which electrons can flow from the cathode to the anode

Emotional: Subject to or involving emotion or emotions; emotion is a generalized feeling or feelings

Imaging program: A 2-year course of study that combines classroom lectures with clinical practice that may equal 40 hours per week with outside homework assignments adding extra time constraints

Joint Review Committee on Education in Radiologic Technology (JRCERT): The recognized body that accredits formal education in radiologic technology to ensure that the education provides the knowledge and skills necessary for quality patient care

Kinesthetic learners: Learn through doing and touching

Mission statement: A published statement that conveys the hospital's purpose and goal for the public

Stress: Physical, mental, or emotional strain or tension

INTRODUCTION

Welcome to the world of diagnostic imaging technology. Beginning a course of studying radiologic sciences might seem like learning a new language would be easier. The challenges to be encountered over the next 2 years may be intimidating, but they can be overcome with due diligence and an eye on the goal of becoming a registered and licensed health care professional.

This chapter is an introduction to some of the elements encountered in other classes that are more specifically related to the in-depth study required to pass the **American Registry of Radiologic Technologists (ARRT)** examination. It is also an inside view of the environment that is about to be entered. The remainder of the book is devoted to different types of patients encountered in the imaging department and how to care for them in a compassionate and professional manner. Patient care becomes a natural way of life as each day of instruction passes and the "language" of medicine becomes a way of life each time the doors of the radiology department are opened and entrance is gained.

IN THE BEGINNING

Although one man is credited with the discovery, there were actually many pioneers who paved the way by using equipment and making improvements on the equipment that eventually led to the actual discovery.

In the early 19th century, many scientists were experimenting with electricity (discovered by Benjamin Franklin) and little else. William Watson demonstrated electrical current. Michael Faraday induced electricity by passing a magnet through the magnetic field of a coil of wire. This led to experimentation with electromagnetic induction and the advent of generators and transformers with higher voltages.

A scientist named William Goodspeed was experimenting with cathode rays and the different energies that they emit. He made the actual first radiograph on February 22, 1890; however, he did not publish his work and was therefore not credited with the actual discovery of x-ray. In the mid-1890s, Sir William Crookes, an English physicist, was studying gas, and in order to continue with his work, he created a vacuum tube. It was a glass tube that contained both positive and negative electrodes and an induction coil (Fig. 1-1). He passed high-voltage electrical currents through the tube, which would allow him to study the conductivity of gases that had been put into the tube. Crookes was able to demonstrate that matter

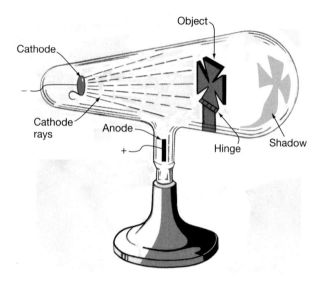

FIGURE 1-1 An early tube created by Dr. Crookes and used by scientists to investigate the nature of light.

emitted from a cathode ray tube had enough energy to turn a wheel that was located in the tube. Shortly afterward, Philipp Lenard, a German scientist, discovered the cathode ray while he was working with a **Crookes tube**. Lenard changed the original tube to include an aluminum window that allowed the cathode rays to pass through to the outside. During one of his experiments, a piece of barium platinocyanide–soaked paper glowed when the rays were directed at it. Unfortunately for him, Lenard failed to further investigate what made the paper glow, thus allowing Wilhelm Conrad Röntgen (spelled Roentgen in English) to make the discovery only a few months later.

A New Kind of Ray

In 1888, Röntgen was head of the physics department at the University of Würzburg in Germany. On the evening of November 8, 1895, he was working with a Crookes tube in his basement laboratory. The tube was sitting on a bench, and across the room lay a plate that had the letter "A" painted on it with barium platinocyanide. Dim lights allowed him to see any change in gas color or electric current through the tube., Röntgen noticed that the plate on the opposite side of the room was "glowing" and he could readily see the letter "A." Röntgen knew that this was not from any kind of light or electricity but had to be caused by the tube. Röntgen did not know what he had produced, but only that it was some type of ray, which he named the "X"-ray because the mathematical symbol for the unknown is "X."

Continuing with his experimentation, he was able to reproduce the fluorescence with each passage of current through the tube despite the various objects that were placed between the plate and the tube. Röntgen held a metal pipe in front of the plate and noticed the fingers of his hand were reflected on the screen. On December 28, 1895, Röntgen submitted his report called "On a new kind of rays" to the Würzburg Physico-Medical Society. Wilhelm Röntgen received the first ever Nobel Prize in Physics in 1901 for this world-changing discovery. He died in Munich on February 10, 1923, just a month shy of his 78th birthday.

Early Uses

In those early years, the scientific world talked of nothing but x-ray and cathode ray tubes. In 1896, less than 1 year after the discovery of x-ray, Thomas Edison developed a handheld Crookes tube with a screen at one end and an eyepiece at the other. He called this new invention a *Vitascope*. It was the first fluoroscope and the forerunner of all of today's fluoroscopy tubes.

Demonstrations were held in Bloomingdale's and Macy's in New York City; entertainment came in the form of x-ray machines that allowed the patron to view the bones of the hand. Portrait studios offered x-rays of hands entwined of newly married couples to give as wedding souvenirs. Women had the upper lip irradiated to remove an unsightly hair line. Even the spiritual world used x-ray as a link to the other side and the fourth dimension. After the discovery of radium by Marie Pierre Curie in 1898, radium parties were held where the cocktails were laced with radium, the lights would be lowered, and the guests could watch their drinks glow in the dark!

X-ray was touted to cure cancer and skin lesions and was used to remove facial hair of women in beauty clinics. However, x-ray did have the most obvious use in medicine. As the negative side of x-ray use became apparent, it was soon realized that hospitals had to take control of the use of x-ray. Boston Hospital was the first by making actual rooms for the use of x-ray and "training" people to take those x-rays. By 1905, Boston Hospital had five full-time technicians operating the equipment and taking medical x-rays.

Advances

The discovery of x-ray has had a significant effect not only on medicine but also on travel, the food industry, industrial equipment, sterilization of products and insects, and other commercial uses.

As the gas tubes were improved and a vacuum was created, the modern tube was born. The newer tubes were stable, more flexible, and safer than the traditional tube used in the past. It was these advances that made possible the invention of the new imaging equipment used today. One such piece of equipment is the computerized axial tomography (now known as CT) machine. In 1972, Godfrey Hounsfield and Allan Cormack created an x-ray tube that encircled the patient who was lying on a table. Although the first scans took hours to complete, the advances have improved the equipment to today's standards that ensure an entire body is scanned in less than 5 minutes.

In similar fashion, the magnetic resonance imaging (MRI) equipment was started in 1946 by Felix Bloch and Edward Purcell. In 1972, Dr. Paul Lauterbur first described the MRI technique in medicine and published the first MRI image in 1973. In 1977, Raymond Damadian showed how MRI could be used on the **whole body**. MRI works similarly to computed tomography (CT) but does not use radiation to image the body. Other advances in the field of x-ray are positron emission tomography (PET), single-photon emission CT (SPECT), mammography, and ultrasound. Not only has the field advanced with new modalities, but x-ray itself has gone from film to digital images. More than a century after it was discovered, the importance of x-ray continues to grow and the technology continues to amaze.

Early Effects of Radiation

The x-ray was seen as a miracle to the world of medicine when it was discovered in 1895. However, the negative side of the miracle was beginning to show itself. In the early 1900s, many problems, such as burns, infections, swelling, and cancer, finally forced the scientists to reinvestigate the whole process of x-ray and how it worked. Thomas Edison's assistant and good friend Clarence Dally lost all of his hair, all of the fingers on both hands, and finally both of his hands before he succumbed to the effects caused by excessive radiation. He was in constant pain and died in 1904. He is the first known fatality of overexposure. Edison himself complained of skin rashes and sore eyes. It was this event that caused Edison to stop his work on radiation and start to look at the problems it caused. X-ray technicians fell victim to its terrible side effects. Twenty-eight Americans suffered fatal effects from x-ray experimentation. The damage that can be done by radiation and how to protect against that damage is a lengthy narrative and is taught in different courses within the training. It is not discussed in this book.

HEALTH CARE ENVIRONMENT

The health care environment is one that is safe, empowering, and satisfying, not only for the patient but for the employee as well. The environment is a major consideration in the health of society. All leaders, managers, health care professionals, and ancillary staff must perform with a sense of professionalism, accountability, transparency, involvement, efficiency, and effectiveness to promote a culture of safety. This can be done through an infrastructure within the following areas:

- Administrative support
- Knowledge and education
- Unbiased reporting
- Nonpunitive feedback
- Planning and strategy
- Continuous assessment
- Effective implementation
- Information and technology
- Evidence-based guidelines and procedures
- Measurement and standardization

Each of these areas is interconnected so that one cannot be fulfilled without the use of another area.

Health Care Settings

When one thinks of the health care environment, hospitals are most often first on the list. This is probably due in part to the large amount of medical care that can be undertaken in a hospital.

Student radiographers most likely spends the majority of their training in a hospital setting; however, smaller clinics might also be a rotation where the radiographer fulfills multiple duties. Clinics are just as important as hospitals, especially in smaller towns and areas where a hospital is not close enough for care that isn't of a life-threatening nature. Many clinics have physicians' offices, laboratory, pharmacy, and radiology. Larger clinics may have a physical therapy department, optometry, and an urgent care (convenient care) center where patients can be attended to. Convenient care centers may be found in areas where there are no hospital services. These centers fill the need when a patient doesn't need the care of an emergency department but does need medical care from a licensed physician. Many convenient care centers have a small radiography room that can provide services for immediate diagnosis such as broken bones, and chest images for pneumonia or other conditions. Freestanding imaging centers that are affiliated with larger medical centers are located in areas that don't have hospitals to make it easier for patients to obtain their imaging studies that have been ordered by their physician.

Other settings that are part of the health care environment include mental health facilities, long-term care facilities (i.e., assisted living), hospice, home health care, and other places that could include jails, prisons, or the medical examiner's office. Although the student radiographer is not normally rotated through these areas, it is important to know that a radiographer could very well be involved in patient care in these areas after graduation.

Payment and Reimbursement Systems

In the past, the rising cost of health care became a major concern of the medical community and of the nation. This gave rise to major changes in the health care delivery system in the United States and has become a major political concern. The belief was that the exorbitant cost of health care and its continued rising cost did not necessarily improve the quality of patient care. On the basis of this belief, many restraints were placed on the institutions and the practitioners of health care. These changes are complex, and it is not within the scope of this book to discuss them at length. However, a very brief outline of the current methods of health care delivery follows.

Medicare: This covers persons 65 years of age and older, permanently disabled workers and their dependents, and persons with end-stage renal disease. There are several parts to Medicare, a few are addressed below:

Medicare, Part A: This covers acute hospital care and home health care service and requires enrollees to pay a deductible for each benefit period for hospitalization.

Medicare, Part B: This covers outpatient care, doctor's services, tests, and preventative treatments, which are medically necessary services. Home health services include limited and only medically necessary part-time care.

Medicare, Part D: This covers prescription drugs from a Part D plan or through a Medicare Advantage program.

All persons paid by Social Security are automatically enrolled in Part A of Medicare. Part B and Part D are optional. Medicare does not cover long-term care and limits other aspects of health care and promotion of health. This encourages elders to enroll in private health care plans called Medigap insurance if they can afford to do so.

It is worth noting that Medicare has an impact on the type of equipment used in radiography because of the reimbursement changes. Medicare reimbursement for radiographic procedures will be affected if the provider does not utilize digital radiography (DR). The reimbursement rate for radiographs done on film will be reduced by 20% to push the use of DR. The reimbursement rate for radiography done with computed radiography (CR) will be decreased by 7% the following year to push CR to DR. In 2023, any provider still obtaining radiographic studies by means of CR will have that reimbursement reduced even further by 10%.

Medicaid: This is a federally funded and state-administered program that provides medical care for families with dependent older adults, children, or otherwise disabled persons who qualify according to income and eligibility requirements.

Prospective Payment System (PPS): Instituted by Medicare, this system uses financial incentives to decrease total charges by reimbursing for medical treatment based on diagnosis-related groups (DRGs). This is a method of grouping for payment dependent on diagnosis. That is, every person with the same diagnosis receives the same financial payment for treatment. The DRGs have resulted in a great deal of controversy in medical circles.

Managed Care Organizations (MCOs): These are divided into two groups that supervise patient care services, namely, Health Maintenance Organizations (HMOs) and Preferred Provider Organizations (PPOs). HMOs are group insurance plans that charge each person insured under their plan a preset fee for care and health care service. This fee is paid by the participant regardless of whether or not they utilize the HMO's services. The HMO attempts to perform preventative health care by education, periodic health care screening (i.e., immunizations, mammograms, and physical examinations), and other preventative methods to reduce the cost of medical care. This type of financial management is called capitation. PPOs gather a group of health care providers who are guaranteed a group of consumers of health care (patients) on the basis of their promise of discounting their fees. The patient is guaranteed health care at lower cost, provided they use the PPO provided.

Point of Service (POS) Plans: A primary care provider is selected from a group of providers. The primary care physician then acts as a gatekeeper for the patient and authorizes any referrals the patient may require, thus reducing unnecessary referrals.

Physician Hospital Organizations (PHO): This evolved as a result of financial concerns of hospitals and physician practices. The PHO creates a corporate structure between a hospital and a group of its physicians; they contract with an MCO to negotiate fees for services for their self-insured employees.

Because of these regulatory bodies, protocols for managing care have been derived. These protocols are known as *guidelines or standards* for managing patient care. *Critical pathways* for diagnoses and procedures to treat particular illnesses have also been developed. Following the course of these pathways is one of several methods used to examine quality of patient care. All of these methods examine and assess morbidity and mortality rates, admissions per year for chronic illness, complications, and patient satisfaction.

In spite of efforts to control the cost of medical care, it continues to be extremely expensive, and there are many who are unable to afford medical insurance or preventative health care of any kind. When there is a medical crisis, these people are left to seek care in city emergency facilities throughout the country. The emergency may be treated; however, there is no follow-up care for these patients.

HEALTH PROVIDER ORGANIZATION

A hospital organizational flowchart may look similar to what is found in Display 1-1. Each facility or health care system has its own organizational flowchart with departments that may have different titles or be supervised under different administrative personnel. Detailed charts

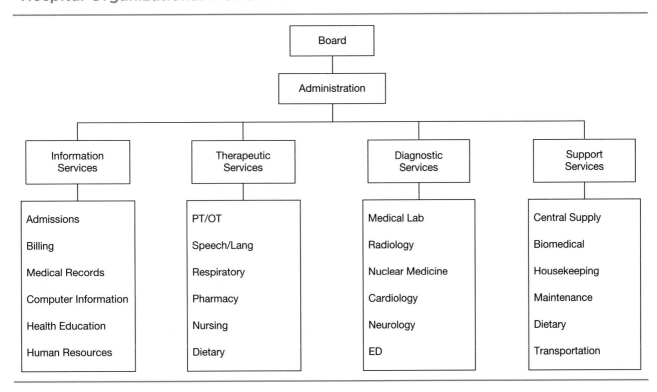

DISPLAY 1-1

Hospital Organizational Flowchart

show the multiple levels of administration as well as each of the service areas being broken down into their own flowcharts. This demonstrates that hospital organizations can be quite large and therefore confusing. To help avoid confusion, the organization starts with a mission.

Mission, Vision, and Values

Health care organizations publicize their mission, vision, and value statements to help potential patients choose where to seek care and employees where to seek employment. The organization has a responsibility to abide by a societally determined standard of care in an ethically sound manner. The mission, vision, and values of the health care organization can create a culture that is one of passion and that results in healthier patients and greater vitality in the community.

Mission statements communicate the health care organization's fundamental purpose. It is a concise explanation of the organization's reason for existence and describes the organization's purpose and overall intentions. The mission statement supports the vision and serves to communicate purpose and direction to employees, customers, vendors, and other stakeholders.

Vision statements highlight what the health care organization sees itself in the future. The mission statement is what the organization is at the present. The vision statement is about the goals. The philosophical ideals of an organization form the heart of the values statement. Words such as "compassion," "cultural sensitivity," and "innovation" are often found in value statements.

Administrative Services

A hospital (or other medical facility) must have services that ensure the smooth operation of the other services that are provided as well as the care of the building itself. Oftentimes, these services are not thought of on a daily basis, but without them, the operation of other departments begins to falter. Some of these areas that could be considered administrative services are:

- Governing board: oversees the management, finances, and quality; set strategic direction; build relationships; establish standards, values, and compliance; and select a CEO
- Administrative services: oversee the day-to-day administrative operations of hospitals and other health care facilities. They plan and supervise all medical services.
- Admissions: determine and implement the best practices, develop and revise both admission and discharge processes. The admissions coordinator is responsible for not only welcoming patients but also collecting their personal and medical information.

- Information systems: a health information system (HIS) that is designed to manage data and that includes collection, storage, management, and transmission of a patient's electronic medical record (EMR)
- Procurement: involves the purchase of products, supplies, equipment, and related services
- Accounting support services: this department is responsible for collecting account payments for services performed, maintaining all staff and patient files, and handling all billing duties.
- Human resources: a department of individuals that is responsible for addressing the many concerns in the health care industry, such as promoting employee retention and ensuring that regulations are being met.

Although the areas in this list could be located in other service areas on other organizational charts, it should be stressed that even though these services may be working behind the scenes and not part of the daily life of a student radiographer, they are as important to the organization as the vice president in charge of them.

Medical Services

There are many and varied medical services that are part of a hospital organization. *Physicians* can be either a doctor of medicine or osteopathy. They often specialize in a specific area of practice and, following licensing, are able to prescribe and supervise the medical care of the patient. *Clinical services* relate to patient care and treatment. They include diagnostic tests and procedures, rehabilitation services, preventative and postoperative care. *Clinical support services* include such areas as pastoral care, ethics committees, and psychological services. Without the interaction of these services, patient care would not be complete.

ACCREDITATION

There is a growing demand for evidence that care provided by health care providers is of high quality as well as cost-effective. Regulatory bodies such as **The Joint Commission (TJC)** and organizations for consumers of health care have been established. Joint Commission accreditation and certification is recognized nationwide as a symbol of quality that reflects an organization's commitment to meeting certain performance standards. It is an independent, not-for-profit organization that accredits and certifies more than 19,000 organizations and programs in the United States such as general, psychiatric, children's and rehabilitation hospitals, critical access hospitals, home care organizations, nursing homes, rehabilitation centers, long-term care facilities, behavioral health organizations, addictive services, ambulatory care providers, and independent or freestanding clinical laboratories.

The **American College of Radiology (ACR)** is recognized as the gold standard of accreditation in medical imaging. The review process is voluntary; however, it is required for outpatient providers that bill for CT and MRI. The ACR currently accredits the following modalities:

- Breast MRI and Breast Ultrasound
- CT and MRI
- Mammography
- Nuclear Medicine/PET
- Radiation Oncology Practices

Facilities that have gone above and beyond the "Gold" standard of ACR receive the coveted "Center of Excellence." ACR offers this award as a way to raise the minimum standard and achieve higher standards toward high-quality patient care.

Programmatic accreditation by the **Joint Review Committee on Education in Radiologic Technology (JRCERT)** ensures that the program provides the knowledge and skills for quality patient care in compliance with JRCERT accreditation standards. Currently, approved and accredited programs operate under six standards, effective January 1, 2021. Included in the six standards are 35 objectives that educational programs must clearly present documentation ensuring compliance. The initial accreditation process for a program takes about 18 to 21 months from the receipt of the application/self-study reports. The accreditation process has several steps, which include a site visit, report of team findings, response to report of findings, and program notification of accreditation.

College-based programs can be accredited by the Council for Higher Education Accreditation (CHEA). Recognition by CHEA affirms that the standards and processes of the college are consistent with quality, improvement, and accountability. CHEA recognizes organizations within different regions of the United States that accredit the college or university. These organizations include:

- Accrediting Commission for Community and Junior Colleges (ACCJC) Western Association of Schools and Colleges
- Higher Learning Commission (HLC)
- Middle States Commission on Higher Education (MSCHE)
- New England Commission of Higher Education (NECHE)
- Northwest Commission on Colleges and Universities (NWCCU)
- Southern Association of Colleges and Schools Commission on Colleges (SACSCOC)
- WASC Senior College and University Commission

PROFESSIONAL CREDENTIALING

A professional credential is used to mark one's knowledge in a particular professional area. Professionals choose to earn and maintain credentials for a variety of personal and professional reasons at different stages of their careers. Various professions offer credentials unique to their industry. In the case of radiologic technology, one cannot practice the chosen profession without the credential.

The American Registry of Radiologic Technologists (ARRT) organization is the national credentialing body in the United States that recognizes qualified professionals in the field of medical imaging. The only way to become certified by the ARRT is to successfully complete an associate degree and an ARRT-approved educational program in radiologic technology. Once the graduate has successfully completed the ARRT examination, the initials RT (R) can be used after the name. These initials stand for "registered technologist" and *not* radiologic technologist. The (R) stands for radiography. As new technologists expand their education and pass additional qualifying examinations, the initials associated with that modality can be added such as RT (R, M, CT) or any other combination. The following modalities are identified by these initials: computed tomography (CT); mammography (M); magnetic resonance imaging (MRI); or cardiovascular interventional (CVI).

In addition to passing the ARRT certification examination, 46 states have licensure requirements that mandate the radiographer not only be certified by the ARRT but also pass an exam administered by the state. Many states are no longer requiring an examination once proof of passing the ARRT is provided and a fee is paid. Radiographers must check the requirements of the state in which they plan on working to determine not only if a license is required but also how to apply for one.

Additional modalities have their own certification credentialing boards. A qualified individual must take a separate examination (separate from the radiography exam) to become certified in that modality. One certified by the Registry for Diagnostic Medical Sonography may use RDMS after the name. Those that pass the Nuclear Medicine Technology Certification Board exam may use NMTCB after their name. If one was registered in both radiography and sonography, they could use RT (R, M), RDMS after their name.

REGULATORY AGENCIES

Health care is governed by regulations set in place to protect both the patients and the providers. There are five federal agencies that have oversight authority of health care facilities. These include the Food and Drug Administration (FDA), the Centers for Disease Control and Prevention

(CDC), the National Institute for Occupational Safety and Health (NIOSH), Centers for Medicare and Medicaid Services (CMS), and the Agency for Healthcare Research and Quality (AHRQ). All health care organizations must answer to the federal and state levels of oversight.

There are state regulatory boards in addition to the federal agencies. These state agencies are responsible for setting licensing requirements, reviewing applications, investigating complaints, and carrying out disciplinary measures. Each state follows one of five regulatory models, which allows full autonomy (Model A) up to a model that has a central agency that retains final decision-making authority (Model E).

PROFESSIONAL ORGANIZATIONS IN RADIOLOGIC TECHNOLOGY

Participation in professional organizations is the responsibility of all practicing professionals, regardless of their field. Membership in professional organizations provides a pathway to continued successful professional development. It also provides comprehensive opportunities to remain current in a constantly changing technologic career. Professional organizations provide pathways for technical growth and the development of leadership skills as well as an arena for professional interaction and problem-solving, especially in career issues. The mission statement of the American Society of Radiologic Technologists (ASRT) is "to advance the medical imaging and radiation therapy profession and to enhance the quality of patient care." ASRT offers many program and member services, including continuing education (CE) opportunities, publications, career information and resources, events, meeting, conferences and seminars, government relations and legislative monitoring and advocacy, group professional liability insurance, and other member benefits and services. In addition, ASRT works with professional certification bodies and accreditation agencies for radiographers. Ultimately, membership in professional organizations enables the radiographer to continue providing quality patient health care in accordance with the standards of the profession.

The radiographer must understand that there are professional societies, certification and licensing boards, and accreditation organizations. The differences might seem obscure; however, it is important to know the difference if one is to be a professional. As an example, a radiographer cannot "belong" to the ARRT as it is not a society, but rather, it is the certification board that determines if an individual is qualified to practice the profession of radiography. If a radiographer joins the society (ASRT) and pays dues, then they belong to the society as long as their dues are current and they have maintained good standing as outlined by the profession.

The different organizations and certification boards that every radiographer should be aware of are listed below. Although this is not an exhaustive list, it gives the student radiographer an idea of the many different acronyms that one hears while involved in the field.

- ACR is the principal organization of radiologists, radiation oncologists, and clinical medical physicists in the United States.
- American Hospital of Radiology Administrators (AHRA) is the professional organization representing management at all levels of hospital imaging.
- American Medical Association (AMA) is a voluntary association of physicians, which sets standards for the medical profession and advocates on behalf of the physician and the patient.
- American Registry of Diagnostic Medical Sonographers (ARDMS) is an independent organization that administers examinations and awards to qualified ultrasound professionals.
- ARRT is the largest credentialing organization that seeks to ensure the highest quality patient care in radiologic technology. Before being allowed to practice radiography, the graduate must pass the credentialing exam.
- ASRT is the professional organization for radiologic science professionals. Membership is voluntary.
- Association of Collegiate Educators in Radiologic Technology (ACERT) is a voluntary organization that was founded to improve the quality of education in radiologic technology. The annual conference normally has three educational tracks: one for the didactic educator, one for the clinical educator, and one for the student radiographer.
- Association of Educators in Imaging and Radiologic Sciences (AEIRS) is another society that was founded to meet the needs of the educator.
- International Society of Radiology (ISR) is a voluntary society with the mission to facilitate the global endeavors of the member organizations to improve patient care and population health through medical imaging.
- The Joint Commission (aka the Commission [TJC]) accredits and certifies health care organizations and institutions in the United States.
- JRCERT is the accrediting board that recognizes the quality of education in radiology. Students graduating from a JRCERT-approved program are allowed to sit for the qualifying certification exam.
- Nuclear Medicine Technology Certification Board (NMTCB) is a certification board that was formed for the purpose of creating and maintaining examinations in nuclear medicine. Once an individual successfully completes this examination, they are given the right to have the initials NMT (nuclear medicine technologist) after their name.

THE HEALTH CARE TEAM

There is a unique interworking within a medical facility and its health care team. There are many departments that make up the whole; and that without those departments, the patient might not receive adequate care. The health care teams have the primary responsibilities for caring for all patients regardless of condition. This means that the lab is just as important as the radiology department. The pharmacy is just as important as the surgical suite. The emergency department is as important as the intensive care unit. Without members of each of the departments within the medical facility, the patient's health could not be managed, illness could not be prevented, research could not be used for the greater good for health. Display 1-2 defines each party of the health care team.

Responsibilities of the Radiographer

Radiology has evolved to meet the criteria of a profession that is oriented toward the diagnosis and treatment of trauma and disease. This means the radiologic technologist, or radiographer, works in intimate contact with people on a daily basis. Patients of all cultures, religions, and socioeconomic backgrounds come to the radiology department and must be treated with dignity and in an unbiased, nonjudgmental manner.

Entry-level radiographers' general requirements include the following skills and abilities:

1. Assist the radiologist or the radiology assistant (RA) in procedures as required.
2. Apply modern principles of radiation exposure, radiation physics, radiation protection, and radiobiology to produce diagnostic images.
3. Demonstrate knowledge of medical terminology, pathology, anatomy, and physiology.
4. Maintain a high degree of accuracy in radiographic positioning.
5. Provide direct patient care.
6. Evaluate recognized equipment malfunctions.
7. Evaluate radiographic images.
8. Correctly document as required.
9. Effectively communicate with other members of the health care team.
10. Provide patient and family education.
11. Demonstrate knowledge of the use of contrast media and drug administration.
12. Follow established practice standards.

It can be seen that the RT is key to the diagnostic and treatment of patient medical conditions. As such, the ASRT has developed a guide for the practice of radiologic technology.

DISPLAY 1-2

Health Care Team

Members of other health care professions with whom the radiographer interacts are:

- **Physicians:** A doctor of medicine or osteopathy. They often specialize in a specific area of practice and, following licensing, are able to prescribe and supervise the medical care of the patient.
- **Registered nurses:** Provide patient care, which is often required 24 hours a day. They also provide home health care and case management, educate, act as a patient advocate, administer medications and treatments as ordered by physicians, monitor the patient's health status, and coordinate and facilitate all patient care when the patient is hospitalized. Advance practice nurses work as clinical nurse specialists and nurse practitioners.
- **Vocational nurses:** Work with patients under the supervision of a registered nurse. The training is the same for these licenses. The term "vocational" nursing is used in the states of Texas and California, whereas the term "practical" nursing is used in the rest of the United States.
- **Occupational and physical therapists:** Members of a profession who work in the rehabilitative area of health care.
- **Pharmacist:** Prepares and dispenses medications and oversees the patient's drug therapy.
- **Respiratory therapist:** Maintains or improves the patient's respiratory status.
- **Laboratory technologist:** Analyzes laboratory specimens for pathologic conditions.
- **Social workers:** Counsel patients and refer them for assistance to appropriate agencies.

There are also many assistive personnel including nursing assistants, ward clerks, pharmacy technicians, ECG technicians, and many more.

The ASRT *Practice Standards for Medical Imaging and Radiation Therapy* is a guide for the appropriate practice, assists in developing job descriptions, and promotes role definition for practitioners. The practice standards define the practice and establish general criteria to determine compliance (Display 1-3). Practice Standards are authoritative statements established by the profession for judging the quality of practice, service, and education. It includes expected and achievable levels of performance against which actual performance can be assessed. Radiographers are the primary liaison between patients, licensed independent practitioners, and other members of the health care team. Radiographers must remain sensitive to the physical and emotional needs of the patient through effective communication, patient assessment, monitoring, education, documentation, and patient safety and care skills. Radiographers use independent, professional, ethical judgment, and critical

---

DISPLAY 1-3

The ASRT Practice Standards for Medical Imaging and Radiation Therapy Effective June 2021

Preface

These practice standards serve as a guide for the medical imaging and radiation therapy profession. These standards define the practice and establish general criteria to determine compliance. Practice standards are authoritative statements established by the profession, through evidentiary documentation, for evaluating the quality of practice, service, and education provided by individuals within the profession.

Practice standards can be used by individual facilities to develop job descriptions and practice parameters. Those outside the profession can use the standards as an overview of the role and responsibilities of individuals within the profession.

The medical imaging and radiation therapy professional and any individual who is legally authorized to perform medical imaging or radiation therapy must be educationally prepared and clinically competent as a prerequisite to professional practice. The individual should, consistent with all applicable legal requirements and restrictions, exercise individual thought, judgment, and discretion in the performance of the procedure. Federal and state statutes, regulations, accreditation standards, and institutional policies could dictate practice parameters and may supersede these standards.

The ASRT Practice Standards for Medical Imaging and Radiation Therapy are divided into five sections:

- *Introduction*—defines the practice and the minimum qualifications for the education and certification of individuals in addition to an overview of the specific practice.
- *Medical Imaging and Radiation Therapy Scope of Practice*—delineates the parameters of the specific practice.
- *Standards*—incorporate patient assessment and management with procedural analysis, performance, and evaluation. The standards define the activities of the individual responsible for the care of patients and delivery of medical imaging and radiation therapy procedures; in the technical areas of performance, such as equipment and material assessment safety standards and total quality management; and in the areas of education, interpersonal relationships, self-assessment, and ethical behavior.
- *Glossary*—defines terms used in the practice standards document.
- *Advisory Opinion Statements*—provide explanations of the practice standards and are intended for clarification and guidance for specific practice issues.

The standards are numbered and followed by a term or set of terms that describe the standards. The next statement is the expected performance of the individual when performing the procedure or treatment. A rationale follows and explains why an individual should adhere to the particular standard of performance.

- *Criteria*—used to evaluate an individual's performance. Each standard is divided into two parts: the general criteria and the

DISPLAY 1-3

The ASRT Practice Standards for Medical Imaging and Radiation Therapy Effective June 2021 (*continued*)

specific criteria. Both should be used when evaluating performance.

- *General Criteria*—written in a style that applies to medical imaging and radiation therapy professionals and should be used for the appropriate area of practice.
- *Specific Criteria*—meet the needs of the individuals in the various areas of professional performance. Although many areas of performance within medical imaging and radiation therapy are similar, others are not. The specific criteria were developed with these differences in mind.

Introduction

Definition

The medical imaging and radiation therapy profession comprises health care professionals identified as a bone densitometry technologist, cardiac interventional and vascular interventional technologist, CT technologist, limited x-ray machine operator, magnetic resonance technologist, mammographer, medical dosimetrist, nuclear medicine technologist, quality management technologist, radiation therapist, radiographer, radiologist assistant, or sonographer who are educationally prepared and clinically competent as identified by these standards.

Furthermore, these standards apply to health care employees who are legally authorized to perform medical imaging or radiation therapy and who are educationally prepared and clinically competent as identified by these standards.

The complex nature of disease processes involves multiple imaging modalities. Medical imaging and radiation therapy professionals are vital members of a multidisciplinary team that forms a core of highly trained health care professionals, who each bring expertise to the area of patient care. They play a critical role in the delivery of health services as new modalities emerge and the need for medical imaging and radiation therapy procedures increases.

Medical imaging and radiation therapy integrates scientific knowledge, technical competence, and patient interaction skills to provide safe and accurate procedures with the highest regard to all aspects of patient care. A medical imaging and radiation therapy professional recognizes elements unique to each patient, which is essential for the successful completion of the procedure.

Medical imaging and radiation therapy professionals are the primary liaison between patients, licensed practitioners, and other members of the support team. These professionals must remain sensitive to the needs of the patient through good communication, patient assessment, patient monitoring, and patient care skills. As members of the health care team, medical imaging and radiation therapy professionals participate in quality improvement processes and continually assess their professional performance.

Medical imaging and radiation therapy professionals think critically and use independent, professional, and ethical judgment in all aspects of their work. They engage in continuing education to include their area of practice to enhance patient care, safety, public education, knowledge, and technical competence.

Radiography

The practice of radiography is performed by health care professionals responsible for the administration of ionizing radiation for diagnostic, therapeutic, or research purposes. A radiographer performs a full scope of radiographic and fluoroscopic procedures and acquires and analyzes data needed for diagnosis at the request of and for interpretation by a licensed practitioner.

Radiographers independently perform or assist the licensed practitioner in the

(*continued*)

DISPLAY 1-3

The ASRT Practice Standards for Medical Imaging and Radiation Therapy Effective June 2021 (*continued*)

completion of radiographic and fluoroscopic procedures. Radiographers prepare, administer, and document activities related to medications and radiation exposure in accordance with federal and state laws, regulations, or lawful institutional policy.

Education and Certification

The individual must be educationally prepared and clinically competent as a prerequisite to professional practice. Only medical imaging and radiation therapy professionals who have completed the appropriate education and training as outlined in these standards should perform medical imaging and radiation therapy procedures.

Medical imaging and radiation therapy professionals performing multiple modality hybrid imaging should be registered by certification agencies recognized by the ASRT and be educationally prepared and clinically competent in the specific modality(ies) they are responsible to perform. Medical imaging and radiation therapy professionals performing diagnostic procedures in more than one imaging modality adhere to the general and specific criteria for each area of practice.

To maintain certification(s), medical imaging and radiation therapy professionals must complete appropriate continuing education requirements to sustain their expertise and awareness of changes and advances in practice.

Radiography

Only medical imaging and radiation therapy professionals who have completed the appropriate education and obtained certification(s) as outlined in these standards should perform radiographic and fluoroscopic procedures.

Radiographers prepare for their roles on the interdisciplinary team by meeting examination eligibility criteria as determined by the ARRT.

Those passing the ARRT radiography examination use the credential RT (R).

Standards
Standard One—Assessment

The medical imaging and radiation therapy professional collects pertinent data about the patient, procedure, equipment, and work environment.

Rationale

Information about the patient's health status is essential in providing appropriate imaging and therapeutic services. The planning and provision of safe and effective medical services relies on the collection of pertinent information about equipment, procedures, and the work environment.

General Criteria

The medical imaging and radiation therapy professional:

- Assesses and maintains the integrity of medical supplies
- Assesses any potential patient limitations for the procedure
- Assesses factors that may affect the procedure
- Assesses patient lab values, medication list, and risk for allergic reaction(s) prior to procedure and administration of medication[*][†]
- Confirms that equipment performance, maintenance, and operation comply with the manufacturer's specifications
- Determines that services are performed in a safe environment, minimizing potential hazards
- Maintains restricted access to controlled areas
- Obtains and reviews relevant previous procedures and information from all available resources and the release of information as needed
- Participates in as low as reasonably achievable (ALARA), patient and personnel safety, risk management, and quality management activities
- Recognizes signs and symptoms of an emergency

DISPLAY 1-3

The ASRT Practice Standards for Medical Imaging and Radiation Therapy Effective June 2021 (*continued*)

Verifies appropriateness of the requested or prescribed procedure, in compliance with the clinical indication and protocol.

- Verifies patient identification
- Verifies that protocol and procedure manuals include recommended criteria and are reviewed and revised
- Verifies that the patient has consented to the procedure
- Verifies the patient's pregnancy status

Specific Criteria

Radiography

- Develops and maintains standardized exposure technique guidelines for all equipment
- Maintains and performs quality control on radiation safety equipment
- Reviews digital images for the purpose of monitoring radiation exposure

Standard Two—Analysis/Determination

The medical imaging and radiation therapy professional analyzes the information obtained during the assessment phase and develops an action plan for completing the procedure.

Rationale

Determining the most appropriate action plan enhances patient safety and comfort, optimizes diagnostic and therapeutic quality, and improves efficiency.

General Criteria

The medical imaging and radiation therapy professional:

- Consults appropriate medical personnel to determine a modified action plan
- Determines that all procedural requirements are in place to achieve a quality procedure
- Determines the appropriate type and dose of contrast media to be administered based on established protocols[*,†]
- Determines the course of action for an emergent situation
- Determines the need for and selects supplies, accessory equipment, shielding, positioning, and immobilization devices

- Employs professional judgment to adapt procedures to improve diagnostic quality or therapeutic outcomes
- Evaluates and monitors services, procedures, equipment, and the environment to determine if they meet or exceed established guidelines, and revises the action plan
- Selects the most appropriate and efficient action plan after reviewing all pertinent data and assessing the patient's abilities and condition

Specific Criteria

Radiography

- Analyzes images to determine the use of appropriate imaging parameters
- Develops, maintains, and makes available optimal exposure technique guidelines for all radiographic and fluoroscopic equipment
- Verifies that exposure indicator data for DR systems have not been altered or modified and are included in the DICOM header and on images exported to media.

Standard Three—Education

The medical imaging and radiation therapy professional provides information about the procedure and related health issues according to protocol; informs the patient, public, and other health care providers about procedures, equipment, and facilities; and acquires and maintains current knowledge in practice.

Rationale

Education and communication are necessary to establish a positive relationship and promote safe practices. Advancements in the profession and optimal patient care require additional knowledge and skills through education.

General Criteria

The medical imaging and radiation therapy professional:

- Advocates for and participates in continuing education related to area of practice, to maintain and enhance clinical competency

(*continued*)

DISPLAY 1-3

The ASRT Practice Standards for Medical Imaging and Radiation Therapy Effective June 2021 (*continued*)

- Advocates for and participates in vendor-specific applications training to maintain clinical competency
- Educates the patient, public, and other health care providers about procedures, the associated biological effects, and radiation protection
- Elicits confidence and cooperation from the patient, the public, and other health care providers by providing timely communication and effective instruction
- Explains effects and potential side effects of medications*,†
- Maintains credentials and certification related to practice
- Provides accurate explanations and instructions at an appropriate time and at a level the patient and their care providers can understand; addresses questions and concerns regarding the procedure
- Provides information on certification or accreditation to the patient, other health care providers, and the public
- Provides information to patients, health care providers, students, and the public concerning the role and responsibilities of individuals in the profession
- Provides pre-, peri-, and postprocedure education
- Refers questions about diagnosis, treatment, or prognosis to a licensed practitioner

Specific Criteria
Radiography

- Maintains knowledge of the most current practices and technology used to minimize patient dose while producing diagnostic quality images

Standard Four—Performance

The medical imaging and radiation therapy professional performs the action plan and quality assurance activities.

Rationale

Quality patient services are provided through the safe and accurate performance of a deliberate plan of action. Quality assurance activities provide valid and reliable information regarding the performance of equipment, materials, and processes.

General Criteria

The medical imaging and radiation therapy professional:

- Adheres to radiation safety rules and standards
- Administers contrast media and other medications only when a licensed practitioner is immediately available to ensure proper diagnosis and treatment of adverse events*,†
- Administers first aid or provides life support†
- Applies principles of aseptic technique†
- Assesses and monitors the patient's physical, emotional, and mental status
- Consults with medical physicist or engineer in performing and documenting quality assurance tests
- Explains to the patient each step of the action plan as it occurs and elicits the cooperation of the patient
- Immobilizes the patient for procedure
- Implements an action plan
- Maintains current information on equipment, materials, and processes
- Modifies the action plan according to changes in the clinical situation
- Monitors the patient for reactions to medications*,†
- Participates in safety and risk management activities
- Performs ongoing quality assurance activities and quality control testing
- Performs procedural timeout
- Positions patient for anatomic area of interest, respecting patient ability and comfort
- Uses accessory equipment
- Uses an integrated team approach
- When appropriate, uses personnel radiation monitoring device(s) as indicated by the radiation safety officer or designee
- Works aseptically in the appropriate environment while preparing, compounding, and dispensing sterile and nonsterile medication*,†

Specific Criteria
Radiography

- Coordinates and manages the collection and labeling of tissue and fluid specimens

DISPLAY 1-3

The ASRT Practice Standards for Medical Imaging and Radiation Therapy Effective June 2021 (*continued*)

- Routinely reviews patient exposure records and rejects analyses as part of the quality assurance program
- Uses appropriate uniquely identifiable pre-exposure radiopaque markers for anatomic and procedural purposes
- Uses preexposure collimation and proper field-of-view selection

Standard Five—Evaluation

The medical imaging and radiation therapy professional determines whether the goals of the action plan have been achieved, evaluates quality assurance results, and establishes an appropriate action plan.

Rationale

Careful examination of the procedure is important to determine that expected outcomes have been met. Equipment, materials, and processes depend on ongoing quality assurance activities that evaluate performance based on established guidelines.

General Criteria

The medical imaging and radiation therapy professional:

- Communicates the revised action plan to appropriate team members
- Completes the evaluation process in a timely, accurate, and comprehensive manner
- Develops a revised action plan to achieve the intended outcome
- Evaluates images for optimal demonstration of anatomy of interest
- Evaluates quality assurance results
- Evaluates the patient, equipment, and procedure to identify variances that might affect the expected outcome
- Identifies exceptions to the expected outcome
- Measures the procedure against established policies, protocols, and benchmarks
- Validates quality assurance testing conditions and results

Standard Six—Implementation

The medical imaging and radiation therapy professional implements the revised action plan based on quality assurance results.

Rationale

It may be necessary to make changes to the action plan based on quality assurance results to promote safe and effective services.

General Criteria

The medical imaging and radiation therapy professional:

- Adjusts imaging parameters, patient procedure, or additional factors to improve the outcome
- Bases the revised plan on the patient's condition and the most appropriate means of achieving the expected outcome
- Implements the revised action plan
- Notifies the appropriate health care provider when immediate clinical response is necessary, based on procedural findings and patient condition
- Obtains assistance to support the quality assurance action plan
- Takes action based on patient and procedural variances

Standard Seven—Outcomes Measurement

The medical imaging and radiation therapy professional reviews and evaluates the outcome of the procedure according to quality assurance standards.

Rationale

To evaluate the quality of care, the medical imaging and radiation therapy professional compares the actual outcome with the expected outcome. Outcomes assessment is an integral part of the ongoing quality management action plan to enhance services.

General Criteria

The medical imaging and radiation therapy professional:

- Assesses the patient's physical, emotional, and mental status prior to discharge
- Determines that actual outcomes are within established criteria
- Evaluates the process and recognizes opportunities for future changes

(continued)

DISPLAY 1-3

The ASRT Practice Standards for Medical Imaging and Radiation Therapy Effective June 2021 (*continued*)

- Measures and evaluates the results of the revised action plan
- Reviews all data for completeness and accuracy
- Reviews and evaluates quality assurance processes and tools for effectiveness
- Reviews the implementation process for accuracy and validity
- Uses evidence-based practice to determine whether the actual outcome is within established criteria

Standard Eight—Documentation

The medical imaging and radiation therapy professional documents information about patient care, procedures, and outcomes.

Rationale

Clear and precise documentation is essential for continuity of care, accuracy of care, and quality assurance.

General Criteria

The medical imaging and radiation therapy professional:

- Archives images or data
- Documents diagnostic, treatment, and patient data in the medical record in a timely, accurate, and comprehensive manner
- Documents medication administration in the patient's medical record[*,†]
- Documents procedural timeout
- Documents unintended outcomes or exceptions from the established criteria
- Maintains documentation of quality assurance activities, procedures, and results
- Provides pertinent information to authorized individual(s) involved in the patient's care
- Records information used for billing and coding procedures
- Reports any out-of-tolerance deviations to the appropriate personnel
- Verifies patient consent is documented

Specific Criteria
Radiography

- Documents fluoroscopic time

- Documents radiation exposure
- Documents the use of shielding devices and proper radiation safety practices

Standard Nine—Quality

The medical imaging and radiation therapy professional strives to provide optimal care.

Rationale

Patients expect and deserve optimal care during diagnosis and treatment.

General Criteria

The medical imaging and radiation therapy professional:

- Adheres to standards, policies, statutes, regulations, and established guidelines
- Anticipates, considers, and responds to the needs of a diverse patient population
- Applies professional judgment and discretion while performing the procedure
- Collaborates with others to elevate the quality of care
- Participates in ongoing quality assurance programs

Standard Ten—Self-Assessment

The medical imaging and radiation therapy professional evaluates personal performance.

Rationale

Self-assessment is necessary for personal growth and professional development.

General Criteria

The medical imaging and radiation therapy professional:

- Assesses personal work ethics, behaviors, and attitudes
- Evaluates performance, applies personal strengths, and recognizes opportunities for educational growth and improvement
- Recognizes hazards associated with their work environment and takes measures to mitigate them

DISPLAY 1-3

The ASRT Practice Standards for Medical Imaging and Radiation Therapy Effective June 2021 (*continued*)

Standard Eleven—Collaboration and Collegiality

The medical imaging and radiation therapy professional promotes a positive and collaborative practice atmosphere with other members of the health care team.

Rationale

To provide quality patient care, all members of the health care team must communicate effectively and work together efficiently.

General Criteria

The medical imaging and radiation therapy professional:

- Develops and maintains collaborative partnerships to enhance quality and efficiency
- Informs and instructs others about radiation safety
- Promotes understanding of the profession
- Shares knowledge and expertise with others

Standard Twelve—Ethics

The medical imaging and radiation therapy professional adheres to the profession's accepted ethical standards.

Rationale

Decisions made and actions taken on behalf of the patient are based on a sound ethical foundation.

General Criteria

The medical imaging and radiation therapy professional:

- Accepts accountability for decisions made and actions taken
- Acts as a patient advocate
- Adheres to the established ethical standards of recognized certifying agencies
- Adheres to the established practice standards of the profession
- Delivers patient care and service free from bias or discrimination
- Provides health care services with consideration for a diverse patient population
- Reports unsafe practices to the radiation safety officer, regulatory agency, or other appropriate authority
- Respects the patient's right to privacy and confidentiality

Standard Thirteen—Research, Innovation, and Professional Advocacy

The medical imaging and radiation therapy professional participates in the acquisition and dissemination of knowledge and the advancement of the profession.

Rationale

Participation in professional organizations and scholarly activities such as research, scientific investigation, presentation, and publication advances the profession.

General Criteria

The medical imaging and radiation therapy professional:

- Adopts new best practices
- Investigates innovative methods for application in practice
- Monitors changes to federal and state law, regulations, and accreditation standards affecting area(s) of practice
- Participates in data collection
- Participates in professional advocacy efforts
- Participates in professional societies and organizations
- Pursues lifelong learning
- Reads and evaluates research relevant to the profession
- Shares information through publication, presentation, and collaboration

---

*Excludes limited x-ray machine operator.
†Excludes medical dosimetry.

thinking. Quality improvement and customer service allow the radiographer to be a responsible member of the health care team by continually assessing professional performance.

The ASRT Scope of Practice is incorporated into the practice standards and is seen in Display 1-4.

It can be seen that the title of radiologic technologist involves a serious commitment to education and the profession.

HEALTH PROFESSIONS IN MEDICAL IMAGING

Once a student has graduated from a radiologic technology program, there are many other areas within the medical imaging department that the new technologist may want to explore. The following list shows the many areas that are available to motivated individuals.

DISPLAY 1-4

Medical Imaging and Radiation Therapy Scope of Practice

Scopes of practice delineate the parameters of practice and identify the boundaries for practice. A comprehensive procedure list for the medical imaging and radiation therapy professional is impractical because clinical activities vary by the practice needs and expertise of the individual. As medical imaging and radiation therapy professionals gain more experience, knowledge, and clinical competence, the clinical activities may evolve.

The scope of practice of the medical imaging and radiation therapy professional includes:

- Administering medications enterally, parenterally, through new or existing vascular access or through other routes as prescribed by a licensed practitioner[*,†]
- Administering medications with an infusion pump or power injector as prescribed by a licensed practitioner[*,†]
- Applying principles of ALARA to minimize exposure to patient, self, and others
- Applying principles of patient safety during all aspects of patient care
- Assisting in maintaining medical records, respecting confidentiality and established policy
- Corroborating a patient's clinical history with procedure and ensuring information is documented and available for use by a licensed practitioner
- Educating and monitoring students and other health care providers[*]
- Evaluating images for proper positioning and determining if additional images improves the procedure or treatment outcome
- Evaluating images for technical quality and ensuring proper identification is recorded
- Identifying and responding to emergency situations
- Identifying, calculating, compounding, preparing, and/or administering medications as prescribed by a licensed practitioner[*,†]
- Performing ongoing quality assurance activities
- Performing venipuncture as prescribed by a licensed practitioner[*,†]
- Postprocessing data
- Preparing patients for procedures
- Providing education
- Providing optimal patient care
- Receiving, relaying, and documenting verbal, written, and electronic orders in the patient's medical record
- Selecting the appropriate protocol and optimizing technical factors while maximizing patient safety
- Starting, maintaining, and/or removing intravenous access as prescribed by a licensed practitioner[*,†]
- Verifying archival storage of data
- Verifying informed consent for applicable procedures[*]

[*]Excludes limited x-ray machine operator.
[†]Excludes medical dosimetry.

1. Application specialist educates and trains radiography professionals to use new software and equipment.

2. Bone densitometry also called Dual Energy X-ray Absorptiometry (DEXA) scans measures bone loss to diagnose osteoporosis.

3. CT produces cross-sectional images of anatomy used for diagnostic and therapeutic purposes.

4. Diagnostic medical sonography is a noninvasive way to visualize internal organs but using sound waves.
   i. Breast sonography uses sound waves to help diagnose breast abnormalities.
   ii. Echocardiography uses sound wave to create moving images of the heart.
   iii. Vascular sonography uses sound waves to evaluate the body's circulatory system and help identify blockages in the arteries and veins and detect blood clots.

5. Diagnostic radiography (medical imaging) uses radiation to produce images of the body to help in the diagnosis and treatment of disease and injury.

6. Education in medical diagnostic imaging is always changing to keep up with the advancing technology. Currently, faculty are aging and there is a need for new people to become interested in educating others.

7. Health physics is a profession that protects people and the environment from radiation hazards. It is, essentially, radiation protection.

8. Imaging informatics is a subspecialty of biomedical informatics. The purpose of this field is to improve efficiency, accuracy, usability, and reliability of imaging services within health care.

9. Interventional radiography is a subspecialty of radiology that uses minimally invasive image-guided procedures to diagnose and treat diseases without the use of surgery.
   i. Cardiac interventional radiography looks at the heart and its blood vessels to diagnose and treat problems without the use of surgery.
   ii. Vascular radiography uses the image-guided minimally invasive procedure to diagnose diseases of the vessels of the body without the use of surgery.

10. MRI uses a magnetic field and computer-generated radio waves to create images of the organs and tissues of the body. There is no radiation involved.

11. Mammography uses low-dose radiation to see the tissues of the breast. It aids in the early detection and diagnosis of breast diseases in both women and men.

12. Medical dosimetry is the field within radiation oncology where a "dosimetrist" performs calculations for the accurate delivery of radiation to cancer cells.

13. Molecular imaging (MI) is a growing biomedical research area of medicine that allows the visualization of processes taking place at the cellular level. It is used to diagnose and manage treatments of cancer, heart disease, Alzheimer and Parkinson disease and many more.

14. Nuclear medicine technology is a specialized area of radiology that uses very small amounts of radioactive material to examine organ function and structure.
   i. Nuclear medicine advanced associate is similar to a radiology assistant. This person works under the supervision of a licensed physician who is authorized to use radioactive materials.

15. Quality management includes all aspects of medical imaging technology such as room and workflow design, equipment selection, purchase and installation, acceptance testing, and other tasks as determined by the facility. It ensures that high-quality images are produced and that ALARA is maintained.

16. Radiation therapy is a cancer treatment using high doses of radiation to kill cancer cells and shrink tumors.

17. Research in radiology is being done at various large facilities such as Stanford, Mayo Clinic, and Johns Hopkins to develop new imaging techniques and equipment for better patient care.

18. Supervisory roles are varied within a department. There is an administrator, manager, lead technologist, shift lead, and others. The radiology organization flowchart seen in Display 1-5 shows some of the supervisors within an imaging department.

RADIOLOGY ORGANIZATION

Because the student radiographer is more involved with the radiology department, it is essential that each component is understood. Knowledge of professional personnel within the imaging department facilitates the student's education. Display 1-5 shows the organization of a radiology department.

The entire radiology department is headed by a *radiology administrator*. Administrators are responsible for budgeting, equipment purchases, policy review as well as many other duties and are the liaison with the institution's administration. The administrator usually hires (or appoints) personnel to be in charge of each of the separate departments within the radiology department. The managers supervise each of their assigned areas and report back to the administrator with whom they work closely to make sure the overall department is a well-run area within the institution.

Radiologists are physicians that have continued their medical education with a focus on looking at radiographic images, assessing the patient's history, and determining a probable diagnosis for the referring clinician. In addition to "reading" the radiographic images, they perform certain radiographic procedures on the patient,

DISPLAY 1-5

Medical Imaging Organizational Flowchart

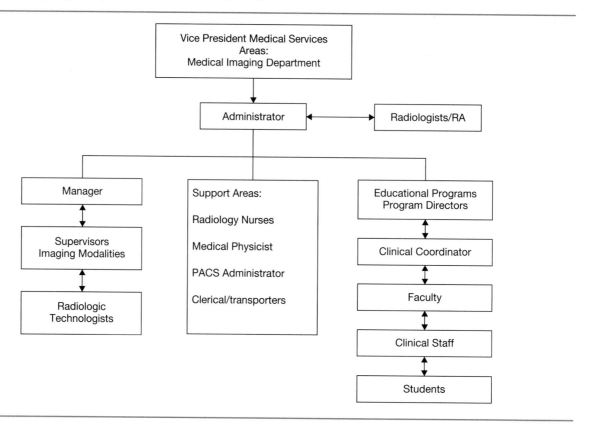

such as interventional cardiac and vascular studies and fluoroscopic studies, with the assistance of a registered radiologic technologist.

Radiologic technologists are individuals that have met the requirements of educational training, passed the national registry examination (ARRT), and are entitled to use the initials "RT" behind their names. It is the RT that performs the procedure on each patient, takes the radiographic images, and prepares it to be sent to the radiologist to be reviewed for diagnosis. Technologists can be further trained in the various modalities within the radiology department such as CT, mammography, or nuclear medicine.

Many departments rely on *radiology physician assistants (RPAs)* to help the radiologist perform the procedures and studies that are done in a large department. They essentially practice radiology medicine under the supervision of a licensed radiologist. All RPAs must be licensed in the state in which they practice as well as being certified by taking the Physician Assistant National Certifying Examination.

Larger departments often hire dedicated nurses to work solely in the diagnostic imaging arena. Radiology nurses assist patients through the use of x-rays, ultrasound,

MRI, and other imaging. They evaluate patients once procedures are complete and care for them until they are discharged. *Radiology nurses* help meet patients' needs and manage their pain levels.

Medical physicists, also known as health science physicists, are often not inhouse employees of a hospital unless the institution is a large health care system. These individuals calculate, operate, and manage the design of equipment, consult with medical professionals, and help ensure that all equipment is operating with all safety precautions in place. Designing new radiographic room configurations and the dosage of radiation that equipment outputs are normal duties of a medical physicist. A master's degree is the standard educational level; however, some positions require a PhD.

Without the *support staff* that work within the department, it would not run. Information technology staff, clerical personnel, transporters, and aides are just a few of the individuals that make a diagnostic imaging department operate with efficiency.

Within the radiology organization of teaching hospitals is the educational aspect. Hospitals may have students from college-based programs or there may be a complete program within the hospital.

Personnel involved with *radiologic technology education* include:

Program director: In a JRCERT-accredited radiography program, the director must have a master's degree. Many university programs are now requiring that the director have (or obtain) a doctoral degree. The director is responsible for the effective organization and coordination of the delivery of radiologic technology education.

Clinical coordinator: To be a coordinator in a JRCERT program, one must have a minimum of a bachelor's degree. The clinical coordinator works closely with the program director to ensure that the program is meeting and maintaining the standards of competency in the clinical setting.

Didactic faculty: Most often, the program director and the clinical coordinator assume the duties of faculty as well as their managerial duties. Didactic faculty are responsible for providing the prescribed curriculum to radiography students in a classroom setting.

Adjunct faculty: In large programs that have many students, part-time faculty members are often hired to work both in the classroom and clinical setting to oversee the education of the student.

Clinical preceptor: Preceptors are individuals who have a supervisory role over students while in the clinical setting. They provide educational training on a one-on-one basis with real patients.

Clinical staff: Every technologist in a teaching facility has an obligation to provide instruction to students in the imaging department. Although they are not in a supervisory role, they must exhibit the critical thinking, problem-solving, and judgment skills so as to be role models for students.

FOUNDATIONS FOR STUDENT LEARNING ACHIEVEMENT

One must consider several essential elements before beginning any course of study to achieve success. Four elements are presented that should be taken into account for achievement in learning. It is recommended that one take time to review all educational, **emotional**, physical wellness, and financial preparedness before beginning the rigor of an **imaging program**. Maintaining a healthy balance with education, family, friends, emotions, physical wellness, and financial obligations is a goal the imaging student should not take for granted. Although the majority of students are successful in completing courses required to begin an imaging program, imaging students often state that they were not prepared for the impact the imaging program has on their entire life. Often cited is the amount of time the successful student must spend each week in lectures, laboratories, clinical hours, and study for 2 consecutive years.

Educational and Emotional Preparedness

There is much to balance in terms of time commitment for the educational demands in attending classes, laboratories, clinical time, and study time, which impacts a student emotionally at one time or another. A full-time load translates into more than 40 hours per week dedicated to attending the required courses and study time. It is important to share with significant family members and friends as much as possible about the new program and career as quality personal time is most likely reduced. Initially, the student does not anticipate the amount of time that is required for the rigors of an in-depth imaging program. These programs are not like taking college courses where one can pick and choose which classes to take and when to go to school. The entire program is laid out in a well-developed and regulated course of study that must be adhered to. Involvement of family and friends is helpful in maintaining a life balance throughout the 2 years.

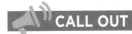 CALL OUT

An excellent opportunity to include a significant other in the educational process is available in practicing positioning skills on willing family members or friends.

In addition to existing support system of family and friends, new relationships are developed with classmates. It is important to inform family that many hours will be spent with classmates in and out of class studying. Some family members and friends realize the importance of collegial studying to facilitate the learning process, and thus they recognize the time spent with classmates is valid.

Physical Wellness and Financial Preparedness

Physical and mental health balance can affect one's ability to be successful as a student and, later, in the workplace. Before beginning a program, students are required to undergo a physical examination conducted by a physician, which includes immunizations, laboratory work, and, in some programs, passing drug testing to ensure health status. By maintaining physical wellness, students will have the energy needed to complete the 2-year program. At times, students relate being tired as a result of the demands of studying, clinical hours, and life in general. Toward the end of the semester, some students feel rundown and tired, and become ill or comment that they are not getting enough sleep. At all times, it is important for the radiography student to keep physical wellness in mind, which includes eating balanced meals, sleeping right, exercising, and managing **stress**.

Financial obligations can be a contributing factor to stress. The amount of savings needed to supplement an income for 2 years is sometimes underestimated. Develop a realistic budget that subtracts housing (rent or mortgage), utilities, transportation/vehicle, clothing allowance, student costs (tuition, texts, supplies, and other fees), child care, food, entertainment, and electronic media (smartphones) from the net income. Remember most students cannot realistically work full-time the entire 2 years they are in the program, and therefore, the income that can be generated as a full-time student must be carefully analyzed to forecast realistically. Students should consider exploring the financial services and resources available through the colleges and universities. Many students are eligible for fee waivers, grants, scholarships, and loans. Taking advantage of the financial resources can help augment a budget plan and reduce financial stress.

How Does the Successful Student Prepare to Begin a Program?

- Taking a learning styles survey inventory test
- Managing stress using a variety of strategies
- Identifying how to effectively manage time for academic and personal growth
- Using study tips best practices that are most effective

Learning Styles

Learning styles are various approaches of understanding and mastering material. Learners are tactile or **kinesthetic learners**, auditory learners, and/or visual learners. These styles can easily be evaluated with an online inventory test. After taking a learning style assessment, the results identify strengths and weaknesses and provide specific strategies to help individuals learn. Knowing what learning style(s) works best translates into effective and efficient learning tools that can be used throughout the program. Identifying strengths and weaknesses with a learning styles assessment has two benefits: taking advantage of strengths for learning and developing coping strategies in areas of weakness.

Managing Stress

Taking a stress management course before beginning the program could be extremely advantageous. Stress occurs at various times throughout the program, whether as an imaging student or in personal life. The ability to

positively control stress by taking action developed as a result of practicing stress reduction strategies alleviates expending unnecessary emotions, time, and energy. Stress reduction activities include physical activities (walking, running, or exercising), yoga, meditation, relaxation, imagination, listening to music, journaling, and spending time with a friend; and even breathing exercises help manage or reduce stress.

Being organized greatly impacts stress reduction. The well-organized student learns better and eliminates a contributing factor to stress. All students can benefit from organization skills as simple as organizing a notebook binder or electronic files for each course with sections for the syllabus, lecture notes, handouts, quizzes and tests, and study notes. Once the course has been completed, the notebook binder or electronic file is organized and ready for review in preparation for the ARRT examination after the program completion.

Organize by developing a master calendar of important dates for quizzes, exams, written report, presentation, or other assignments for each course for the semester or quarter. This provides an overview of what is expected and assignment due dates. Knowing and reviewing the calendar periodically leaves no room for surprises and therefore, less stress. Keeping track of all grades in terms of points and/or percentage for each course provides an exact view of successful standing in each course. It is important to compare calculations with the instructor of record for validation. By knowing a grade at any given time, stress can be alleviated. In some cases, the grade may be higher than perceived, but the student may be experiencing undue stress from not knowing the actual grade. If a grade needs improvement, setting goals to do what it takes to meet higher benchmarks for passing grades also reduces the stress of not having a plan.

Time Management

The ability to manage time to allocate sufficient and appropriate time to activities for both personal and academic life is essential for the successful student. Learning or study time is a valuable commodity, and, therefore, maximum use of available time must be fundamentally managed. The time management grid seen in Display 1-6 can help students sort out how their time is spent. Students have full lives, jobs, families, and other responsibilities and obligations in addition to full-time academic commitments. Priorities must be established before the start of the program, and once established, these priorities should be honored by removing obstacles that get in the way. Eliminate distractions by finding ways to free up time for what is important.

DISPLAY 1-6

Time Management Grid

Time	Monday	Tuesday	Wednesday	Thursday	Friday	Saturday	Sunday
5:00 AM							
6:00 AM							
7:00 AM							
8:00 AM							
9:00 AM							
10:00 AM							
11:00 AM							
12:00 AM							
1:00 PM							
2:00 PM							
3:00 PM							
4:00 PM							
5:00 PM							
6:00 PM							
7:00 PM							
8:00 PM							
9:00 PM							
10:00 PM							
11:00 PM							
12:00 AM							
1:00 AM							
2:00 AM							
3:00 AM							
4:00 AM							

Be realistic when estimating the time spent on the following activities:

- Sleeping
- Eating
- Working
- Caring for children or other family members
- Performing school activities (class and study time)
- Running errands
- Traveling to and from destinations
- Conducting personal activities (personal hygiene, shopping, exercising)
- Social media and gaming activities
- Performing household chores (meal preparation, cleaning, and laundry)
- Socializing (church, clubs, etc.)

The weekly overview of the time spent in a typical week hour by hour helps determine if there is adequate time to undertake and accomplish day-to-day activities with the additional responsibility of being a successful full-time student. Typically, adjustments are made after having a visual of how time is being spent for a week. Some find that they can successfully complete all responsibilities and still have time left over. This scenario reduces anxiety and stress, especially if there was a perception of not having enough time before tracking daily activities. On the other hand, if the time management results show not enough time is spent on the highest priorities, adjustments to the time spent on specific activities can be made. It is important to ensure that once a workable schedule is made, stick to it. It is also recommended to reassess this time management schedule every so often according to short- and long-term goals.

Study Tips Best Practices

To complete a radiologic technology program, the successful student must keep the goal of becoming an imaging technologist first and foremost. Being persistent, realistic, and conscientious in pursuing this important and life changing goal is accomplished with the right attitude and practices. Some of the fundamentals for successfully completing a program include using methods that are well known to provide the greatest impact for student learning. Good examples of study tips best practices are listed on Display 1-7. These activities support results for course completion and overall program completion.

DISPLAY 1-7

Study Tips Best Practices

1. Read the reading assignments before the class session at least once.
2. Know what are the overall course objectives and specific class session objectives to use as a road map for studying.
3. Take notes during the class sessions and use color highlighters to emphasize topics.
4. Ask questions during class or make an appointment to meet with the instructor to ask questions.
5. Make notations in textbooks, whether hard copies or e-texts.
6. Study at least 2 hours for each class hour, breaking the time into smaller segments. Example: a 3-hour class would require 6 hours of study. This can be broken down to 1 hour a day for the week.
7. Meet with the instructor to clarify any material.
8. Join a study group and meet once a week. The recommendation is a maximum of three participants. Each participant should come prepared to contribute to the study session and to keep on task.
9. Independent study time should take place in a comfortable environment as identified in the learning styles assessment.
10. Play music in the background if that helps in focusing on the material.
11. Determine whether writing or word processing the information is the best learning method.
12. Keep material organized to minimize the time it takes to get organized before beginning to study.
13. Plan on studying every day instead of studying once or twice a week for 10 to 12 hours at a time.
14. Develop acronyms or statements to recall information.

CASE STUDY

Pasha is a 31-year-old single parent who was just accepted into a radiography program. In addition to taking care of her 9-year-old daughter she is responsible for the care of her mother who is in assisted living and suffering from dementia. Pasha has been working at a local hospital in the dietary department. She takes the food trays to the patients in their hospital rooms. In fact, this is how she became interested in furthering her education and becoming a radiographer.

As part of the introductory class, all students were required to do a time study management assessment and find three other students with whom they would form a study group and have a standing weekly session. Pasha did her assessment and found that she had extra time on Wednesday after clinical at 3:30 until 5 PM when she had to get her daughter from after-school day care, and also Saturday evenings. She was sure that she could have the study session at her home as she rarely went out.

The first 2 months of the program seemed to be okay, but as more time went by, Pasha was finding herself exhausted at the end of the weekend and was dreading going to classes on Monday. The first class, 8 to 11 AM, was physics class and then anatomy, and positioning was noon to 3 PM. She hated physics as she was a visual learner and because she couldn't "see" how x-ray was made, she was having a hard time understanding it. To top it off, her study group was falling apart because the other students were much younger than she and didn't want to meet on Saturday night. In addition, her mother's dementia was becoming a problem at the assisted living facility and administration there was suggesting it was time to move her to a memory care unit. However, Pasha has not been able to see her mother on a regular basis like she did before entering school, so she is not sure how her mother is actually faring at the facility.

By the end of the semester, Pasha was calling off ill in order to stay home to study. Her study group had disbanded and she was failing the physics class. Her daughter was being neglected and became belligerent and she was falling behind on paying the bills. Pasha is considering taking a semester leave of absence in order to work double shifts to catch up but that would mean she would not graduate with her classmates.

ITEMS FOR CONSIDERATION

1. What would be the first thing that Pasha should do to try to get back on track with her grades?

2. How best should Pasha handle studying? Is calling off from clinical practice appropriate? Why or why not?

3. Her financial health is at risk. What could Pasha do to try to alleviate that stress?

4. With whom should Pasha communicate in order to establish an action plan so that she might be able to continue in the program: Her mother? The program director? The clinical coordinator? The physics instructor? A counselor? The administration at the assisted living facility? Her daughter? Suggest possible scenarios for each of these conversations.

Summary

1. Discovery of x-rays
   a. Wilhelm C. Roentgen discovered x-ray in November 1895 while working with a Crookes tube and barium platinocyanide.
   b. He named it "X" for the mathematical symbol for the unknown.
   c. He received the first Nobel Prize in Physics in 1901 for his work.

2. Uses
   a. Thomas Edison developed the "Vitascope," the forerunner of today's fluoroscopy.
   b. Marie Curie discovered radium in 1898.
   c. Radiation was novel in the early years and was used for entertainment, souvenirs, and spiritual seances. It was touted to cure cancer and skin lesions.

3. Early effects
   a. The effects were not understood in the early days of x-ray. Clarence Dally was the first fatality of radiation exposure in 1904. He was a good friend of Thomas Edison who stopped his work in radiation upon the death of his friend.
   b. Radiation was burning patients to the point that amputations were being performed. Twenty-eight Americans died from the effects of experimentation.
   c. Boston hospital opened the first school to try to teach the proper and safe use of radiation.

4. Advancements
   a. Commercial uses like sterilization
   b. CT in 1972 with the first scans taking several hours to complete
   c. MRI in 1946 and perfected for medicine in 1977 on the whole body
   d. Ultrasound was beginning to be used in medicine in 1974.
   e. Other areas include PET and SPECT scanning, mammography, and sonography.
   f. The way imaging is done has changed drastically in the last few decades. Film was replaced by computerized images that quickly led to digital imaging.

5. Health care settings
   a. Many facilities can make up the health care system. They can be large organizations like an HMO or a small community setting located in a rural setting. Different facilities within a health care system include:
      i. Hospitals and clinics/pain clinics
      ii. Mental health and long-term care facilities
      iii. Hospice and home health care
      iv. Convenient care centers
      v. Freestanding imaging centers
      vi. Jails, prisons, medical examiner
   b. Students may not be rotated through all of these areas but should be familiar with them. Patients may question the student about certain clinics or home health care and the student should be knowledgeable enough to answer general questions.
6. Payment and reimbursement systems
   a. Medicare covers persons over the age of 65, permanently disabled workers and their dependents, and patients with end-stage renal disease. There are different parts of Medicare that cover different services.
   b. Medicaid is a federally funded and state-administered program for families with dependent older adults, children, or disabled persons.
   c. MCOs include HMOs and PPOs. Each of these groups tries to lower cost to the patient.
   d. POS plans allow the patient to choose a physician that acts as a gatekeeper to authorize all referrals.
   e. PHOs create a corporate structure between the physicians and the hospital.
7. Health provider organization
   a. The organization of a hospital is set up to provide leadership at all levels, which provide quality patient care. Without patients, there is no need for the many physicians, therapists, and technologists that are employed in a hospital.
      i. Mission statements are published to let people (patients and employees) know the focus of the organization.
      ii. Vision statements highlight where the organization sees itself in the future.
      iii. Value statements are about the philosophical ideals of an organization.
   b. Administrative services and medical services are made up of individuals necessary to help keep the hospital functioning smoothly to meet patient needs. This is accomplished by staying focused on the philosophy defined in the mission and values statements.

8. Accreditation
   a. TJC is the accrediting agency of health care institutions.
   b. ACR is recognized as the gold standard of accreditation in medical imaging. It is a voluntary process, but is so well thought of that most facilities try to attain it.
   c. Educational programs in radiography are accredited by JRCERT. The ARRT recognizes programs that have this accreditation as those who follow the regimented curriculum. College-based programs can also be accredited by the CHEA, which then recognizes different regional agencies within the United States, such as Western Association of Schools and Colleges Senior College and University Commission (WSCUC).
9. Professional credentialing
   a. Obtaining a credential in the profession marks the individual as one who has been educated and is knowledgeable to perform the particular work.
   b. The ARRT is the national credentialing body in the United States. In order to work in the United States, one must have passed the ARRT credentialing exam.
   c. A total of 46 states in the union also have licensure requirement.
10. Regulatory agencies
    a. Federal agencies that have oversight authority of health care facilities are
       i. FDA
       ii. CDC
       iii. NIOSH
          1. CMS
       iv. AHRQ
    b. State agencies also have authority and are responsible for such things as licensing requirements, reviewing applications, investigating complaints, and carrying out disciplinary measures.
11. Professional organizations in radiologic technology
    a. All radiographers are encouraged to join and participate in the professional organizations on both the state and national level. These organizations write the rules and codes that apply to the profession. Participation allows one to keep abreast of technologic changes and alterations in professional standards.
    b. The strength of the profession is promoted as well as prevention of infringement from groups that desire to assume parts of the professional responsibilities of the radiographer.
    c. There is a difference between societies (to which a person can belong) and certification boards (to

which a person must pass an examination). Accreditation agencies review different aspects of a facility or an educational program and determine if certain criteria are being met.

12. Health care teams
    a. Teams are dedicated individuals that meet the needs of the patient and provide service in a hospital or clinical setting. It is important for all teams to work as an integrated unit for the support of the patient's health care delivery.
    b. The personnel involved as part of the health care team include:
        i. Physicians and physician assistants
        ii. Registered nurses, licensed vocational nurses, and certified nursing assistants
        iii. Therapists
            1. Physical, occupational, and respiratory
        iv. Pharmacists
        v. Technologists work in many departments such as radiology, cardiology, and the laboratory.
        vi. Social workers, support staff, and assistive personnel are critical in all health care environments.

13. Responsibilities of the radiographer
    a. Radiographers are responsible for many components of the field. Only five are listed here but these encompass the majority of the profession.
        i. Assist the radiologist or RA.
        ii. Apply principles of radiation safety.
        iii. Maintain a high degree of accuracy in radiographic positioning.
        iv. Provide direct patient care.
        v. Follow established practice standards and the scope of practice.
    b. The radiographer must also follow the ASRT Practice of Standards for Medical Imaging and Radiation Therapy. These standards include the expected level of performance from the radiographer.

14. Health professions in medical imaging
    a. There are many areas that the radiographer can become interested in and possibly employed. Not only are there the subspecialties such as nuclear medicine, CT, MRI, sonography, and interventional radiography, but there are those areas that are not often thought of as being affiliated with medical imaging such as
        i. Applications specialist
        ii. Education
        iii. Health physics
        iv. Imaging informatics
        v. Quality management
        vi. Therapy
        vii. Research

15. Radiology organization
    a. The radiology administrator is the liaison with the hospital administration and the imaging departments.
    b. Managers or lead technologists supervise each area of the imaging department and report back to the administrator. CT, MRI, ultrasound, nuclear medicine, interventional imaging, and diagnostic imaging all have a supervisor that meets with the administrator. These individuals help keep the entire department running smoothly by helping disperse communication from the staff to the administration and vice versa.
    c. Radiologists are the physicians that interpret the radiographic images and provide a probable diagnosis to the referring clinical physician. Although radiologists are employees of the hospital (either individually or as a group) they are often included in a different section of the organizational chart for the radiology department. They work closely with the administrator to ensure that the procedures and various departments meet the needs of the physicians and the patients.
    d. Some facilities may have an educational program affiliated with the organization. As such, the radiographers within the department become educators of those students while in the clinical setting.

16. Student learning
    a. There are many ways that a student learns things. Visual, audio, or tactile (doing) are different styles of learning where students best understand the material. Many students are a combination of two of these styles.
    b. Once understanding what style facilitates learning, a time line should be established for daily activities. The student should analyze how time is spent in a typical week in order to determine what is crucial and what can be deleted from a schedule.
    c. One of the most crucial factors in being a successful learner is to be organized. Organize all course materials and keep them separate from other courses. They become a useful study guide for the ARRT.
    d. Find a study group that will help in understanding topics that do not come easily. Spend at least 2 hours of study time for each 1 hour of class time. Meeting as a group makes this time go quickly and allows for all members of the group to have

the material presented differently than from the instructor.

e. Find ways that alleviate stress. Talk to family members and friends to have them be a support system. Involve family in studying to help them understand the critical nature of what each topic covers.

f. Reassess goals as the program advances and make changes as needed. The program itself is dynamic and the way a student progresses should be as well. Change as the courses change and study habits adjust to the nature of the assignments.

CHAPTER 1 REVIEW QUESTIONS

1. Who is credited with the discovery of x-rays and when?

2. Who discovered fluoroscopy and when?

3. Who was the first known American fatality from radiation exposure?
   a. Thomas Edison
   b. Benjamin Franklin
   c. Michael Faraday
   d. Clarence Dally

4. What type of tube was used when x-rays were discovered?
   a. Calvin tube
   b. Coolidge tube
   c. Catcher tube
   d. Crookes tube

5. Which of the following are modern-day advances that came from x-ray? (Circle all that apply)
   a. SPECT
   b. PET
   c. Ultrasound
   d. Mammography
   e. CT

6. Match the type of services on the left with the correct description on the right

   a. DRGs   1. Covers acute hospital care for persons aged over 65

   b. POS   2. Provides medical care for children or disabled

   c. Medicare   3. Groups payment by medical diagnosis

   d. HMO   4. Decreases costs by preventative medicine

   e. Medicaid   5. Primary care provider is a gatekeeper

7. What is the purpose of a mission statement?

8. Name four elements to consider for student success.

9. Clinics are considered a health care environment.
   a. True
   b. False

10. What is the purpose of the time management grid?

11. Name two professional societies in radiologic technology.

12. After completing a radiologic technology program, you are employed at the local community hospital in the diagnostic imaging department. You are approached by a colleague who asks you to become a member of the local chapter of your professional organization. You know that you are expected to pay yearly dues. What would be your best response to your colleague?

    a. You explain that you have just begun your first job and money is in short supply at this time.

    b. You laugh and say, "No, thanks, I've had all of the organization I can take for a while."

    c. You join in 1 or 2 years when your financial status improves.

    d. You join at once because you feel that it is an obligation to be a member of your professional organization.

Professionalism and Related Issues

2

After studying this chapter, the student will be able to:

1. Describe how to develop professional attitudes.

2. Discuss career opportunities and advancement for the radiographer.

3. Identify the benefits of continuing education as related to improved patient care and professional development.

4. Explain the importance of the Health Insurance Portability and Accountability Act (HIPAA).

5. Describe the special needs of the terminally ill or grieving patient as they present in imaging.

6. Explain death and dying from the view point of both patient and radiographer.

7. Define advance directives for medical care and differentiate between the various types of advance care documents.

KEY TERMS

Advance directives: Directions given by a person while in a healthy mental state concerning wishes at time of death

Anticipatory grieving: That which makes a problem worse (aggravating) or better (alleviating)

Anxiety: A feeling of unease

Basic needs: Those conditions which are necessary for human life

Continuum: Elements that make up process wherein the adjacent elements have very little differences but the elements from one end to the other have a large difference

Continuing education (CE): Professional education received following completion of a training program to maintain skills

Do-not-resuscitate (DNR): An order on the patient's medical record and signed by the patient's physician that orders the staff not to perform cardiopulmonary resuscitation or call the emergency team if the patient expires

Ethical: Conforming with the rules governing personal and professional conduct

"Full code": The opposite of DNR. It orders the staff to exhaust all possible efforts to keep the patient alive. This is also called a "code blue" in a hospital or clinical setting.

In-service: Training given to employees in connection with their work or profession to update or maintain knowledge

Mentor: A teacher, coach, or adviser of conduct

"No code": The same as a do-not-resuscitate order; a written medical order must follow this request for the patient to be allowed to expire without emergency assistance

Practitioner: Any individual practicing in a specific area or discipline

Profession: A calling that requires specialized knowledge and intensive academic preparation

Radiographer: A radiologic technologist who uses critical thinking, problem-solving, and judgment to perform diagnostic images

Regulatory compliance: Control of a situation or group of laws that supervise a profession

Stress: The result of anxiety or tension

INTRODUCTION

A **profession** is defined as a body of work that meets specific criteria and characteristics. Any profession can be said to

- contain a unique body of knowledge;
- have relevance to social values;
- require long specialized education;
- be motivated to serve the needs of the community versus the needs of oneself;
- be organized into associations that help guide the profession;
- have set performance standards;
- maintain a level of public trust and confidence; and
- be made up of people who are motivated by a strong service desire and commitment to competence.

As in all professions, **radiographers** are expected to adhere in conduct and behavior to the particular **ethical** and legal standards of the field. Any person who does not adhere to this code may lose their license as well as the privileges of the profession.

Students who have made the decision to enter the profession of radiologic technology need to understand that they are making the commitment to accept the code of ethics of this profession and must work within the scope of practice. They must also understand that they are accountable for how they perform as a radiographer and may be held legally liable for any errors made while caring for patients. The legality of radiography is discussed in-depth in Chapter 4.

Anyone contemplating a career in radiologic technology needs to examine the reasons why this profession was chosen. As in other health care professions, such as nursing, the radiographer works intimately with the patient who may be very ill. In recent years, the COVID-19 pandemic was extremely hard on health care workers, and for many, it signaled the end of a career. If a person is not willing to be subjected to deadly viruses and work many hours overtime during times of extreme illness, it might be wise to rethink this profession as a career choice. Once in the field and employed, it is not an option to refuse working on certain patients or in circumstances that put oneself in harm's way. Before spending 2 years studying a rigorous course of classes, one needs to seriously consider the ability to be selfless; otherwise, this career choice should be reconsidered.

CRITERIA FOR A PROFESSION

Radiologic technology has evolved from an undereducated workforce of x-ray technicians in the early 1900s to its continued advances as a profession in the 21st century. This progression took place over decades with the efforts and dedication of the persons who worked in this field. These dedicated people, known as **practitioners**, are united by criteria that identify them as a profession. These criteria are summarized as follows:

1. A vital human service is provided to the society by the profession.
2. Professions possess a special body of knowledge that is continuously enlarged through research.
3. Practitioners are expected to be accountable and responsible.
4. The education of professionals takes place in institutions for higher education.
5. Practitioners have an independent function and control their own practice.
6. Professionals are committed to their work and are motivated by doing well.
7. A code of ethics guides professional decisions and conduct.
8. A professional organization oversees and supports standards of practice.

All professions have a code of ethics and professional organizations that control the educational and practice requirements of its members. The two organizations that assume these roles for radiographers are the American Society of Radiologic Technologists (ASRT) and the American Registry of Radiologic Technologists (ARRT). The professional radiographer is certified by ARRT and, if applicable, is licensed by the state where employed.

Radiologic technology fulfills the basic requirements of a profession and is becoming increasingly autonomous in professional practice. The status of a profession demands certain responsibilities and educational requirements that former "x-ray technicians" did not possess. An individual contemplating radiologic technology as a profession must examine the criteria of a profession to make certain that there is a willingness to uphold the high standards of a professional. These standards include responsibility, accountability, competence, judgment, ethics, professionalism, and lifelong learning. The professional radiographer is expected to demonstrate all these qualities.

BECOMING A PROFESSIONAL

After reviewing the requirements of the radiography program and the commitment that this undertaking requires, students must also realize the emotional component that a professional undergoes. Chapter 1 discussed the different diseases that have Chapter 4 discusses the ethical dilemmas that arise when working with patients with communicable diseases. Students must be self-aware of their capability to work with individuals suffering from these infections. Professionals do not have the choice of saying "no" to working with the ill. Going into the health field requires self-regulation and the motivation to come to work, day after day, in the face of catastrophic illness; students and professionals should remain empathic for the patient and practice the social skills that are necessary to provide quality patient care, no matter the reason for being in the medical imaging area.

Developing Professional Attitudes

Students are continually told that the clinical aspect of the program is like a 2-year-long job interview. They are also told to learn from everyone and take the best of what they have learned from that individual and make it their own. Students interact with radiographers that have years of experience or have just graduated. There may be a difference between how these technologists work with their patients. The seasoned technologists have learned skills over the years that may seem like shortcuts to the student, whereas the new graduate's training is still fresh and every step seems deliberate. No matter how long a radiographer has been in the field, it must be remembered that professional attitudes must not only be learned but also practiced on a daily basis throughout the career.

Teamwork is a quality that is often found on a resume of an applicant for a position. Putting the word on the resume is not the same thing as actually being a team member. Being a professional means that working overtime to cover a shift when a coworker has a legitimate reason for being late. Conversely, teamwork means that one is on time for the start of the shift so that coworkers can leave when their shift is over. This might also be considered to be a work ethic, as is being on time, being dependable by not calling off ill needlessly, or not asking for days off excessively.

Other attitudes that are needed to become a professional include sympathy and compassion. Showing sympathy needs to be done with care so as not to overstep the bounds of being a health care professional. Chapter 3 discusses communication that will help the student learn how to deal with issues that require a sympathetic tone but not be overly sensitive to the patient's condition. This is where compassion may be more appropriate. Compassion is defined as the sympathetic consciousness of others' distress with a desire to alleviate that distress. Compassion can be demonstrated by listening to the patient and answering any questions. Not all questions can be answered for legal reasons, but listening to the patient may provide the emotional support that is needed.

Be a health role model for the patient and others within the department. This can be accomplished by the attitudes listed earlier (teamwork, work ethic, sympathy, and compassion), but a professional should know when and when not to be assertive. This doesn't mean being aggressive. Being assertive means communicating

with others in a direct and honest manner without intentionally hurting anyone's feelings. Assertiveness is a skill that anyone can learn and should be practiced not only with patients but also with coworkers. This type of direct communication with others in the department can reduce conflict and enhance work relationships. The knowledge to become a competent and independent radiographer is gained as the student nears the end of the educational process.

As a radiographer becomes more experienced, they possess all of the qualities and abilities listed earlier. With continued experience and training, radiographers may also obtain the abilities to:

1. supervise, evaluate, and counsel staff;
2. plan, organize, and administer professional development activities;
3. utilize superior decision-making and problem-solving skills to assess situations and identify solutions for standard outcomes;
4. promote a positive, collaborative atmosphere in all aspects of radiography;
5. act as a **mentor**; and
6. provide knowledge in areas of **in-service** and/or continuing education (CE), and **regulatory compliance**.

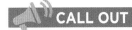
CALL OUT

Developing professional attitudes in all areas such as teamwork, a good work ethic, good role model, sympathy and empathy, and willingness to perform less desirable aspects of the job identifies the radiographer for advancement.

Professional Development and Advancement

Developing professional skills and advancing in the career takes time and effort. Many times, students want to continue within the field of imaging and go directly into a subspecialty. There are advantages and disadvantages to that. Students feel like they are on "a roll," that they are in school and it is easier to continue with their education than it would be to stop for a year or two and then return to the classroom setting. Conversely, if a student is not sure where employment might be found, it may be more logical to gain experience in the field before continuing with education. This scenario may also allow the student to change the direction of what was originally desired. Perhaps computed tomography (CT) was the student's original goal but after working for a year in the radiography field on the night shift, the student now realizes how exciting that work actually is and decides to remain a radiographer.

As a health care professional, one must acquire and maintain current knowledge to preserve a high level of expertise. **Continuing education (CE)** provides educational activities to enhance patient care, knowledge, skills, performance, and awareness of changes and advances in the field of radiologic technology. CE supports professionalism, which fosters quality patient care.

Previously voluntary for radiographers, CE became a mandate in 1995 for all those certified by ARRT. The radiologic technologist is required to earn 24 CE credits every 2 years. The credits are verified by both the ARRT and any state licensing board before renewal. CE credits, such as seminars, conferences, lectures, departmental in-service education, directed readings, home study, and college courses, may be achieved by participating in educational activities that meet the criteria set forth by the ARRT and approved by the ASRT. By participating in CE activities, professional knowledge and professional performance are enhanced, which ensures a higher standard of patient safety and care. Twenty-four credits may also be earned by taking an entry-level examination in another eligible discipline that was not previously passed. The entry-level examinations are in radiography, nuclear medicine, or radiation therapy. Another way to earn 24 credits is by passing an advanced-level examination in the field after proving eligibility. The advanced-level examinations are in mammography, cardiovascular interventional technology, magnetic resonance imaging (MRI), CT, quality management, bone densitometry, and sonography.

The ARRT implemented Continuing Qualification Requirements (CQR) for all technologists that were certified in 2011 and after. The ARRT stresses that this is not a test but a structured self-assessment that evaluates the abilities and knowledge of the radiographer based on the examination content of that current year. The candidate has 3 years to complete the requirements. Although the 24 CE requirements remain, most of the prescribed CQR units serve as the required biennium CE.

EMPLOYMENT AND ADVANCEMENT CONSIDERATIONS

Once the student passes the ARRT, employment is the next step. Issues to consider include financial ability to move, salary of new position, family situation, viability of the new position, educational opportunities, and current capability of the applying technologist.

As a new technologist gains experience, opportunities may open up in supervisory positions such as a lead technologist, department manager, or radiology administrator (discussed in Chapter 1). Educational positions are becoming more available as "graying of the faculty"

continues and more educators retire. To fill a position as clinical coordinator, one must have a bachelor's degree and have a master's degree to become a program director. These positions require a minimum of 3 years of experience in the clinical setting in addition to the degree.

If a radiographer likes the more technical aspect of the field, opportunities exist in commercial positions such as sales or equipment applications. This allows the technologist to travel to other facilities and may be to other states. One might be more interested in the maintenance and repair of the equipment, which would allow the technologist to remain in-house at one facility or health group. Research and development are other commercial career opportunities that may open up in large corporations.

Many facilities may recruit technologists from within to perform CT or MRI and help with training. After completing a formalized training in nuclear medicine or ultrasound, many technologists are hired within the facility where clinical training was completed. As in training for diagnostic radiography as an entry-level technology, one must remember that clinical training has been likened to a job interview. Being professional, reliable, and providing the best quality patient care one can within their ability is the best means for employers to determine the best fit for the job.

RELATED ISSUES

Confidentiality is a requirement under the ASRT Practice Standards. Professional conduct is key when dealing with patients that may say or do things that would not be appropriate for others to be aware of if they are not directly related to the patient's care.

Professional skills are key for the radiographer to deal with patient issues that are not directly related to the field of radiography but are presented while the patient is in the department. Realizing that patients may be experiencing emotions related to issues that cannot be seen, the radiographer provides more compassionate health care.

Confidentiality, Privacy, Health Insurance Portability and Accountability Act

In 1996, Congress recognized the need for national patient record privacy standards. For this reason, the Health Insurance Portability and Accountability Act (HIPAA) was enacted. The law included provisions designed to save money for health care businesses by encouraging electronic transactions, but it also required new safeguards to protect the security and confidentiality of information.

In November 1999, the Department of Health and Human Services (DHHS) published proposed regulations to guarantee patients' new rights and protections against the misuse or disclosure of their health records. All medical records, including radiographic images of any type, and other individually identifiable health information, whether electronic, hard copy, or verbal, are covered by the rule. The rule requires appropriate safeguards to protect the privacy of patients' health information. In addition, the rule gives patients the right over their health information.

The radiographer must abide by the same rules concerning confidentiality, security, and privacy of patient information with electronic records as with previous systems. Written consent by the patient is the only legitimate reason to obtain and pass on confidential material.

Before entering the clinical setting, the student radiographer must learn about confidentiality, security, privacy, and HIPAA compliance practices. There are state and federal regulations that impose financial penalties and fines for patient data breaches. At the federal level, the Health Information Technology for Economic and Clinical Health (HITECH) Act was enacted as part of the American Recovery and Reinvestment Act of 2009 and signed into law on February 17, 2009. HITECH further addressed patient health information privacy and security concerns and strengthened the civil and criminal enforcement of the HIPAA rules.

Health and Illness Continuum

All persons seek to maintain a high level of health and a feeling of well-being. Health can be defined as the status of an organism functioning without any evidence of disease or disfigurement. Unfortunately, a perfect state of health is rarely achieved; therefore, health is seen as on a **continuum** (Fig. 2-1). All persons are in various places on this continuum depending upon a state of physical and mental health.

Stress in its various forms affects a person's ability to maintain their health status at a high level. Stressors may take many forms, from a simple change in living area or beginning a new job to a major life change such as diagnosis of a potentially terminal illness or losing a significant person in one's life. Any change in life requires adaptation to that change with its accompanying stressors.

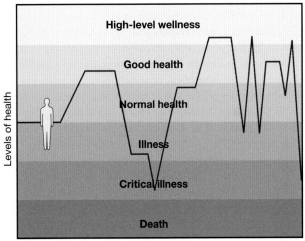

FIGURE 2-1 Drawing of health-illness continuum.

CASE STUDY

Students in radiologic technology often find themselves in situations that are unusual and exciting. Social media is a huge factor in communication and is prevalent in today's society. A senior student is doing a night rotation and is called to the emergency department to take mobile images on a trauma patient who has been bludgeoned with a hammer to the head. The patient died of injuries during the shift. This was the first death that the student had encountered. Wanting to share the experience, the student posted on social media about what had happened. There were no names used but the cause of death was identified. Many people knew where this student was doing clinical rotation, and may have known the patient from the description. A fellow student saw the post and reported it to the clinical instructor. In the inquiry process of this incident, it was revealed that the student had also posted information about another patient with interesting images, where the patient's name was used.

ISSUES TO CONSIDER:

1. Is this a violation of HIPAA? Why or why not?

2. As a fellow student, how would you handle this incident? Talk to the offending student? Report it? Keep quiet? Explain the reasons for your choice.

3. As a fellow student, how do you think the program should handle this incident knowing that there were two known offenses?

All persons have **basic needs** that must be met. When basic needs are met, one aspires to higher needs. When a person who is in a state of prolonged stress eventually finds that their basic needs are unable to be met, illness may result.

Abraham Maslow, a renowned psychologist, visualized humans as governed by a hierarchy of needs. These needs are viewed as a "building block" in a pyramidal structure. At the base of the pyramid are the basic physiologic needs; at the top is self-actualization, which is the end result of growth of the human spirit. At the lowest end are basic needs to maintain the body (Fig. 2-2).

Persons whose state of mental and physical health is at the most positive end of the health-illness continuum have their basic needs met and have no stressful events affecting their well-being. They are able to begin to pursue higher goals. When illness—whether physical or emotional—overtakes a person, the state of well-being is no longer a perception of one whose basic needs for food, water, air, shelter, love, belonging, and self-esteem are being met. Illness may mean the loss of ability to maintain social and economic status. The person's place in a social group is threatened. As illness progresses, the awareness of unmet basic needs increases, and a feeling of great **anxiety** overwhelms the ill person.

Patients are often in a state of anxiety by the time the radiographer comes into contact with them. Persons who are in need of imaging procedures may present themselves for diagnosis and treatment after a long period of feeling unwell. Others may come to the department immediately after a serious accident has destroyed, or threatens to destroy, their state of well-being. These situations result in a state of severe stress. When one's level of wellness has been compromised, regressive behavior may result. A person in such a state may have difficulty communicating effectively. The patient may resort to aggressive demands, or may withdraw in silence and not be able to make any needs known at all.

When assigned to care for any person, the radiographer must be able to determine that person's state of health or illness and must understand that the fulfillment of the patient's most basic needs may have been compromised by the stress of illness or trauma. Stressful life events may result in unpleasant patient behavior.

While providing care to a patient, there may be some instances in which the professional radiographer may become involved with emotional responses from the patient that were not expected. Being aware of how patients of different ages, genders, cultures, religious affiliations, and physical conditions may react is important. Women more than men are likely to be expressive. Men, on the other hand, become more stoic when bad news has been delivered.

Younger patients tend to be more emotionally expressive than older adults. Patients who have had the advantage of life experiences are more likely to reflect on the situation before reacting with an emotional outburst. Patients that have a solid marital or family status tend to handle grievous situations better than individuals that have no support system. The same holds true for those patients that have support through their religious affiliation.

It is also important to remember that some patients may feel frustrated when they are no longer able to move as they used to do because of a limiting physical condition. As a professional, allow patients to do what they are able, but ask if assistance is needed. Physical conditions are not mental conditions and patients should not be treated as an incompetent individual.

Loss and Grief

Grief is a normal response to the loss of a loved one, a prized possession, social status, a bodily function, or a body part. It is also to be expected when a person is faced with the possibility of imminent death. This is called **anticipatory grieving**. Unfortunately, the process of grieving is often a long and difficult one. One may never fully recover from a serious loss, but learn to live without the person or object of that loss.

How one manages the process of grieving depends largely on cultural, ethnic, religious, and economic factors as well as on the value placed on the loss. Grief reactions are often more severe for children and the elderly, especially if they have lost a person on whom they have depended.

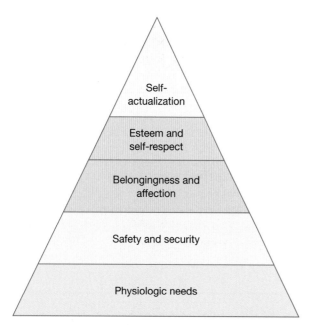

FIGURE 2-2 Drawing of Maslow's hierarchy of needs. (Modified from Hinkle JL, Cheever KH. *Brunner & Suddarth's Textbook of Medical-Surgical Nursing.* 14th ed. Wolters Kluwer Health/Lippincott Williams & Wilkins; 2018.)

In all health care professions, exposure to the loss and grief of others is common. Radiologic technology is no exception. Before being exposed to persons who are in various stages of the grieving process, the student must examine personal feelings and attitudes concerning death and loss. It is not unusual for a health care worker to be filled with emotion when caring for a person who has suffered a tremendous loss; however, these emotions must not prevent one from caring for the grieving patient. If the radiographer feels that they may have difficulty in this aspect of patient care, it may be wise to seek counseling or discuss these fears with a respected colleague.

Scholars have presented many concepts and theories that may be used to facilitate understanding of persons who are grieving. Each theory identifies phases in the process of grieving. It must be remembered that grieving is a human process and, as such, does not follow an orderly sequence. The grieving person may go from one phase of grief to another and then return to a previous phase. It is possible to be in more than one phase of grief at a time or may entirely omit one phase in the described grieving process. There may also be gender variations in the manner in which a person grieves.

Dr. Elisabeth Kübler-Ross was among the first to study the process of grieving and summarized this process in a concise manner. Remember that the picture of the grieving person presented in this text is general and varies with each individual. The radiographer's ability to care for the grieving patient may be enhanced by some understanding of the grieving process. The phases as described by Dr. Kübler-Ross are listed in Display 2-1.

DISPLAY 2-1

Phases of the Grieving Process

Phase 1: Denial

The patient who is facing imminent death or loss often responds by not accepting the truth. This is a defense mechanism that allows the person receiving the loss to become accustomed to the idea. The physician is the person who must inform the patient of approaching death or loss. If questioned by the patient, the radiographer may respond in a reflective manner.

Phase 2: Anger

The patient may become angry preceding death or disfigurement. Criticism and abuse may be hurled at family members or at health care workers because it may be felt that a serious injustice has occurred and hopeless rage is the only defense. In this instance, the radiographer who is the object of this type of anger should be matter-of-fact and understanding. Releasing anger is therapeutic for the patient and should be permitted.

Phase 3: Bargaining

The patient feels that by becoming the "good and submissive patient," a miraculous cure may occur. During this phase, the patient may seek alternative modes of treatment, some of which may be unusual or even nontherapeutic.

Phase 4: Depression

The patient accepts the impending loss and begins to mourn for a past life and all that is to be lost. The patient may be very silent and unresponsive at this time. Quiet support is the best response of the health care worker during this period.

Phase 5: Acceptance

The patient accepts the loss and loses interest in all outside occurrences. There may be interest only in the immediate surroundings and the support of persons close at hand. The patient deals with pain and begins to disengage from life. The health care worker should be quietly supportive and allow the patient to discuss whatever is wished.

During the phase of acceptance, if the patient is facing permanent disability, this is the time that there is a first attempt at rehabilitation. The disabled person may have a longer grieving period than the person suffering the loss of a loved one because of the constant reminder of the change.

The radiographer must stand by to assist, rather than taking the lead. A matter-of-fact approach in the disabled patient care is recommended with compliance to the patient's request for assistance.

When caring for a person who has suffered a serious loss, the radiographer must be supportive and allow the patient to retain hope for attaining any short- or long-term goals. All patients have the right to be treated as persons with dignity and worth until they have taken their last breath.

Patient Rights Related to End-of-Life Issues

The science of medical care has advanced to the point at which life can be maintained by mechanical means to at least long after the quality of life has deteriorated. This may not be in the patient's best interest and would probably not be the patient's wish if a decision was able to be made. The public's wishes to make its own determination in this matter were resolved when the Patient Self-Determination Act (PSDA) was made law in 1990. PSDA establishes guidelines concerning patients' wishes when confronted with serious illness. It creates clear understanding of the patient's desires when an illness cannot be cured or if the illness causes a life without quality.

Advance directives are legal documents that are formulated by a competent person and provide written information concerning the patient's desires if the patient is unable to make the decision. All health care institutions are required to provide written information to all patients informing them of their right to make an advance health care directive and to inquire if such a directive is already established. The patient's admission records should state whether such directives exist. These directives dictate preferences for the type of medical care and the extent of treatment desired. These directives become effective if the patient is unable to make health care decisions. There are three instruments through which the patient's wishes are dictated. They are as follows:

A Living Will: Expresses the patients' wishes concerning future medical care. These may be altered by a

CASE STUDY

Missy, RT, works the 3:30 to 11 PM shift at the convenient care down the block from where she lives. Missy is single and has no children so she usually takes the Christmas holiday shifts so that her colleagues who have families can spend time celebrating with them. On a particular Christmas eve, at 10 minutes to 11 PM, an elderly woman checks into the registration desk with a sore wrist. Missy is called by the staff and told not to leave as this patient may probably require radiographic images.

At 11:10 PM, the order comes through for a wrist radiograph on the patient and Missy walks over to get her. As Missy is taking the images, she is conversing with the patient to get a history as to how she hurt her wrist. Edna, the patient, explains that she did not hurt it at all and that it has been painful for about 3 months. Edna stated she thought it was probably just arthritis. Missy left the imaging room to view the images on the computer screen muttering about how "some people have no concept of how they impact those of us who have to work late at night and on holidays . . . ."

When Missy returns to take Edna back to her bed in the convenient care area, she found her crying. When asked if her wrist was hurting that much, Edna stated that no, it wasn't her wrist at all, but that her husband had passed away on Christmas eve 2 years ago. She had no family and just couldn't stand sitting at home by herself on this particular holiday.

Although many questions could be asked about this scenario, students are encouraged to think about how the grieving process affects not just the person suffering the loss but others as well. In Chapter 3 communication will be discussed and that area of patient care that is affected in this situation. Certainly, professionalism plays a role as does compassion and understanding. Students should reflect on all the issues presented in this case study to determine how best to handle situations like this that may arise in their career.

competent patient at any time. Each state has different rulings concerning changes in a living will by an incompetent patient. Living wills help patients understand the definition of death. Quality of life is determined by the patient, and living wills allow the patient to state what should be done when that quality is no longer able to be maintained.

Durable Power of Attorney for Health Care: Appoints an agent that the person trusts to make decisions if the patient is unable to do so.

There may be a combination directive called *Five Wishes* that may be used and that specifies the following:

1. The person that is wanted to make care decisions
2. The level of medical treatment desired
3. Level of comfort desired
4. Type of treatment desired
5. Level of knowledge to be given to family

A sample of a combination directive is illustrated in Display 2-2. When copies of these documents have been completed, they should be copied and given to the agent appointed and included in the patient's hospital medical records.

DISPLAY 2-2

Sample Advance Health Care Directive

Part 1: Power of Attorney for Health Care

_____ I designate the following individual as my agent to make my health care decisions for me:

NAME _____

PHONE HOME _____ WORK _____ CELL _____

ADDRESS _____

ALTERNATE AGENT: If I revoke my agent's authority or if my agent is not willing or able, or reasonably available to make a health care decision for me, then I designate and appoint the following person(s) to serve as my agent, in the order listed as follows, to make health care decisions for me, as authorized in this document:

First Alternate Agent:

NAME _____

PHONE HOME _____ WORK _____ CELL _____

ADDRESS _____

Second Alternate Agent:

NAME _____

PHONE HOME _____ WORK _____ CELL _____

ADDRESS _____

Part 2: Instructions for Health Care

END-OF-LIFE DECISIONS (initial applicable line)

_____ **Choice not to prolong life.** I do not want my life to be prolonged with life-sustaining treatment if I have an incurable and irreversible condition that will result in my death within a relatively short time; I become unconscious; and, to a reasonable degree of medical certainty, I will not regain consciousness OR

(continued)

DISPLAY 2-2

Sample Advance Health Care Directive (*continued*)

_____ **Choice to prolong life.** I want my life to be prolonged as long as possible within the limit of generally accepted health care standards that my doctor recommends.

_____ Other wishes: _____

_____ **Relief from pain.** I direct that treatment for alleviation of pain or discomfort should be provided at all times, even if it hastens my death OR

_____ Other wishes: _____

ARTIFICIAL NUTRITION AND HYDRATION

_____ I do not want artificial nutrition and hydration started in order to keep me alive OR

_____ I want artificial nutrition and hydration to keep me alive

_____ Other wishes: _____

Part 3: Donation of Organs at Death (Optional)

Upon my death (initial applicable line)

_____ I do not donate any of my organs, tissues, or parts and do not want my agent, conservator, or family to make a donation on my behalf OR

_____ I will donate any needed organs, tissues, or parts

_____ I will donate only the following organs, tissues, or parts: _____

Part 4: Primary Physician (Optional)

PHYSICIAN NAME _____

PHONE HOME _____ WORK _____ CELL _____

ADDRESS _____

_____

Part 5: Execution

OPTION 1: Sign before two qualified witnesses
FIRST WITNESS:

DATE _____ SIGN YOUR NAME _____

PRINT NAME OF WITNESS _____

ADDRESS _____

_____

STATEMENT OF WITNESS:

I declare that the individual who signed or acknowledged this advance health directive is personally known to me, that the individual signed or acknowledged this advance directive in my presence, that the individual appears to be of sound mind and under no duress, fraud, or undue influence, that I am not related to the person, that I am not the individual's health care provider or an employee of the health care provider who is now, or has been in the past, responsible for the care of the person making this advance directive.

DISPLAY 2-2

Sample Advance Health Care Directive (*continued*)

SECOND WITNESS:

DATE _____ SIGN YOUR NAME _____

PRINT NAME OF WITNESS _____

ADDRESS _____

_____

Part 6: Date and Signature of Principal

I hereby sign my name to and acknowledge this Advance Health Care Directive:

Dated: _____   Name: _____

(Signature)

The radiographer may find a **do-not-resuscitate** (**DNR**) order on the patient's record. This may also be called a "**no code**" order. This is often included as part of the patient's advance health care directive; however, the radiographer must have a written medical order to follow this request. The standard of care dictates that health care professionals must attempt resuscitation if the patient stops breathing or is in a state of cardiac arrest, and there is no signed DNR order to the contrary. The radiographer must determine their institution's policies concerning all health care directives and orders pertaining to these issues.

There are persons who do not wish to have a DNR inclusion in their desires for end-of-life care. In this case, there often is an order for a "**Full Code**," which means that a full cardiopulmonary resuscitation is called. In most institutions, this is referred to as a "Code Blue." The radiographer must be familiar with the manner of calling this emergency if the patient becomes lifeless.

CALL OUT

Any time that a patient becomes lifeless in the diagnostic imaging area, a "Code Blue" should be called. The emergency team does what is necessary. The radiographer does not have time to look in the patient's chart to determine if a DNR is listed!

All patients are entitled to pain control despite the nature of their illness. This includes persons who are at the end of life. The objective of pain control for a dying patient is to block pain at a level that does not suppress consciousness. Pain medication should be administered at a level that permits a plateau level of control. This maintains the patient's comfort and prevents the agony and exhaustion that comes with severe pain.

Summary

1. A profession is defined as a work body that contains unique knowledge, requires specialized education, is motivated to serve the needs of the community, has performance standards, and employs individuals that are motivated and have a commitment to service.

2. Becoming a professional radiographer requires emotional intelligence that is achieved through self-awareness, self-regulation, motivation, empathy, and social skills.

   a. The attitudes of a professional include teamwork, an excellent work ethic, sympathy, compassion, assertiveness, and being a worthy health role model.

3. Radiologic technology has evolved to meet the criteria of a profession by extended education requirements and clinical practice.

   a. It has a theoretical body of knowledge and leads to defined skills, abilities, and action.

   b. It also provides a specific service, and its members have a degree of decision-making autonomy when working within their scope of practice.

c. CE is mandatory and can be earned in several ways, such as professional journals, conferences, in-services, or passing another modality exam.

4. Employment in diagnostic imaging should be thought out in terms of economic considerations, where there is a need and the radiographers' ability to move to another location.

    a. Areas that are available for a professional radiographer include supervisory roles, education (after obtaining specific degrees and experience), industrial arenas, research, sales and applications, and computer informatics.

5. HIPAA compliance ensures protection for the patient's privacy.

    a. Hospitals must have some policy in place in regard to the release of patient information. Patients must provide permission to have information released to a third party.

    b. Patients have the right to restrict the sharing of any of their information and if this is violated, the patient has the right to file a complaint.

6. All human beings have basic needs. Threats to those human needs create stress, and severe stress may lead to illness. The patient who seeks medical cares does so because basic needs are no longer being met as a result of illness. The radiographer must understand that a person in poor health may relate to people in an unpliant manner. If this is understood, the radiographer s able to care for the patient in a sensitive and caring manner regardless of patient behavior.

7. Patients who are grieving need special consideration.

    a. The radiographer must not let personal emotions regarding the patient affect how care is delivered.

8. Radiographers must respect the patient's right to make choices concerning health care.

    a. Advance directives provide directions on how a patient wishes to be treated if unable to make that decision.

    b. Living wills and durable power of attorney for health care also dictate the patient's choice regarding health care and must be followed.

    c. DNR and a "no code" mean that the patient does not want to be resuscitated upon expiration.

CHAPTER 2 REVIEW QUESTIONS

1. Which of the following is an example of privileged (confidential) information?

    a. Your friend buys a new car and asks you not to tell anyone about it yet.

    b. A colleague discusses their stock market holdings with you.

    c. You assist with a diagnostic study and a large adherent mass is discovered in the colon.

    d. A fellow student is told that they have the highest grades in the class.

2. Information about a patient's condition or prognosis:

    a. May be freely discussed with close relatives

    b. Must always remain confidential

    c. Should always be open discussion, because "a well-known fact is no secret"

    d. Should be discussed only on a coworker/interdepartmental basis

3. The process of grieving, though painful and difficult, is normal and the patient follows the various stages in order before finding relief.

    a. True

    b. False

4. Lee, a 56-year-old male, was diagnosed with cancer 6 weeks ago. He was told it is inoperable and, thus, incurable. He has decided to seek treatment in another country that promises instant cures with natural herbs. One might conclude the Lee is in which stage of the grieving process?

    a. Denial

    b. Anger

    c. Bargaining

    d. Acceptance

    e. Depression

5. An elderly woman loses her spouse of 40 years. Shortly after his death, she becomes ill and requires hospitalization. One might consider that her illness might be related to

    a. Relief

    b. Fear

    c. Stress

    d. Hope

6. Which of the following is NOT an example of invasion of privacy?

    a. Touching a patient against their will

    b. Sending a patient's records to another health care provider without consent

    c. Refusing to discuss a patient's diagnosis with a family member

    d. Leaving a patient's chart open so that anyone can see what is on it

7. CE that is a requirement for all radiographers who graduate after 2011 is known as:
   a. CEU
   b. CQR
   c. Attending seminars as a means for obtaining the required CE
   d. Radiographers must pass an exam in another modality
8. Which of the following is NOT a professional attribute?
   a. Sympathy
   b. Compassion
   c. Work ethic
   d. Aggressiveness
9. Criteria for a profession includes which of the following? (Circle all that apply)
   a. A vital human service is provided.
   b. Education is obtained in institutes of higher education.
   c. Supervisors are accountable for a practitioner's actions.
   d. There is a code of ethics.
   e. The federal government oversees the actions of the profession.
10. Career advancement should not be considered until at least 2 years after graduation for a program in order to obtain a full understanding of what the field involves.
    a. True
    b. False

Communicating for Successful Patient Interactions

3

OBJECTIVES

After studying this chapter, the student will be able to:

1. Identify methods for determining the correct patient for a given procedure.

2. Determine how to collect information from the patient prior to an examination.

3. Describe how critical thinking skills must be used for effective communication.

4. Explain the problem-solving process in patient education.

5. Describe age/generation-specific communication.

6. Interpret medical abbreviations and symbols.

7. Define medical imaging terms.

8. Define verbal and nonverbal communication.

9. Describe the challenges that affect communication.

10. Define therapeutic communication and demonstrate its techniques.

KEY TERMS

Adverse effects: Unfavorable happenings

Aggravating or alleviating factors: That which makes a problem worse (aggravating) or better (alleviating)

Anterior posterior (AP): The central ray that travels through the body entering on the anterior side and exiting at the posterior side

Associated manifestations: Symptoms that occur concurrently with the disease.

Attention deficit hyperactivity disorder (ADHD): A common neurodevelopmental disorder that causes trouble in paying attention, controlling impulsive behaviors, or is overly active

Attitudes: A manner of feeling or thinking; opinions

Autism spectrum disorder: A developmental disability that affects how individuals communicate, interact with others, and experience the world

Biases: Prejudices

Central ray (CR): Refers to the path of the main beam of x-ray leaving the collimator housing

Cerebral palsy (CP): A disorder that affects the brain and spinal cord; also affects movement, muscle tone, reflexes, posture, balance, and coordination

Chronology: The arrangement of events in time

Communication: Expressing information that is accurate and clear so that the listener understands the message and can respond

Critical thinking: Assessing one's thinking to make it clearer, more accurate, or more defensible

Culture: A set of beliefs and values common to a particular group of people

Evaluate: To make a judgment as to the value of something; to size up

Feedback: A response that indicates that the message delivered was correctly or incorrectly perceived

Global: Complete; worldwide

Intellectual disability (ID): A general term for any type of significant cognitive or intellectual impairment that impacts an individual's ability to function in everyday life

Interpret: To explain or to make understandable

Learning disabilities: Affect the brain's ability to receive, process, store, and respond to information; not a mental illness but rather a neurologic disorder

Linear: Easy to comprehend because it is basic or logical

Location: The exact area of origin

Nontherapeutic relationship: An association with another person that is unpleasant or unsatisfactory

Nonverbal: Unspoken

Onset: Time of beginning

Paralanguage: Tone of voice, gestures, and facial expressions that accompany speech

Posterior anterior (PA): The path of the central ray as it enters the body posteriorly and exits anteriorly

Quality: The measurement of something poor (bad) to excellent (good)

Rapport: A sense of harmony or agreement

Stress: Pressure or weight placed upon oneself that creates either physical or mental strain

Therapeutic: Healing; curative

Therapeutic communication: Speaking and listening in a manner that makes the receiver of the communication feel improved or restored

Validate: To confirm; to justify or establish as true

INTRODUCTION

Communication is one of the most critical components of the patient care experience. It is the radiographers' first opportunity to establish a good **rapport** with the patient. Communication is affected by the **attitudes** of all the people involved in the exchange of information. Patients can exhibit a wide range of emotions before coming to the imaging department and may not receive the intended message by the radiographer. Radiographers who can understand not only the patients' emotions but also those of their own will be a more active and compassionate health care provider. The patient expects the radiographer to be concerned and articulate. The patient also expects to be the focus of concern, to the exclusion of any personal concerns of the radiographer. Case study—Amelia illustrates these various points.

FIRST INTERACTIONS

Communication begins the first time the patient and the radiographer meet. Although the patient is the focus of the communication, the patient's family and friends must also receive attention. Many times, a family member may ask questions about the care of the patient. As a professional, the radiographer must make the visitors feel confident that the best care is being provided to the patient. If necessary, the family should be directed to speak with the referring physician; however, it is important that the family does not feel like they have been "brushed off." Remember to smile and provide a brief explanation that will not compromise the patient's confidentiality. Oftentimes, this brief communication assures everyone that the patient is in good hands. Any delay this may cause is offset by the rapport that has been established between patient and radiographer.

Patient Identification Methods

The first interaction that a radiographer has with a patient is when the patient is being brought to the imaging room. Before proceeding with any procedure, the radiographer must make certain that the correct patient has been taken to the work area and that the procedure has been properly explained. The patient must be properly identified as the correct patient by the radiographer; this must be done every time, regardless of the number of times the patient has been seen in the imaging department. The proper method for identification is through interviewing and questioning the patient in a precise manner. "Please tell me your last name and date of birth" is the only correct and legal method to ensure that the correct patient is about to have radiographs. Do not say "Is your last name Ryan? Were you born on Christmas day in 1950?" It is too easy to misunderstand and have the patient reply "yes" to the questions.

If the patient is an inpatient, the radiographer must look at the wrist band in addition to asking for the patient's last name and birthdate. Review the imaging order and the patient's chart to confirm the procedure or x-ray that is to be done. The radiographer should include this in the conversation by saying, "I am going to x-ray your right elbow. Is that your understanding?"

Once the patient and procedure have been verified, the radiographer must explain the procedure to the patient so that there is an understanding of the length of time that will be spent in the department, the different devices that may be used in imaging the part, and any immobilization devices that may be necessary. All of these interactions can be done within a few minutes and prevents mistakes from being made. It also allows the patient and the radiographer to establish a rapport that facilitates the remainder of the examination.

Patient History

The goal of a patient history is to obtain necessary information to perform a safe and comfortable procedure. Frequently, the radiographer may not need to take a complete health history because it has been accomplished by the patient's physician or nurse before the patient arrives in the imaging department.

On many occasions, the radiographer must obtain information from the patient that is personal and confidential. Obtaining this information accurately demands sensitivity and critical thinking on the radiographer's part.

As the interviewer, the radiographer asks direct, personal questions of a relative stranger. During the history-taking process, the radiographer must convey a professional image to ensure the patient's confidence.

Rules to follow to complete a successful patient history are:

- Provide an atmosphere that is private and as quiet as possible.
- Establish rapport with the patient by being friendly but respectful.
- Inform the patient why the information is needed.
- Use open- and closed-ended questions as necessary to elicit information concerning the patient's medical condition.

There is information that is of the utmost importance in the imaging department that must be included in a patient history. These include:

- For female patients of childbearing age: last menstrual period and possibility of pregnancy when particular examinations are being performed (i.e., lumbar spine or pelvis). This must be done in a thoughtful and professional manner, keeping in mind cultural as well as age considerations. Asking a young woman in the presence of her family may not provide the appropriate answer and may also insult the family.
- Confirmation with the patient of the imaging examination to be performed. Be certain that the correct side and body part has been requested. If there is any question, a call to the requesting provider must be made.

The radiographer must gather the information necessary for a successful examination. To compile a complete history, the radiographer must listen, observe, reply, and question in an organized and analytic manner. The items necessary in a complete history must include the following:

- **Localization** of the problem (Where is the problem or area of pain?)
- **Chronology** (When and for how long has the problem been present?)
- **Quality** (How severe is the problem or pain?)
- **Onset** (When did the problem begin?)
- **Aggravating or alleviating factors** (What makes the pain or problem worse or better?)
- **Associated manifestations** (What else happens during the pain episodes?)

An example of a complete history of a patient for a chest image would include the following items:

"Do you have a cough?

Is it a dry cough or do you cough up anything?

How long have you had it?

When do you cough more, in the morning or at night?

Is there anything that you notice makes the cough worse?

Do you have any pain in your chest when you cough?"

This information is then conveyed to the radiologist to provide a complete understanding of why the images were requested. This helps in the reading of the images and what the requesting physician is looking for.

Patient Record

A medical record is kept for each patient who seeks medical treatment whether as an outpatient or as an inpatient. The medical record may be electronic or a hard copy, is commenced the moment the patient arrives or is admitted for care, and is kept until the patient is discharged from the hospital. The medical record is kept for a number of reasons, including the following:

1. To transmit information about the patient from one health care worker to another
2. To protect the patient from medical errors and duplication of treatments
3. To provide information for medical research
4. To protect the health care worker in cases of litigation
5. To provide information concerning quality of patient care for institutional evaluation teams such as The Joint Commission

A patient's medical record is usually in the form of a computerized chart (known as an e-chart) that has replaced the paper charts of the past. The medical records contain the patient's identifying data, documentation of all physician's orders, physician's consultation notes, patient progress notes, medications and treatments received, around-the-clock nurse's notes, all patient visits for outpatient or ambulatory care, laboratory and radiology reports, medical history and physical examination, admitting and discharge diagnosis, results of examinations, surgical reports, consent forms, education received by the patient, discharge planning, health care team planning, nursing care plans, and discharge summary. All members of the health care team are expected to document the care they have rendered for the patient in the medical records.

With a computerized format, there are clear tabs that can be clicked on for easy access to the section that is needed. When a patient arrives in the imaging department, the radiographer should check the e-chart for pertinent information regarding the examination that is about to be done. Radiography reports can be reviewed if the case is a follow-up. If the patient is about to have a study involving contrast media, it is important to determine if there is any documentation of an allergic history from a past experience. However, this should not replace a contrast allergy history for each and every study!

Documentation in the patient's chart may be required. For example, a radiographer should document in the chart when a patient has received contrast media. Documentation must include what contrast was used, the amount, any reactions that occurred, and any treatment that was done while in the imaging department, even if it was just giving the patient oxygen.

Many imaging departments have their own documentation forms that are used in addition to documenting in the patient's record. This may be the only documentation found for outpatients that go to a free-standing imaging center. Any documentation made in these centers should be forwarded to the patient's physician to become part of the permanent record.

Procedure Orders and Requests

In imaging departments, a requisition from a physician contains the orders for specific procedures to be performed on patients. In addition, the requisition includes the following data: the patient's name, gender, date of birth, diagnosis, and other patient information that the radiographer uses to verify the correct examination to be performed on the correct patient. With Medicare billing, if the clinical indication or patient history does not match the examination that is being ordered, Medicare may not pay for the procedure. This process is usually ascertained in the physician's office but may not be found until the patient arrives at the registration desk of the radiology department. Certainly, it is the responsibility of the radiographer to ensure that the patient's history confirms the examination being ordered. Many times, upon reviewing the clinical history, the request states a history that does not coincide with the x-ray that is ordered. As an example, the request might state that the patient has gallstones, yet the order is for a left shoulder x-ray. It is incumbent on the radiographer to get the correct history as to why the shoulder x-ray is requested.

Nurses and physicians who participate in diagnostic imaging examinations or treatments are also responsible for documentation. Any item that has not been documented on the medical record is considered as "not performed" in a court of law. All entries on medical records must list the time and date of the procedure and be signed by the qualified person who administered it. The credentials of the person must be listed.

Certain documentation is specific to radiographic imaging. The radiographer is accountable for the documentation or record keeping according to departmental protocol of any radiographic images taken, including the number of images or exposures (including repeated images), the exposure factors, the radiographic room or equipment, and the amount of fluoroscopic time used during a procedure. The radiographer must also document any patient preparation for procedures that were made, medications that were administered, and any adverse reactions to medications or treatments received.

Medical record formats are also made and approved by each institution; however, the contents of the record are reviewed and approved, disapproved, or changed according to recommendations made by the accreditation bodies inspecting the records.

If an error is made while writing an entry into a medical record, *mistaken entry* is documented next to the error, and the person making the error initials the documentation

Diagnostic Reports

Many times, a radiographer needs to review a previous diagnostic report if the current order is a follow-up to what was done previously. If this is the case, the radiographer must understand any of the pathology or technical parts of the report. Diagnostic reports contain the examination that was done, when it was done, and the radiologist's findings. This is usually where the radiographer finds any information that may be helpful for the current study.

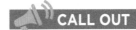 **CALL OUT**

Under no circumstances should the radiographer tell the patient what the previous report states!

PROCEDURE EXPLANATION

A patient who comes to the imaging department for treatment or diagnosis has a right to expect to be instructed in the procedure that is to be received and that the care or instruction following the procedure is complete. The radiographer is often the health care worker who must provide this education. Instruction must include the following:

- A detailed description of the preparation necessary for the procedure or examination
- A description of the purpose and the mechanics of the procedure and what is expected of the patient; for instance, frequent position changes, medications to be taken or injected, and any contrast agent to be administered
- The approximate amount of time the procedure takes
- An explanation of any unusual equipment that will be used during the examination, including the use of immobilization devices
- Any follow-up care necessary when the procedure or examination is complete

The patient who is hospitalized before imaging procedures may receive preexamination preparation. The radiographer's obligation as a member of the health care team is to communicate the preparation needs for imaging procedures in the department to other members of the health care team who are preparing the patient. The member of the health care team who usually prepares hospitalized patients for imaging examinations is part of the nursing staff.

The radiographer must be certain that the staff who prepare the patient have explicit and current preparation instructions for each procedure to be performed. Scheduling of imaging procedures with other members of the health care team must be planned so that the examinations are performed in a logical sequence that meets the patient's health care needs and accomplishes the diagnostic goals in the most time- and cost-efficient manner.

The possible **adverse effects** of a procedure should be addressed by the patient's physician before the patient is left in the radiographer's care. The radiographer is responsible for determining the extent of the patient's knowledge of the procedure and understanding of what is to occur. The techniques of therapeutic communication can be used to explore this with the patient. If the patient does not completely understand the purpose of the procedure or has concerns about it, the radiographer should not begin the examination until the patient's concerns have been addressed by the technologist/supervisor or in some cases by the patient's physician. Informed consent forms must be correctly signed if they are required. If a patient refuses an examination, the patient's physician must be notified.

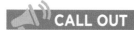

CALL OUT

If the patient questions an examination or a procedure, do not begin until the problem is resolved by the patient and the department supervisor/technologist.

In addition to providing information regarding the examination, it is sometimes necessary to answer questions pertaining to other modalities in the imaging department. Perhaps the patient is scheduled for a nuclear medicine scan and is fearful of how the examination may affect the body's organs. Patients may associate nuclear medicine with nuclear power and assume the same concepts are used for medical purposes. Regardless of which modality is being asked about, the radiographer must be able to answer these questions. Chapter 14 addresses these other modalities to allow the student some insight as to what these are before a clinical rotation is commenced in that area.

Establishing a Plan for Patient Education

Assessment skills, **critical thinking** skills, problem-solving skills, and therapeutic communication skills are required to establish the patient's need for instruction and the method to be used to accomplish this task. Patient assessment should include:

- The patient's previous experience with the procedure to be performed
- Knowledge of the preparation needed for the procedure
- The patient's age, culture, ethnicity, and educational level
- The patient's health status
- The patient's anxiety level and ability to assimilate instruction

Each of these may contribute to either the understanding of the message or the misunderstanding of it. Patients who are in poor health and anxious may not fully comprehend the message that the radiographer is trying to convey.

Patients, like radiographers, have different styles and ways of learning. Chapter 1 discussed the different styles of learning (visual, auditory, and kinesthetic). Another type is:

- **Global** versus **linear:** Some people look at the entire picture and the details (global), whereas others look at each component of the material before looking at the whole (linear).

The radiographer must plan a method of evaluation to be certain that the patient has understood any instruction. This may be done by obtaining verbal or written feedback or by a return demonstration. The plan is then implemented and **evaluated**.

When an examination or a procedure is complete, the radiographer must reinforce to the patient what was initially taught concerning follow-up treatment or care. The patient may be anxious and somewhat forgetful of previous instruction. Written instruction and verbal instruction are beneficial.

AGE-SPECIFIC COMMUNICATION

Health care members should learn about communicating with children at all levels of development as this may improve delivery of care to the patient and the relationship with the parent. Just as with adults, listening is key to providing care for the child as well as the parent. Remember that the parent has the choice to take the child elsewhere for treatment or procedures. One would not use the same communication skills with a young child as would be used with an adult. This does not mean the tone of voice and speech pattern, such as "baby talk," but rather the sentence structure and choice of words used to convey a message.

Neonates are infants under the age of 28 days and will react to the tone of voice of the radiographer. Touch is also important during this time frame. Involve the parents with the study, making sure to communicate every aspect of what is being done.

As children age from *infant to toddler*, they begin to communicate with small sentences that may be merely two or three words strung together to convey their wants. Toddlers like to explore as they are naturally curious about their environment and this can be used to the radiographer's advantage. Incorporating the child into the process of having a "picture taken" may allow the examination to progress more smoothly. Playing "games" with the child by having them "blow out the light" on the collimator housing can be enough of a distraction that images can be obtained relatively easily. Allowing a favorite toy to be held during the process may also help put the child at ease.

Adolescents prove to bring challenges to the health care provider. Barriers are encountered when involving the patient's sensitive and personal aspects of life. Keep in mind that modesty and privacy are extremely important to patients in this age group. It is wise not to ask the patient certain preparatory questions in front of the parent. For example, asking a 15-year-old female if there is any possibility of pregnancy in front of her parents might bring an outburst of denial and negativity from the parent and complete silence from the patient. Be sensitive to the patient's possible situations that are not known to the parents. The next case study shows what may happen in this type of situation. Provide a complete explanation about the procedure and any assurances that may be necessary to both the patient and the parent if necessary. Do not talk about the patient to the parent but involve the patient in all discussions.

CASE STUDY

John, RT, imaging director, convened a session with Jacob, RT. The session was to address a written patient complaint from a patient's mother. Mrs. Nelda Garcia complained on behalf of her 18-year-old daughter, Lupe. According to the mother, Jacob questioned Lupe asking if there was any chance of her being pregnant before he x-rayed her lumbar spine. The mother heard Jacob's question because she was in the area when her daughter was questioned. She answered "no" for her daughter and stated that Lupe was a virgin. In the complaint, the mother requested an apology from the RT to her daughter.

ISSUES TO CONSIDER

1. Being culturally sensitive, how could the technologist have questioned the patient?
2. How could the technologist have prepared the patient for such a question?
3. In light of the mother's answer for the daughter, what course of action should the technologist take?

The *young adult* patient (under the age of 45) is able to make their own decisions about what is being done and should be addressed with respect and a caring attitude. Middle-aged adults may be starting to see the loss of their previous ability to be mobile. Radiographers must be mindful in instructing these patients about moving and turning. Do not push the patient into position but explain what is necessary for them to do in order to achieve the image necessary. Allow the adult patient to make their own choice on how to best comply with instructions.

Communicating with patients that are less than 65 but over 45 is virtually the same as with middle adults. The following are good tips for communication with patients:

1. Minimize distractions.
2. Make eye contact.
3. Listen without interrupting.
4. Speak clearly using short sentences.
5. Speak about one topic at a time.
6. Give the patient time to ask questions and express themselves.

Older adults, age 65 and above, are seen the most in the medical institutions and may require more care in the imaging department than other age groups. Patients in this age group are more likely to experience hearing and vision loss and require slower speaking rates and closer distances to communicate well. It is also important not to shout at a patient simply because of age. Not all elderly patients are hard of hearing. Cognitive ability may also begin to decline in this age group. Keep communication simple and factual. Ask for feedback that involves the patient repeating directions rather than using questions that can be answered with a "yes" or "no."

GENERATION-SPECIFIC COMMUNICATION

Different generations approach their health care much differently and, as such, tend to communicate at different levels with the health care provider.

Silent Generation (those born before 1942) are often called the "greatest generation" because of the hardships that they endured through the financial collapse in 1928, the "Dust Bowl" and WWII. This generation defers to their physician's opinion. They have firm beliefs in good service, as they grew up in a time when the customer was considered to be right. This generation considers only physicians and nurses to be health care professionals and follows the advice of these individuals. Assure the patients in this generation that the physician will be getting the report of the images and that they can communicate with their physician, which is whom they trust.

Baby Boomers were born between the years 1943 and 1960. This generation wants to be engaged in their medical care. They investigate specialists and providers. Many Boomers are responsible for the medical care of their aging parents as well as their children. Because of dealing with three generations of medical data, Boomers may cause some challenges in communication for the health care provider. This generation may have a tendency to be argumentative or question why things are being done. Baby Boomers are extremely busy so communication about delays and education about the length of time for the study is important to them.

Generation Xers were born between 1961 and 1981. This group of individuals are relatively healthy and actively seek information on how to remain so. Generation X individuals are not loyal to their physicians or health care environment. They are more likely to change based on the most recent experience they had. This generation is not so impressed with certificates hanging on the wall but want to see the proof of competence in action. Communicating directly with them and answering questions in a matter-of-fact manner is best. This group is not in the imaging department for humor or conversation. Perform the study and release the patient. Most of them have researched the study and have a sense of what is being done.

Millennials were born between 1982 and 1996. These individuals usually do not use inpatient services unless they come through the emergency department. They listen to the verbal instructions but are not as likely to ask questions about their concerns. Rather, they research it online. Remember that this group grew up using their phone as a means of communicating through text messages. It may seem like they are not able to put the phone down as it is a source of entertainment, communication, news, and weather. Many facilities have signs now that ask the patient to refrain from using the phone while in the department, but this fact may need to be reiterated while in the imaging department.

COMMUNICATION

It can be seen by the previous narrative that there is more to communication than just speaking! There is more still to the process. The following sections provide general information on medical terminology that was most likely learned in a prerequisite course and information that is encountered in the clinical aspect of training.

Medical Communication

Most radiologic technology programs require a course in medical terminology before entering the actual program whereas others incorporate terminology within the program. These courses teach the student the word-building process of the root word with prefixes or suffixes that gives the meaning of the term. It must be remembered that the correct pronunciation of the terms is important when speaking with other health care workers and that medical terms are translated into layman's terms when communicating with the patient. The section on abbreviations is meant to be strictly an overview of subject matter learned in other courses.

Medical Abbreviations

The student radiographer encounters radiographic abbreviations taught in other courses of the program, such as mA (milliamperage) or SID (source to image distance). However, all radiographers come across abbreviations and symbols in physicians' orders and other documentation that must be understood. Because these are not always seen in the beginning of a 2-year program, it is well to provide an overview found in Display 3-1. These abbreviations are only a small list that the radiographer encounters over a career; however, knowing what they mean helps in the critique of orders, requests, and diagnostic reports.

Abbreviations must be approved by the institution in which the radiographer is employed. A list of acceptable abbreviations must be on record at that institution and learned by those using them. No others are acceptable.

In 2001, The Joint Commission identified a list of abbreviations that are not to be used and should not be seen in any medical facility. Abbreviations can be mistaken for other letters and change the meaning of the abbreviation. The abbreviation "U" can be mistaken for a zero and must now be written out as unit. "IU" can be mistaken for IV so now must be written out as "International Unit." When an amount was written out for injection purposes, oftentimes the decimal point was missed. Now, all amounts must be clearly written out as 2 mg instead of 2.0 mg as this last entry may have been perceived as 20 mg, a 10-fold difference in the amount! With the use of e-charts, there are fewer misreading than there were with handwritten notes.

Procedure and Terminology

Standard terminology is used to describe positioning a patient for various examinations and procedures that physicians order for the diagnosis and treatment of injuries or illness. The American Registry of Radiologic Technologists (ARRT) has defined radiographic position and radiographic projection. The radiographic position refers to a specific body position, such as supine, prone, recumbent, erect, or Trendelenburg. These terms refer to the patient's physical position and describe the way the patient is placed to achieve an outcome radiographic image. Radiographic projection is defined as the path of the **central ray** (CR) of the x-ray beam. The CR enters and exits the patient before the image

DISPLAY 3-1

Common Medical Abbreviations

ALOC	altered levels of consciousness
Ba	barium
BUN	blood urea nitrogen
BX	biopsy
CA	cancer, carcinoma
CAP	chest-abdomen-pelvis (such as in a CT scan)
CHF	congestive heart failure
COPD	chronic obstructive pulmonary disease
CT	computed tomography (CTA is computed tomography angiogram)
DOB	date of birth
DVT	deep vein thrombosis
ECG	electrocardiogram
ED	emergency department
ENT	ear, nose, and throat
FT	follow-through (as is SBFT, which is small bowel follow-through)
F/U	follow-up
Fx	fracture
GI	gastrointestinal
GSW	gunshot wound
GU	genitourinary
Hx	history
LOC	loss of consciousness
NE(T)	nasoenteric (tube)
NG(T)	nasogastric (tube)
NKA	no known allergies
NPO	nothing per oral (nothing to eat or drink)
NVD	nausea, vomiting, diarrhea
PPE	personal protective equipment
RBC	red blood cells
Rx	prescription
SOB	short of breath
TIA	transient ischemic attack
UA	urine analysis
WB	weight bearing
WBC	white blood cells
XR	x-ray

is captured, which is the radiographic position. **Posterior anterior** (PA) is an example of radiographic projection, because the CR would be entering the patient's back, or posterior, and exiting the patient's front side, or anterior, thereby forming a PA projection. Just the opposite would be an **anterior posterior** (AP) projection. Other radiographic body positions used for various examinations include lateral, obliques (right and left), decubitus (ventral, dorsal, right, and left lateral), axial, and tangential. The obliques are further described as right and/or left anterior obliques or right and/or left posterior obliques. Figure 3-1, from the ARRT handbook, demonstrates these definitions. Figure 3-2

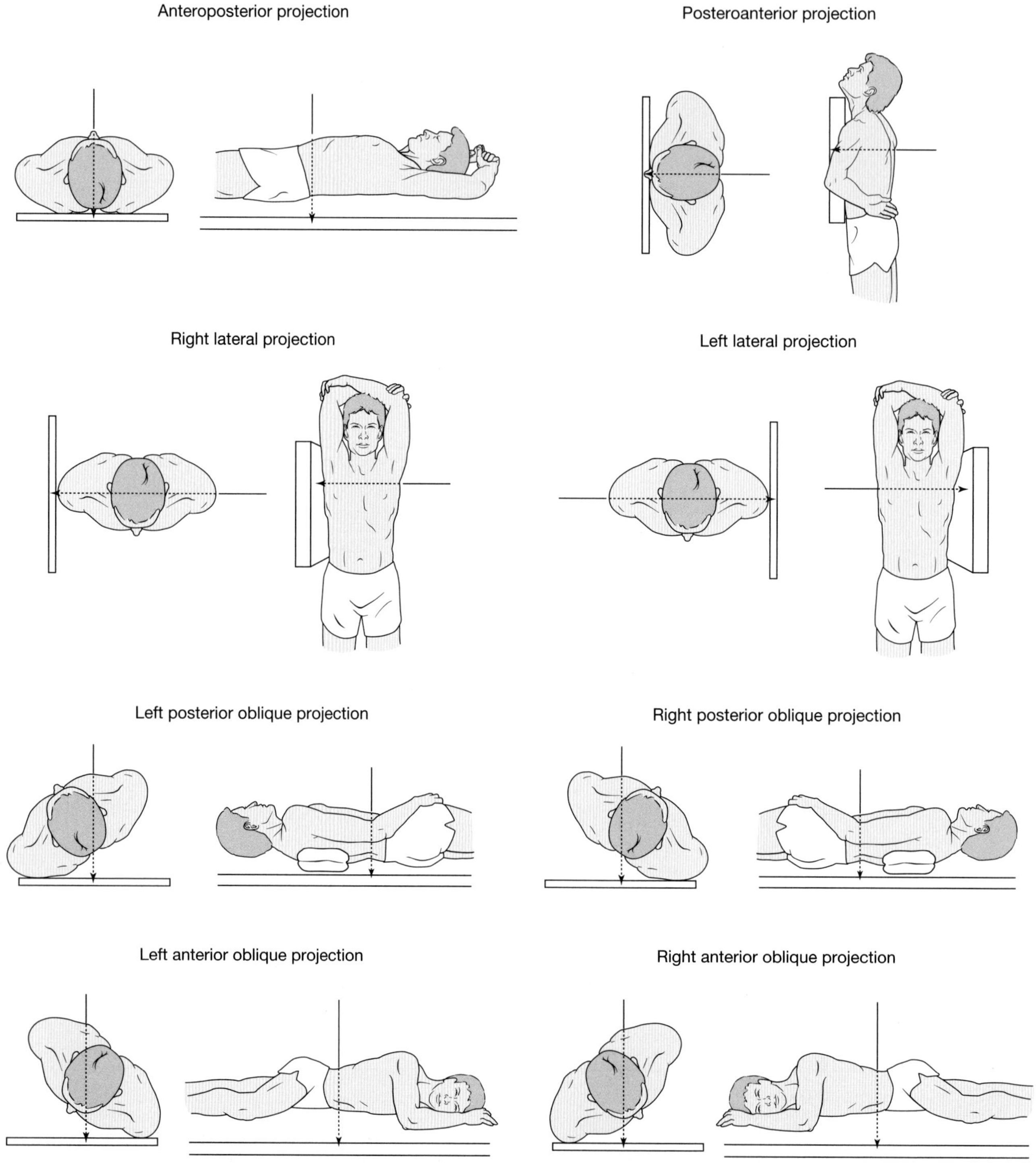

Anteroposterior projection

Posteroanterior projection

Right lateral projection

Left lateral projection

Left posterior oblique projection

Right posterior oblique projection

Left anterior oblique projection

Right anterior oblique projection

FIGURE 3-1 Projections and positions. (From Kronenberger J. *Lippincott Williams & Wilkins' Clinical Medical Assisting.* 5th ed. WK/LWW; 2016: Figure 10-3 (p 260). ISBN: 9781496302380.)

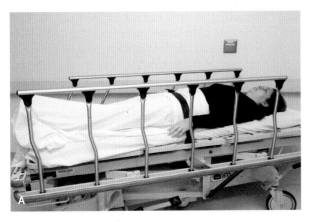

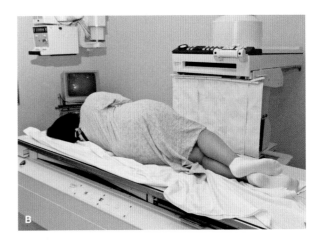

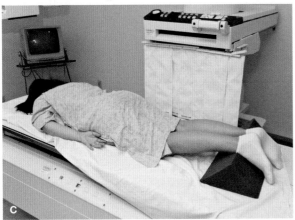

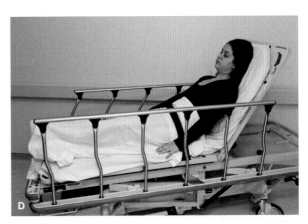

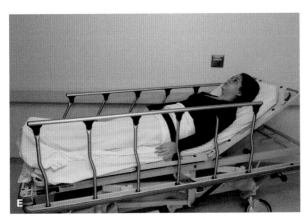

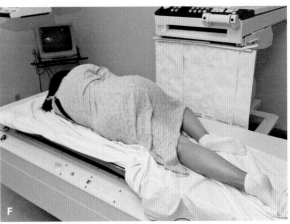

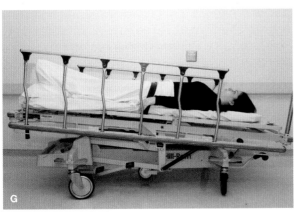

FIGURE 3-2 **(A)** Supine position. **(B)** Lateral position. **(C)** Prone position. **(D)** High Fowler position. **(E)** Semi-Fowler position. **(F)** Sims position. **(G)** Trendelenburg position.

shows the different positions utilized in health care settings. Students must memorize these different terms.

The student radiographer encounters other terminology throughout the clinical rotation in other imaging modalities, oncology and surgery. If a term is not familiar, ask someone at an appropriate time so as to become educated as to their meaning.

TYPES OF PATIENT COMMUNICATION

Communication can be defined as the exchange of information, thoughts, and feelings. Clear communication establishes a respectful and professional relationship with the patient. This helps the patient feel more comfortable to ask questions.

Verbal Communication

Communication is a two-way process. The patient conveys concerns to the radiographer. The radiographer utilizes this information to make the best plan of action to perform the radiographic study. This communication requires skill and experience by the radiographer to obtain the information needed to make an assessment. In order to be a successful communicator, the radiographer must study communication and interpersonal relations in education. The various aspects and application of communication must be understood.

The radiographer must be able to convey messages in an organized and logical manner. Any problem of communication, whether major or minor, has an impact on the patient's health care. If a patient leaves a health care situation feeling confused or misunderstood, the choice not to continue care that is necessary may be reached. On the other hand, the patient who leaves feeling that treatment was handled with dignity and respect probably continues the needed treatment.

Most patients' feelings about health care, whether positive or negative, are, in part, the result of communication between the health care worker and the patient. The radiographer must receive, **interpret**, implement, and give directions in the daily work routine. Consolation and reassurance must be offered while caring for a patient. An empathetic attitude is a must when the radiographer is dealing with any patient. Being able to communicate effectively is as important as knowing the correct use of the complex equipment in the department.

Becoming a successful communicator requires developing skills in listening, observing, speaking, and writing. The student may feel that hearing, seeing, talking, writing, and using a computer are all skills in the art of communication. This is not necessarily the case. The ability to accept others with an open mind and to interact with people in a perceptive manner is based on learned attitudes and self-understanding.

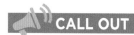 **CALL OUT**

Skills in listening, observing, speaking, and writing are required of the successful communicator!

CASE STUDY—AMELIA (PART 1)

Amelia is scheduled for a 2:00 PM appointment in the radiology department of a world-renowned health facility. Amelia is to have an injection into the hip joint with ultrasound guidance, and although she is familiar with ultrasound, she is not certain what this procedure entails or what the pain level will be on a hip that has already been detrimental to her mobility.

Amelia lives almost 300 miles away from this facility and it takes 4 hours to drive this distance. Parking is a challenge, and a spot to park was finally found almost five blocks away. Once arriving at the reception desk 5 minutes early, she is unable to check in at reception as her electronic chart is open and locked by someone else. After waiting for a few minutes, the receptionist tries to call the department to have the chart closed so she could check Amelia into the system as being present for her appointment. All phone lines were busy, and finally the receptionist suggested that Amelia have a seat and if further information is required, it can be obtained after the appointment.

Thirty minutes goes by. Amelia returns to the reception desk asking if she had, in fact, been entered into the system as it was now past her appointment time. After confirming that she was showing as active, Amelia tracked down someone coming out of the radiology department for another patient, and asked if they knew when she would be taken back. She was informed that they would check to see what the progress was on her appointment as it was a subspeciality and they did not work in that area. When she was finally called back into the area for her procedure, Amelia witnessed four people sitting at computers or standing around "chatting."

ISSUES TO CONSIDER

1. what mood would Amelia be in after a long drive, no parking, walking on a poorly functioning hip, not being able to be checked in, and waiting 30 minutes past her appointment?

2. Is it reasonable etc.

3. What might happen to Amelia's stress at seeing so many people in the hall—if they aren't with patients, why was she called back so late for her appointment?

Critical thinking skills must be used to assess how the radiographer thinks about those with whom interaction occurs. Critical thinking requires the radiographer to interpret what the patient is saying and to evaluate it in a manner that is not filled with personal bias. After answering the patient, it is wise to reflect and see if the communication was successful. In order to become a skilled and thoughtful communicator, an honest analysis of beliefs and **biases** must be made by the radiographer.

Modes of Communication

There are various ways to communicate with another individual that seem commonplace to the non–health care person. Speaking and writing are the most common forms that first come to mind. The use of interpersonal devices, such as a cell phone, tablet, or computer, is simply that—devices used for a person to speak (phone) or text (write) messages to another. Nonverbal communication is critical in the health care profession because it may convey more than intended or may cause the individual that is receiving the message to believe the opposite of the spoken word because of nonverbal cues.

Speaking has layers within it that can convey different meanings to what is actually said or enhance the actual words. The pitch and tone of the voice can do either. As an example, a frustrated radiographer might say to a mischievous patient, "I am having a difficult time with these x-rays because you keep moving." The use of terse, firm, and strong voice conveys to the patient that the radiographer is no longer tolerating any misbehavior that the patient might be displaying. However, the use of a light voice higher in pitch might convey the message to the patient that the radiographer knows that the patient is moving but hasn't reached the "end of the rope" yet.

Writing is an important tool in communication, especially between different teams of health care providers. Documentation is absolutely critical so that others included in the patient care are able to determine what has transpired and make informed decisions regarding aspects of the patient care for which they are responsible. In legal terms, if there is no documentation regarding an incident, the aspects of that incident didn't happen. It is extremely important that all adverse occurrences are fully documented, not only for other health care personnel that might be caring for the patient but also for any legal considerations that might occur.

Nonverbal Communication

There is more to communication than the spoken word. The unspoken, or **nonverbal**, aspects of communication can be defined as all stimuli other than the spoken word involved in communication. To understand nonverbal communication, one must depend on what one sees the patient doing as one speaks, what one hears in speech other than the spoken words, and what is felt if the patient is being touched during the communication. The unspoken messages can often indicate how the patient feels more quickly than any words spoken. Nonverbal communication functions in the following ways:

- It may repeat or stress the spoken message.
- The face or body movement may be in agreement with what is said, or it may contradict what is being said.
- It may accent the spoken word. An emphasis on words spoken may occur with the shake of a fist or a hand placed on the arm of the listener.
- It may regulate the spoken word. A receiver may nod their head or look interested in the spoken word and, therefore, encourage further communication.
- It may substitute for verbal communication. A nod, a smile, or a frown may suffice for words.

The perceptive health care worker can learn a great deal about a patient by other forms of nonverbal communication. For instance, the manner in which a person's body moves or facial expressions may say a great deal. The set of one's jaw may determine anger. The patient who does not look the receiver in the eye may feel insecure or mistrustful. Body carriage may indicate the patient's self-concept and mental status. Nonverbal cues may also suggest social and economic status. Clothing worn and posture, or the manners in which a person enters a room or addresses those in the room are often indicators of this type of status.

The radiographer must make certain that the verbal and nonverbal messages that are sent match. If the patient suspects that the radiographer is not sincere in the interaction, anxiety may increase. The work being done on a patient may force movement into the patient's personal space. This may result in feelings of discomfort for the patient as well as for the health care worker. Informing the patient before entering any personal space may alleviate anxiety.

The patient who comes to the imaging department for a difficult procedure may be fearful but may not wish to express this verbally. The sensitive radiographer is able to detect the patient's nonverbal expression of fear and anxiety. By using therapeutic communication techniques, a trusting relationship is established with the patient. This allows the patient to express any feelings, thereby reducing fear and anxiety.

Cultural Variations in Communication

The radiographer must be aware of cultural differences in verbal and nonverbal communication in order not to offend or be offended; nor misunderstand or be misunderstood. In some **cultures**, it is considered courteous to place one's body close to the body of another person during communication. In the United States, people are very protective of the space close to their bodies and might be offended if a person with whom they are not on very friendly terms invades this "personal space."

Nonverbal symbols such as a nod, meaning "yes," or a shake of the head, meaning "no," do not mean the same thing in all cultures. Symbols also have different meanings to different age groups. People of one age group may not understand the symbols of another. A safe rule when communicating with a patient is to use speech instead of symbols if there is any possibility of being misunderstood. Another common cause of cultural misunderstanding is the use of humor. Although humor is often an effective communication tool, it must not be used if there is a possibility of it being misunderstood. Humor can be an effective means of releasing tension or conveying a difficult message, but it should not be used in life-threatening situations, when there is a possibility of legal action, or when there may be a cultural misunderstanding. In addition, a patient's age may affect a common understanding of humor. If there is any doubt concerning the appropriateness of humor, it should not be used.

Cultural variations don't have to occur just with patients from other ethnicities or races. The area where the patient grew up may have different colloquialisms and slang that may not be familiar to the radiographer. A very common example is the term "pop" (Midwest states) or "soda" from the Southwestern states. Although this is a very simple example, it illustrates the differences between different regions.

FACTORS THAT MAY AFFECT COMMUNICATION

There are a number of variables that may affect the way a patient receives and understands the message sent by the radiographer. The following paragraphs are challenges that can be experienced in both verbal and nonverbal communication. Students and seasoned radiographers need to be mindful that not all patients speak English well, understand it, can hear well, have the ability to cognitively assess what is said, or have the same medical beliefs about the procedure.

English as a Second Language Patients

Patients identified as English as a second language (ESL) may have a limited command of the English language in that they understand some of what is being said but not all of it. They may not be able to respond with correct answers, if they did not entirely understand what was being said. There has been federal legislation that guarantees the patient's right to have effective communication in all health care institutions, regardless of the language barrier. Large facilities have interpreter service available either via a phone-in system or from other staff that have been certified to provide communication in the patient's language. The use of webcam services on a computer allows the interpreter to see and hear the patient for the full communication experience (both verbal and nonverbal).

Although it may delay the procedure until an interpreter is located and is able to help the patient, it is of the utmost importance that a friend or family member not be used to assume this role. The interpreter is trained to translate only what is being said in the manner that it was spoken. A family member may add or delete information that is not deemed important to what is thought to be happening. Although family members and friends are trying to be helpful, it is not in the best interest of the patient or the radiographer to allow this form of communication to occur.

Gender Factors

The radiographer must be aware that the manner of communication varies depending on the gender of the patient. The male radiographer and the female radiographer may tend to deliver and receive messages in an altered manner based simply on their gender. Men tend to be reticent in their expression of feelings. Women tend to feel comfortable in discussion rather than in activity as a means of interaction. Whatever the gender of the patient or the radiographer, it is necessary to avoid sexual innuendoes and denigration of or use of gender as a means of humor.

The radiographer must also be sensitive to the issue of gender in professional interactions with coworkers. A nonbiased and nonjudgmental attitude in manner and speech and in sexual references and avoidance of sexual innuendoes must always be used. Avoidance of relating in a flirtatious manner prevents many uncomfortable interpersonal or legal problems in relationships with coworkers or patients.

Patients that identify themselves as gender neutral and transgender should never be treated differently than any other patient that is seen in the imaging department. If the radiographer needs to explain any procedure, it must be done in the same caring manner as it would be with any patient of the age group of the patient.

Patient Impairments

Not all patients come to the imaging department able to communicate in a manner that is the same as the radiographer. Hearing, vision, and speech impairments as well as impaired neurologic function, developmental impairments, and altered levels of consciousness affect the communication that is so critical to the success of the procedure.

Hearing Loss

Hearing loss becomes more common as patients age; however, this is not always the case. Children may have a congenital hearing loss or they may have acquired it through chronic otitis media or other infections. Traditionally, patients who are hard of hearing have poor communication in the health care setting, particularly in imaging, as there is a lack of sign language interpreters. Patients with mild hearing loss pick up some information that may lead the radiographer to believe that the message being sent was understood. Elderly patients may ask to have the information repeated, but this should not be assumed. They may smile or nod their heads as if the message was heard but they might not fully understand the meaning of the instruction or information.

Good communication strategies must be utilized when communicating with a patient that may have hearing loss, even if the patient utilizes hearing devices. Ask the person how they prefer to communicate. Face the patient on the same level and in good light if possible. Do not talk from another room, and when giving breathing instructions,

explain to the patient while in front of them what is going to be said. The patient may be able to lip-read (speech read) so speak clearly, slowly, and distinctly. However, be natural. Shouting distorts the sound of speech and makes it more difficult to understand. It is best not to ask closed-ended questions that require a simple yes or no answer. Ask the patient leading questions rather than "do you understand what I have said" as it is the best way to ensure that the patient has received the message. Whenever possible, provide pertinent information in writing. Pay attention to the patient's facial expressions. A puzzled look may indicate misunderstanding.

Visually Impaired

Interacting with a patient who is visually impaired is not as challenging as the hearing impaired. There are points of communication that should be kept in mind that facilitates the patient's experience. Gently touching the arm or shoulder of patients to make introductions lets them know that the message is meant for them. Speak directly to the patient, not through a companion. Remember that the patient is not hearing impaired, so natural conversational tones are normal for the patient. Be precise and descriptive when explaining what the procedure is that the patient is about to have. Use language that refers the patient's orientation such as "I need to have you move slightly to your left." Communicate what is required of the patient rather than pushing or pulling the patient while on the radiographic table. Let the patient know when exiting the room to make an exposure or to review the image. Always announce a return to the room. Offer assistance to patients by allowing them to hold onto your arm.

Speech Impaired

Difficulties communicating with patients with speech impairments may cause **stress** for both the patient and the radiographer. Patients that have suffered a stroke may be required to have more radiographic procedures than others. The radiographer who can understand the special needs of these patients is able to complete the study with little or no anxiety on the part of the patient. Stroke patients may not be able to communicate physically, but cognitively, they know what they want to say, it is just not possible to have the brain make the mouth form the words. This is frustrating for the patient requires additional patience and compassion from the radiographer. Tips to help communicate include:

- Reduce any distractions that may be happening. Remove the patient from a crowded waiting room or hallway before beginning any explanation about the procedure.
- Use shorter, less complicated sentences. Rather than saying, "I am going to take an x-ray of your

abdomen after I get you on the x-ray table," try simply saying, "I am going to take a picture of your abdomen."

- The use of nonverbal communication such as facial expressions, gestures, or writing is an effective way to support what is being said.
- Ask the patient what kind of help they need. Don't assume that the patient does, or does not, need help to perform what is being asked.
- If the patient uses a communication device, such as a manual or electronic communication board, ask the patient the best way to make sure it stays safe during the procedure.
- Be honest. Health care professionals don't always know the answer. They don't always understand a message from a patient. If this is the case, tell the patient. Pretending can make the patient frustrated if the radiographer's response doesn't correspond with a question that was asked.
- Develop a specific communication strategy that is consistent with the person's abilities such as nodding or shaking of the head to indicate agreement or disagreement.
- Other skills addressed in therapeutic communication techniques such as rephrasing or repeating should be used as appropriate.

Patients that have had laryngeal cancer may have lost the ability to speak in a normal manner. In these instances, patients may communicate through the use of artificial speech using a device known as an electrolarynx. This small, battery-operated device is placed directly on the neck, under the chin. The patient pushes a button on the device causing the electrolarynx to produce a vibration that is transferred through the skin to the throat. The patient shapes the sound into words with the mouth, tongue, lips, and teeth. The sound is quite metallic but can be understood.

Neurologic Impairments

Neurologic impairments are exhibited in patients that have lost the use of memory, cognitive function, sensory and/or motor skills, speech, language, organizational skills, information processing, affect, social skills, or basic life functions. These types of impairment occur with patients that have suffered a traumatic brain injury. Communication with patients that have neurologic impairments can be frustrating for both the radiographer and the patient. The following tips may help in communication:

- Use clear, specific language.
- Be patient and allow the patient time to express any needs.
- Use short, concise instructions.
- Communicate at a relatively slow pace with pauses as needed.

- Use pictures or visual aids to reinforce information if needed.
- Ask the patient what is needed.

Developmental Impairment

There are five types of developmental disabilities, which include **autism spectrum disorder (ASD), cerebral palsy (CP), intellectual disability (ID), attention deficit hyperactivity disorder (ADHD),** and **learning disabilities**. Individuals with developmental disorders are able to effectively communicate their needs through a wide variety of communication skills and abilities. Patients that are nonverbal can communicate with gestures and/or body language. Many individuals with developmental disabilities are capable of informed consent for medical procedures. When communicating with the patient, speak to the patient, rather than through their caregiver or the sign language interpreter. If the caregiver needs to be involved in the conversation, ask the patient's permission. The following tips facilitate communication with a developmentally impaired patient:

- Be interested in communicating with the patient. Act and speak naturally.
- Communicate about what is happening at the moment.
- Make the patient the most important part of the communication. Listen, clarify, and restate as necessary.
- Respond appropriately to all communicative attempts by the patient. Respond at the patient's level.
- If the patient is an adult, treat them like an adult. Don't shout at any patient.
- Don't pretend what the patient said is understood. If the radiographer does not understand the patient, be honest and ask for clarification.

Altered States of Consciousness

Level of consciousness (LOC) is a medical term for identifying how awake, alert, and aware of their surroundings someone is. It also describes the degree to which a person can respond. Altered or abnormal levels of consciousness (ALOCs) describe states in which a person either has decreased cognitive function or cannot be easily aroused. Most medical conditions affect the brain and impair consciousness when they become serious or life-threatening, and an altered state of consciousness usually signals a serious medical problem. Sometimes impaired consciousness is reversible, whereas other times it is not.

Communicating with individuals that are unconscious may seem unreasonable; however, it is important to know that patients still have the ability to hear and remember conversations that occurred while they were in a coma or unconscious. Radiographers performing diagnostic imaging with patients who are unable to respond and appear to be in a coma should treat the patient as if every conversation is heard. Explain to the patient what is being done during the procedure.

Other causes of ALOC may be alcohol or drug induced. The technologist caring for an intoxicated patient must keep communication simple, direct, and nonjudgmental. Do not become involved in patients' attempt to argue. If the patient refuses treatment or becomes difficult to manage, call for help immediately. Don't attempt to complete the assignment until adequate assistance has arrived. It may be best to simply stop the procedure. Before doing so, get direction from the referring physician. Do not leave the patient alone, and observe at all time to prevent falls.

Other Factors That Affect Communication

Patients that are undergoing a stressful situation, such as the grieving process, may need more compassionate communication than other patients. The radiographer may be asked questions of a sensitive nature or ones that might be uncomfortable. Responses in this situation require the radiographer to use therapeutic skills such as rephrasing the patient's question or statement to allow the patient to talk about the circumstances that brought about the initial statement or question. When faced with these situations, it is common for anyone to respond with denial statements, such as "You are going to be fine" or "Don't say such things." These types of statements block any further communication. Patients in this situation may not necessarily be seeking a response but just a supportive listener.

The rate at which one speaks, the volume of the voice, fluency, and vocal patterns are combined into one category called **paralanguage**. Paralanguage has to do with the sound of speech rather than the content. The correct pauses and inflections are extremely important if communication is to be understood. If one speaks without proper inflection, a question will not sound like a question. If words run together, they are difficult to sort out. Poor knowledge of correct grammatical usage may also make it difficult to understand what is being said. Speech that is too rapid, too slow, too soft, or too loud may also be a problem. Another problem could be the use of various words with multiple meanings. "Stool" to the health care worker means something different than it does to the patient who might think the radiographer is talking about something to sit on. The use of words like "thigh" versus "femur," or "lower leg" versus "tibia" makes more sense to the patient. When communicating with the patient and/or the family, be sure to include an explanation of any medical terms that seem to be confusing.

Feedback

To be certain that the transmitted message has been correctly received, it is necessary to obtain **feedback**.

Feedback is the patient's response that enables the radiographer to evaluate the effectiveness of the message. Feedback is essential so as to know whether the patient has understood the message in the same terms as intended by the sender. In interactions between the radiographer and the patient, it is effective to have the patient repeat the directions that have been given, or simply observe the patient to be certain that the instruction is being followed. If the patient understands the message, an appropriate response occurs. If the patient does not respond correctly, it is the radiographer's responsibility to restate the message in a manner that is understood.

Therapeutic Communication

There are a series of communication techniques that, if cultivated, assist the radiographer in becoming a therapeutic member of the health care team. The useful therapeutic communication techniques are listed in Display 3-2.

Establishing Communication Guidelines

Many relationships between the radiographer and the patient are brief, and it is essential to make the best use of the time. Establishing guidelines for the interaction is essential. Guidelines should include introducing oneself to the patient, giving an explanation of the examination to be performed, and giving an explanation of what is expected of the patient and what the patient can expect from the imaging staff. Delivery of instructions to the patient should be clear, concise, and nonthreatening in manner. This requires careful, organized thought. If the patient understands the message, it is easier to comply with the plan. Successful communication requires critical thought on the part of the radiographer. The following paragraphs aid the technologist in providing therapeutic communication.

DISPLAY 3-2

Therapeutic Communication Techniques

- Establishing guidelines
- Reducing distance
- Listening
- Using silence
- Responding to the underlying message
- Restating the main idea
- Reflecting the main idea
- Seeking and providing clarification
- Making observation
- Exploring
- Validating
- Focusing

Reducing Distance

Physical distance between the patient and the radiographer must be reduced in order for communication to be effective. Proximity makes the patient feel included and involved. Physical barriers and a noisy environment should be avoided. Face the patient directly and make eye contact when speaking and being spoken to. Crossed arms or legs by the radiographer convey a lack of receptiveness. Performance of other tasks while speaking to the patient indicates disinterest in the patient.

Listening

Listening in a therapeutic manner requires that the radiographer overcome personal biases. To do this, one must think critically about one's biases and learn to dismiss them, and assume a totally nonjudgmental attitude as one is listening to the patient. To compare or interpret what the speaker is saying, one must listen without anticipating a response. The goal must be to gather accurate information and to understand the feeling and meaning of the message the patient is trying to convey.

Using Silence

There are two types of silence, constructive and destructive. Constructive is used in therapeutic communication and moves a conversation or discussion forward. This type of silence is reflective and respectful. The radiographer should wait for the patient to answer and not rush to fill the silent void. The patient needs time to gather thoughts and responses. Additionally, this gives the radiographer time to assess the patient's nonverbal cues such as body language and facial expressions.

Responding to the Underlying Message

When a patient expresses a feeling of frustration, anger, joy, or relief, it is helpful if there is a response that lets the patient know that any feelings about the situation have been understood. An example of this type of response might be as follows:

> PATIENT: *I'm really discouraged. I'm not sure that these procedures are worth it.*
> RADIOGRAPHER: *You are feeling disheartened because you don't feel the procedures are doing any good.*

Restating the Main Idea

Restating or repeating the main idea expressed by the patient is a useful communication technique. It **validates** the radiographer's interpretation of the message and also informs the patient that what is being said is being heard. Consider the following:

> PATIENT: *I am having a lot of pain in my left hip, and I might need help getting up on the examining table.*

> RADIOGRAPHER: *You think that you'll need help getting up on the table because of pain?*

Reflecting the Main Idea

Reflecting or directing back to the patient the main idea of what was stated is another useful communication technique. It keeps the patient as the focus of the communication and allows the patient to explore any feelings about the matter. In this instance, the radiographer helps the patient make a decision. For example:

> PATIENT: *Do you think that I really need this procedure? It's really expensive, and I'm not sure it helps.*
> RADIOGRAPHER: *Do you feel that you should refuse this procedure?*

Seeking and Providing Clarification

Seeking clarification is another useful therapeutic technique one might use. It indicates to the patient that the radiographer is listening to what is being said but is not sure that the message was fully understood. In such a situation, the radiographer should simply state that the message was clearly heard. The radiographer may clarify directions by using different terminology. For instance:

> RADIOGRAPHER: *In preparation for this procedure, you must drink this full glass of fluid.*
> PATIENT: *How much of this do I have to drink?*
> RADIOGRAPHER: *Before we begin the procedure, you must drink all of it.*

Making Observations

Making observations or verbalizing the perceived feeling of another person is a useful communication technique. For example:

> RADIOGRAPHER: *You seem to be very tense, Mr. Smith. Are you concerned about this examination?*

Exploring

The radiographer must direct questions relating to the problems of the patient directly to the patient, not to a caregiver or other individual. When the patient relates personal information, it may be helpful to pursue the problem by exploring further. An example of this technique might be as follows:

> PATIENT: *Every time I receive that type of injection, I feel sick.*
> RADIOGRAPHER: *Can you tell me what it feels like when you have this type of injection?*

Validating

When speaking to a patient, the radiographer may wish to verify what the patient has reported. This is called validating the message.

> RADIOGRAPHER: *Mr. Angelo, are you saying that you have difficulty breathing when you are lying flat?*
> PATIENT: *Yes, I must be in a sitting position in order to breathe well.*

Focusing

The guiding principle of therapeutic communication is to keep the communication focused on the patient by asking open-ended questions that allow the patient to expand answers to questions. Avoid "what" and "why" types of questions or those that require only a yes or no response. It is important for the conversation to be focused on the patient. The radiographer's verbal responses should be kept to a minimum, and the communication should always be redirected to the patient. For example:

> PATIENT: *Do you have other patients that have the same problem?*
> RADIOGRAPHER: *I am sure that I have, but right now I am concerned about how you feel.*

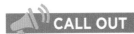
CALL OUT

Respond to the feeling and the meaning of the patient's verbal expression!

Nontherapeutic Communication

An atmosphere of discontent is created primarily through communication and is called a **nontherapeutic (or disruptive) relationship**. This can occur between the radiographer and patient or between the radiographer and coworkers.

BLOCKS TO THERAPEUTIC COMMUNICATION

Several factors actually block or destroy the possibility of creating a therapeutic atmosphere in communication. Rapid speech, complex medical terminology, and distracting environments such as a noisy waiting room or crowded hallway are serious barriers to communication. Radiographers should deliver messages to the patient in a quiet area of the department in a simple and direct manner and make sure that the patient understands English. If this is not the case, an interpreter of the appropriate language must be provided.

Obtaining incomplete answers or failing to explore the patient's description of a problem can also be detrimental to communication. The radiographer must listen to what the patient is saying. If the message is not clear, the radiographer must explore by further questioning until certain that the message is understood. Failure to do this may result in harm to the patient.

Using nontherapeutic communication techniques may also block communication. Some of the common nontherapeutic communication techniques are listed in Display 3-3.

Judgmental statements place the patient in the position of feeling that the approval of the health care worker must be received in order to receive care. These statements can be as simple as saying, "that's good" or "that's bad." They may also take the form of cliché statements such as "We have to take the bad with the good, you know." Another nontherapeutic communication is false reassurance to the patient who expresses fear or anxiety by making a comment such as "Now don't you worry. Everything will be just fine."

Just as silence can be therapeutic so that the patient can gather thoughts, it can also be destructive, or nontherapeutic. When a radiographer fails to respond to a question or acknowledge a statement made by a patient, the patient may assume that the radiographer is not listening, or that the radiographer does not care enough about the conversation to respond. This may lead the patient to stop communication.

DISPLAY 3-3

Nontherapeutic Communication Techniques

Judgmental statements
Cliché statements
False reassurance
Silence
Defending
Changing the subject
Giving advice
Subjective interpretation
Disagreeing
Probing
Demanding an explanation

Defending is another block to therapeutic communication. This type of communication rejects the patient's opinion and prevents the patient from continuing to communicate. For instance:

> PATIENT: *I'm not sure Dr. Jay knows what to do for me.*
> RADIOGRAPHER: *Dr. Jay is an experienced physician, and he has taken care of many people with problems just like yours.*

This type of nontherapeutic response ends the communication with the patient feeling rejected and unworthy.

How much better it would be if the radiographer simply restated the patient's comments and allowed the completion of any expression of concern.

Changing the subject while the patient is speaking is a means of informing the patient that what is being said is unimportant. The radiographer must also avoid giving advice, offering subjective interpretations of a patient's statements, disagreeing, probing, or demanding explanations. All of these responses interfere with therapeutic communication. The following case study demonstrates how nontherapeutic communication is destructive to patient care.

CASE STUDY—AMELIA (PART 2)

Amelia followed a person in a uniform to the dressing area. She had to assume it was the ultrasound technologist as the person never introduced herself. The technologist spoke with a very pronounced accent. Because of the COVID-19 pandemic, all persons in the facility were required to wear a mask covering their nose and mouth, which made it difficult for Amelia to understand the technologist. She had to ask several times for the information that was being given to be repeated. Amelia had not seen the type of garment that was required of her to wear for the procedure and didn't know how to put it on. Both the technologist and Amelia were obviously frustrated and the technologist looked at Amelia saying, "It doesn't matter. Just put it on and the doctor will fix it if he needs to." Having said that, she left Amelia to change and await the doctor's arrival.

ISSUES TO CONSIDER

Remember that the appointment was for midafternoon, which may have been the last case for the ultrasound technologist. Because there was a delay of over 30 minutes, this technologist may have been working overtime.

Remember also that Amelia had to walk a significant distance to get to the building, had to wait in the waiting room for that extended time, and was also unable to understand the directions that were being given to her.

1. How did this last interaction affect Amelia's emotional status?
2. How could the technologist have communicated better to help Amelia put on a special garment that was necessary for the procedure?

PATIENT INTERACTIONS DURING COMMUNICATION

Communication requires the focus to be on the patient. Trying to multitask by setting the control panel at the same time questioning the patient to gain a history might seem like a way to get the patient completed in a timely manner but actually gives the patient a feeling of not being important. When obtaining a patient history or providing patient education, it is important to give the patient the feeling of being the most important aspect of the interaction, which, of course, is true. Make eye contact to ensure that the patient is listening and understanding what is being said. Remember the volume and speed of speech (paralanguage) affects the way the message is delivered and received. Be a good listener. Effective listening is done by focusing completely on what the patient might be saying, not on what must be done next to get the job done, or what a response might be. In order to make sure that the messages have been understood, get feedback. When the patient and the radiographer work together to send and receive messages, effective communication can be accomplished in just a few minutes.

Summary

1. Clear communication is critical for successful patient care. It helps the patient feel confident, comfortable, and at ease. It also demonstrates a professional demeanor on the part of the radiographer.

2. Methods of identifying the patient:

   a. Interviewing and questioning by asking for the last name and date of birth should be done every time the patient comes to the imaging department, even if the patient is known to the radiographer.

   b. Inpatients should also have the wrist band looked at in addition to answering the questions from above.

   c. The patient's chart and the requisition must also be checked against the patient's verbal information and the wrist band.

3. Obtaining a patient history may require asking sensitive questions. This requires tactful communication from the radiographer. Patient history can also be found in the patient chart.

4. Communication also involves the patient's record (chart).

   a. Elements within a patient's chart may be off-limits to the technologist for confidentiality reasons.

   b. If it is necessary to open the patient's chart, be sure to log off once finished so that others are not able to look into the patient's information. Retrieve the information that is needed and then close the computer.

   c. Remember to document in the chart as is necessary. This includes any contrast media or medication that was given and also any unusual incident that may have happened while in the department and any care that may have been needed and provided.

5. Patient education is part of the scope of practice of a radiographer. Make sure the patient understands the language. Pre- and postexamination information is important.

   a. Information preprocedure must include what the study entails, the different positions that may be used, and the length of the study. Be able to answer any questions the patient may have regarding the study. Any adverse effects must be stated.

   b. Use critical thinking skills to establish a plan for educating the patient postexamination.

   c. Radiographers must be able to answer basic questions regarding other modalities such as mammography, ultrasound, nuclear medicine, computed tomography (CT), magnetic resonance imaging (MRI), or invasive procedures.

6. The age and generation of the patient affect communication styles on both sides, and the radiographer must become skilled in communicating with all ages.

7. The student radiographer becomes skilled in medical terminology and radiographic terminology as education in the clinical setting progresses.

   a. Abbreviations are most often seen on the radiography request or report and students need to spend time familiarizing themselves with these.

8. Verbal communication includes listening, observing, speaking, and writing.

   a. It is a two-way process and includes paralanguage, which is the rate of speech and the tone of voice.

9. Nonverbal communication conveys attitudes and demeanor and may communicate a completely different message than the verbal message.

   a. Body language, clothing worn, posture, facial expressions, and gestures are all forms of nonverbal communication.

10. Cultural variations can affect communication. Be sure to identify potential issues that might arise from inappropriate communication.

11. Communication can be altered by variables such as language, gender, and patient impairments. Be sure to get feedback to make sure the message was received correctly.

12. Therapeutic communication is that which encourages the patient to provide answers to any questions that may arise. There are multiple methods that can be utilized and these must be practiced in order to use them effectively.

13. Blocks to therapeutic communication (nontherapeutic) are those statements that close a conversation immediately or within a few minutes. These blocks are often offensive to the patient or are rude statements that are made without considering how the words sound to the patient. Inappropriate communication is a good cause of patients going elsewhere for their medical care.

CHAPTER 3 REVIEW QUESTIONS

1. List the skills required of a successful communicator.

2. The concerns of the radiographer preparing to take a history on a patient must include:
   a. Privacy and a quiet environment
   b. Ensuring confidentiality
   c. A professional demeanor and appearance
   d. Establishment of rapport with the patient
   e. All of the above

3. Mary is scheduled for an MRI procedure. She tells the radiographer that she is afraid she may not be able to tolerate this examination. The radiographer states, "Don't worry, it will be simple and over quickly." This is an example of:
   a. Verbalizing the implied and therapeutic
   b. Reflecting and therapeutic
   c. Changing the subject and nontherapeutic
   d. False reassurance and nontherapeutic

4. When directions are given to a non-English-speaking patient, it is best to:
   a. Speak English slowly and loudly
   b. Use a family member such as a child to interpret for you
   c. Draw pictures
   d. Get a trained and accepted interpreter

5. When dealing with children in the imaging department, it is best to:
   a. Talk "baby talk" to the child to make them do what you want
   b. Talk like an adult and speak to only the parents, the child is not important
   c. Incorporate both parent and child in the communication and, if necessary, into the imaging process
   d. Have the child sedated so you can get the examination over with

6. What is the best communication skill to use for cognitively impaired patients?
   a. Assume that the patient understands what you are saying if they don't ask any questions.
   b. Use shorter and less complicated sentences.
   c. Pretend that you don't notice anything about the patient.
   d. Write everything down and don't speak to the patient.

7. Your last patient on Christmas eve at 11:30 is a widow who says her wrist has hurt for 3 weeks. In conversation, you discover that her husband died over Thanksgiving. What is the best therapeutic communication skill you can use?
   a. Your wrist has been hurting for 3 weeks and you come in here at 11:30 on Christmas eve?
   b. What took you so long to see what was wrong with your wrist?
   c. I imagine that you are missing your husband very much at this time of year.
   d. Use silence. You just want to go home to your family.

8. Which of the following statements is a form of destructive communication?
   a. "You feel like you are not getting any better after all of these treatments?"
   b. "If you would just follow the doctor's orders, I am sure you would feel much better."
   c. "I am going to sit you upright now, are you feeling well enough to do that?"
   d. "Tell me where the pain is most often located."

9. Paralanguage is considered to be a form of:
   a. Nonverbal communication
   b. Nontherapeutic communication
   c. Humor
   d. Verbal skills

10. Patient education concerns all of the following except?
    a. Pre- and postexamination descriptions
    b. Follow-up care
    c. How to pay the bill
    d. Any questions about examinations in other modalities

11. Which of the following can be either a therapeutic or nontherapeutic communication skill?
    a. Observing
    b. Listening
    c. Demanding
    d. Silence

12. You are taking the history of a male patient before placing him on the examining table. He tells you that he has difficulty moving from a sitting to a standing position. The radiographer says, "You feel that you need help to stand?" This therapeutic communication technique is called:
    a. Exploring
    b. Silence
    c. Making an observation
    d. Verbalizing the implied
    e. Validating

Ethics and Law in Medical Imaging

4

OBJECTIVES

After studying this chapter, the student will be able to:

1. Describe the basis of ethics.

2. Explain the characteristics of ethical behavior.

3. Explore theoretical situations relating to the ethics of medical imaging.

4. Discuss the basis of law.

5. Discuss the major ethical/legal concerns in health care.

6. Describe documentation in health records, particularly in medical imaging.

7. Explain the types of consent.

KEY TERMS

Attribute: Quality or characteristic of a person or a profession

Bias: An inclination or temperament based on personal judgment; prejudice

Bioethics: Moral issues dealing with the ethical issues of human life, health care, and death

Common law: Decisions and opinions of courts that are based on local customs and habits of an area within a particular country or state

Defaming: To attack or injure a person's reputation

Diagnostic imaging: Current terminology used to encompass all areas devoted to produce an image of a body part

Ethical: Conforming to the standards of conduct of a given profession or group

Holistic: The view that an organic or integrated whole has a reality independent of and greater than the sum of its parts

Immoblizing device: A piece of equipment that ensures restricting patient movement

Liable: Something that a person is obligated to do or an obligation required to be fulfilled by law; usually an obligation of financial nature

Litigation: The process of taking legal action

Moral reason: The logical process of determining whether an action is right or wrong when faced with a decision over what to do

Statutory law: Established law that is enacted by a legislative body and punishable by the court system

Unethical: Not conforming to the standards of conduct of a particular profession or group

INTRODUCTION

For health care professionals, most **litigation** comes from not following the standard of care as set forth by the profession. Breaking state and federal laws also leads to lawsuits. It is imperative that radiographers understand that they can be sued for **unethical** or illegal acts. Gone are the days where only the radiologist or the hospital was held accountable. As radiologic technology gained recognition as a profession, it took on the responsibility to practice with the patient's best interest in mind, while doing no harm; and to always act within the scope of practice.

ETHICS AND ETHICAL BEHAVIOR

Ethics may be defined as a set of moral principles that govern one's course of action. *Moral principles* are a set of standards that establish what is right or good. All individuals have a personal code of ethics that evolves on the basis of their cultural and environmental background—the same background that has taught us to place *values* on behaviors, as well as on objects in our environment, that is, to assign a judgment of either good or bad to an action, behavior, or object. Ethics is a combination of the **attributes** of honesty, integrity, fairness, caring, respect, fidelity, competence, and accountability. The terms "ethics," "principles," and "values" are closely linked and may be used interchangeably from time to time.

Bioethics is a branch of ethics that was established because of the advanced technical methods of prolonging life. Bioethics blends philosophy, law, history, and theology with medicine. It refers to complex and controversial choices that range from difficult decisions to prolong life or honor a "do not resuscitate" order, to stem cell research. An individual in the field of radiology may not be called upon to act upon these "bioethical decisions" that are found in health care; however, the radiographer's exposure to these ideas in the medical field may influence one's own beliefs and ethics.

Origins and History of Ethics

There were many **ethical** theorists who created or professed a particular ethical model in health care. The earliest writings on medical ethics are attributed to Hippocrates who gave medical practitioners their first and most important rule: "to help and not to harm." There are two principles involved in this statement. The first is beneficence (i.e., to help others). The second is nonmaleficence (i.e., to avoid harming others). These principles have held as the foremost priorities of medical providers for thousands of years. Other individuals contributed to the theories of ethics in medicine that are relevant to radiology through today.

In the 1930s, medicine was a paternalistic profession. Doctors gave advice, and patients were expected to follow along. Patients did not have many rights. They could even be enrolled in experiments without their knowledge, which was widely condoned. After World War II, the world learned the horrors of German doctors working in the concentration camps and conducting deadly scientific experiments in which the subjects had no say. Efforts to right these wrongs, enshrined in the Nuremberg Code, signaled the beginning of modern medical ethics. The 1960s brought several reforms in bioethics that emphasized patient autonomy in all areas of health care. The National Patient Safety Foundation was founded in 1997 to "create a world where patients and those who care for them are free from harm." In 2005, the Patient Safety and Quality Improvement Act encouraged medical professionals to voluntarily and confidentially report issues that compromise patient safety and quality service. In May 2017, the Institute for Healthcare Improvement and the National Patient Safety Foundation combined forces to better promote patient safety in many health care fields. Although laws and guidelines are written and amended to address new ethical concerns, it is the moral duty of the individuals in the medical community to apply ethical guidelines to difficult or uncertain challenges.

Ethical Philosophies

There are three basic ethical philosophies from which ethical principles are derived. These are *utilitarianism*, *deontology*, and *virtue*. Utilitarianism is often called *consequentialism* and advocates actions are morally correct or right when the largest number of persons is benefited by the decision made. For example, a large accident occurs and a number of persons are critically injured. The triage team assigns a higher priority to the less injured patients and, because the chance of survival is less for the most severely injured, attends last to those who are critically injured. This is an acceptable philosophy if one benefits from the decision.

Deontology upholds the philosophy that rules are to be followed at all times by all individuals. Deontology comes from a Greek word meaning "duty"; therefore, deontology requires that one judge an action by deciding if it is an obligation. When making decisions using this school of thought, one generally does not take consequences into consideration even if it proves to be beneficial to the patient. Following the rules at all times may be too restrictive, especially when specific circumstances surrounding a situation do not fit in a set of rules. An example of deontology is illustrated by the accident portrayed earlier. Because the health care provider has the duty to "do no harm," assigning a low priority number to the most critical patients would be wrong. Deontology and utilitarianism being more or less opposite, the more critically injured patients would get the highest priority and the most likely to survive would be attended to last, with the assumption that they would survive longest without care.

Virtue is a philosophical belief that focuses on using wisdom rather than emotional and intellectual problem solving. With the popularity of **holistic** medicine, virtue ethics incorporates certain principles of both utilitarianism and deontology to provide a broader view of issues. Analysis, review of consequences, and societal rules are essential to forming decisions using virtue. Again, using the accident example to illustrate, with virtue ethics, the triage of the patients would take into account the significance of each individual. How the family and friends of the victims would be affected by the triage decisions would be the deciding factor in who gets first treatment.

Ethical Principles

When one is confronted with an ethical dilemma, it is best to use a set of moral principles that can be judged and weighed against each other within the scope of practice of radiography. There are many articles that are written about ethical principles and may include variations of the principles listed here. Principles that are relative to radiology include the following:

Autonomy: All persons have the right to make rational decisions free from external pressures. Patients have the right to make decisions concerning their medical treatment, and all health care workers must respect those decisions. In practice, the radiographer acts as the liaison between the radiologist and the patient. In these circumstances, the radiographer must act on behalf of the patient.

Beneficence: Health care practitioners should act to attain a good result or to have a beneficial result for the patient. The radiographer must always plan patient care to ensure safe outcomes and avoid harmful consequences. Beneficence requires action that either prevents harm or does the greatest good for the patient. This may require one to side with the patient and against coworkers.

Confidentiality: All patients have the right to have information concerning their state of health kept in confidence without disclosing it to others unless it is of benefit to the patient or unless there is a direct threat to society if not disclosed. The radiographer must not disclose facts concerning the patient's health or other personal information to anyone not involved with the patient's care.

Justice: All persons are to be treated equally or receive equal benefits according to need. One patient must not be favored over another or treated differently from another, regardless of personal feelings. It is fairness and equality.

Nonmaleficence: The health care worker's duty is to abstain from inflicting harm and also preventing harm. The radiographer is obligated to practice in a safe manner at all times. "First, do no harm."

Paternalism: An attitude of acting like a parent sometimes prompts health care workers to make decisions regarding a person's care without consulting the person affected. Within the scope of practice, the radiographer is justified in taking action in instances in which not acting would do more harm than the lack of patient input into the decision-making process.

Veracity: Truthfulness and honesty should be in all aspects of one's professional life. One must be honest with patients, coworkers, and oneself.

Other principles that can be brought to bear in the study of ethics include double effect (an action having both a good and a bad effect), fidelity (loyal or keeping a promise), sanctity of life (life is of the highest good), and respect for property (not intentionally damaging or wasting property).

Moral Reasoning

Moral reasoning refers to the logical process of determining whether an action is right or wrong. Through the process of moral reasoning a person is able to evaluate a situation and choose a course of action that corresponds to moral values. It may lead to greater moral behavior.

Personal Behavior Standards

All individuals have a personal code of ethics or sense of morality that evolves on the basis of their cultural and environmental background—the same background that has taught us to place *values* on behaviors, as well as on objects in the environment, that is, to assign a judgment of either good or bad to an action, behavior, or object. These manners, customs, and beliefs continue with an individual to help formulate an important role in decision-making. These decisions play an important role in health care and with the use of guidelines determine outcomes when situations are encountered concerning legal issues.

Professional Attributes

As a professional, an individual must be open to learning more and advancing a set of skills that demonstrate integrity and moral values, in other words, demonstrating an ethical behavior. These personal attributes include honesty, accountability, and competence. Professional attributes include competence, integrity, and competence as well as others. Although the attributes were discussed at length in Chapter 1, they are discussed again as they are tied to personal and professional ethics.

Professional ethics is defined as a set of rules that govern the conduct of a professional group. These ethics set the standards by which practitioners' actions can be regulated. Ethics and morals are often used interchangeably;

however, morals are generally a personal practice as an individual relates to the customs of their conscience.

Standards of Professional Ethics

Medical ethics is a set of principles set up to act as a guide for health care practitioners to make informed choices about the care that is given to patients. The behavior that each medical professional exhibits should be based on these ethical guidelines.

The Standard of Ethics for Radiography is made up of two parts: the Code of Ethics and the Rules of Ethics. The Code of Ethics was developed, revised, and adopted by the American Registry of Radiologic Technologists (ARRT) on September 1, 2021. It serves as a guide in maintaining ethical conduct in all aspects of the radiologic sciences. Considered to be mandatory and enforced by the ARRT, the Rules of Ethics are designed to ensure protection, safety, and comfort of the patient (Display 4-1).

DISPLAY 4-1

American Registry of Radiologic Technology Standards of Ethics

---

Last Revised: September 1, 2021
Published: September 1, 2021

Preamble

The *Standards of Ethics* of the ARRT shall apply solely to persons holding certificates from ARRT that are either currently certified and registered by ARRT or were formerly certified and registered by ARRT (collectively, "Certificate Holders"), and to persons applying for certification and registration by ARRT in order to become Certificate Holders ("Candidates"). Radiologic technology is an umbrella term that is inclusive of the disciplines of radiography, nuclear medicine technology, radiation therapy, cardiovascular interventional radiography, mammography, computed tomography, magnetic resonance imaging, quality management, sonography, bone densitometry, vascular sonography, cardiac interventional radiography, vascular interventional radiography, breast sonography, and radiologist assistant. The Standards of Ethics are intended to be consistent with the mission statement of ARRT, and to promote the goals set forth in the mission statement.

Statement of Purpose

The purpose of the ethics requirements is to identify individuals who have internalized a set of professional values that cause one to act in the best interests of patients. This internalization of professional values and the resulting behavior is one element of ARRT's definition of what it means to be qualified. Exhibiting certain behaviors as documented in the Standards of Ethics is evidence of the possible lack of appropriate professional values. The Standards of Ethics provide proactive guidance on what it means to be qualified and to motivate and promote a culture of ethical behavior within the profession. The ethics requirements support ARRT's mission of promoting high standards of patient care by removing or restricting the use of the credential by those who exhibit behavior inconsistent with the requirements.

a. **Code of Ethics**
   The **Code of Ethics** forms the first part of the *Standards of Ethics*. The Code of Ethics shall serve as a guide by which Certificate Holders and Candidates may evaluate their professional conduct as it relates to patients, health care consumers, employers, colleagues, and other members of the health care team. The Code of Ethics is intended to assist Certificate Holders and Candidates in maintaining a high level of ethical conduct and in ensuing the protection, safety, and comfort of patients. The Code of Ethics is aspirational.

   1. The radiologic technologist acts in a professional manner, responds to patient needs, and supports colleagues and associates in providing quality patient care.
   2. The radiologic technologist acts to advance the principal objective of the profession to provide services to humanity with full respect for the dignity of mankind.

DISPLAY 4-1

American Registry of Radiologic Technology Standards of Ethics (*continued*)

3. The radiologic technologist delivers patient care and service unrestricted by the concerns of personal attributes or the nature of the disease or illness, and without discrimination on the basis of race, color, creed, religion, national origin, sex, marital status, status with regard to public assistance, familial status, disability, sexual orientation, gender identity, veteran status, age, or any other legally protected basis.
4. The radiologic technologist practices technology founded upon theoretical knowledge and concepts, uses equipment and accessories consistent with the purposes for which they were designed, and employs procedures and techniques appropriately.
5. The radiologic technologist assesses situations; exercises care, discretion, and judgment; assumes responsibility for professional decisions; and acts in the best interest of the patient.
6. The radiologic technologist acts as an agent through observation and communication to obtain pertinent information for the physician to aid in the diagnosis and treatment of the patient and recognizes that interpretation and diagnosis are outside the scope of practice for the profession.
7. The radiologic technologist uses equipment and accessories, employs techniques and procedures, performs services in accordance with an accepted standard of practice, and demonstrates expertise in minimizing radiation exposure to the patient, self, and other members of the health care team.
8. The radiologic technologist practices ethical conduct appropriate to the profession and protects the patient's right to quality radiologic technology care.
9. The radiologic technologist respects confidences entrusted in the course of professional practice, respects the patient's right to privacy, and reveals confidential information only as required by law or to protect the welfare of the individual or the community.
10. The radiologic technologist continually strives to improve knowledge and skills by participating in continuing education and professional activities, sharing knowledge with colleagues, and investigating new aspects of professional practice.
11. The radiologic technologist refrains from the use of illegal drugs and/or any legally controlled substances that result in impairment of professional judgment and/or ability to practice radiologic technology with reasonable skill and safety to patients.

b. **Rules of Ethics**

The **Rules of Ethics** form the second part of the *Standards of Ethics*. They are mandatory standards of minimally acceptable professional conduct for all Certificate Holders and Candidates. Certification and registration are methods of assuring the medical community and the public that an individual is qualified to practice within the profession.

Because the public relies on certificates and registrations issued by the ARRT, it is essential that Certificate Holders and Candidates act consistently with these Rules of Ethics. These Rules of Ethics are intended to ensure protection, safety, and comfort of patients. The Rules of Ethics are enforceable. Radiologic technologists are required to notify ARRT of any ethics violation, including state licensing issues and criminal charges and convictions, within 30 days of the occurrence or during their annual renewal of certification and registration, whichever comes first. Applicants for certification and registration are required to notify ARRT of any ethics violation, including state licensing issues and criminal charges and convictions, within 30 days of the occurrence.

Certificate Holders and Candidates engaging in any of the following conduct or activities, or who permit the occurrence of the following conduct or activities with respect to them, have violated the Rules of Ethics and are subject to sanctions as described hereunder:

(continued)

American Registry of Radiologic Technology Standards of Ethics (*continued*)

The titles and headings are for convenience only, and shall not be used to limit, alter, or interpret the language of any rule.

1. Employing fraud or deceit in procuring or attempting to procure, maintain, renew, or obtain or reinstate certification and registration as issued by ARRT; employment in radiologic technology; or a state permit, license, or registration certificate to practice radiologic technology. This includes altering in any respect any document issued by ARRT or any state or federal agency, or by indicating in writing certification and registration with ARRT when that is not the case.

2. Engaging in false, fraudulent, deceptive, or misleading communications with any person regarding the individual's education, training, credentials, experience, or qualifications, or the status of the individual's state permit, license, or registration certificate in radiologic technology or certificate of registration with ARRT.

3. Knowingly engaging or assisting any person to engage in, or otherwise participating in, abusive or fraudulent billing practices, including violations of federal Medicare and Medicaid laws or state medical assistance laws.

4. Subverting or attempting to subvert ARRT's examination process, and/or the structured self-assessments that are part of the Continuing Qualifications Requirements (CQR) process. Conduct that subverts or attempts to subvert ARRT's examination and/or CQR assessment process includes, but is not limited to:
   i. disclosing examination and/or CQR assessment information using language that is substantially similar to that used in questions and/or answers from ARRT examinations and/or CQR assessments when such information is gained as a direct result of having been an examinee or a participant in a CQR assessment or having communicated with an examinee or a CQR participant; this includes, but is not limited to, disclosures to students in educational programs, graduates of educational programs, educators, anyone else involved in the preparation of Candidates to sit for the examinations, or CQR participants; and/or
   ii. soliciting and/or receiving examination and/or CQR assessment information that uses language that is substantially similar to that used in questions and/or answers on ARRT examinations or CQR assessments from an examinee, or a CQR participant, whether requested or not; and/or
   iii. copying, publishing, reconstructing (whether by memory or otherwise), reproducing or transmitting any portion of examination and/or CQR assessment materials by any means, verbal or written, electronic or mechanical, without the prior express written permission of ARRT or using professional, paid or repeat examination takers and/or CQR assessment participants, or any other individual for the purpose of reconstructing any portion of examination and/or CQR assessment materials; and/or
   iv. using or purporting to use any portion of examination and/or CQR assessment materials that were obtained improperly or without authorization for the purpose of instructing or preparing any Candidate for examination or participant for CQR assessment; and/or
   v. selling or offering to sell, buying or offering to buy, or distributing or offering to distribute any portion of examination and/or CQR assessment materials without authorization; and/or
   vi. removing or attempting to remove examination and/or CQR assessment materials from an examination or assessment room; and/or
   vii. having unauthorized possession of any portion of or information concerning a future, current, or previously administered examination or CQR assessment of ARRT; and/or

DISPLAY 4-1

American Registry of Radiologic Technology Standards of Ethics (*continued*)

viii. disclosing what purports to be, or what you claim to be, or under all circumstances is likely to be understood by the recipient as, any portion of or "inside" information concerning any portion of a future, current, or previously administered examination or CQR assessment of ARRT; and/or

ix. communicating with another individual during administration of the examination or CQR assessment for the purpose of giving or receiving help in answering examination or CQR assessment questions, copying another Candidate's, or CQR participant's answers, permitting another Candidate or a CQR participant to copy one's answers, or possessing unauthorized materials including, but not limited to, notes; and/or

x. impersonating a Candidate, or a CQR participant, or permitting an impersonator to take or attempt to take the examination or CQR assessment on one's own behalf; and/or

xi. using any other means that potentially alters the results of the examination or CQR assessment such that the results may not accurately represent the professional knowledge base of a Candidate, or a CQR participant.

5. Subverting, attempting to subvert, or aiding others to subvert or attempt to subvert ARRT's *Continuing Education (CE) Requirements*, and/or ARRT's CQR. Conduct that subverts or attempts to subvert ARRT's CE or CQR Requirements includes, but is not limited to:

    i. providing false, inaccurate, altered, or deceptive information related to CE or CQR activities to ARRT or an ARRT-recognized recordkeeper; and/or

    ii. assisting others to provide false, inaccurate, altered, or deceptive information related to CE or CQR activities to ARRT or an ARRT-recognized recordkeeper; and/or

    iii. conduct that results or could result in a false or deceptive report of CE or CQR completion; and/or

    iv. conduct that in any way compromises the integrity of the CE or CQR requirements such as sharing answers to the posttests or self-learning activities, providing or using false certificates of participation, or verifying credits that were not earned.

6. Subverting or attempting to subvert ARRT's certification and registration processes by:

    i. making a false statement or knowingly providing false information to ARRT; or

    ii. failing to cooperate with any investigation by ARRT.

7. Engaging in unprofessional conduct, including, but not limited to:

    i. a departure from or failure to conform to applicable federal, state, or local governmental rules regarding radiologic technology practice or scope of practice; or, if no such rule exists, to the minimal standards of acceptable and prevailing radiologic technology practice;

    ii. any radiologic technology practice that may create unnecessary danger to a patient's life, health, or safety.

8. Engaging in conduct with a patient that is sexual or may reasonably be interpreted by the patient as sexual, or in any verbal behavior that is seductive or sexually demeaning to a patient; or engaging in sexual exploitation of a patient or former patient. This also applies to any unwanted sexual behavior, verbal or otherwise.

9. Engaging in any unethical conduct, including, but not limited to, conduct likely to deceive, defraud, or harm the public; or demonstrating a willful or careless disregard for the health, welfare, or safety of a patient. Actual injury need not be established under this clause.

10. Performing procedures that the individual is not competent to perform through appropriate training and/or education or experience unless assisted or personally supervised by someone who is competent (through training and/or education or experience).

(continued)

DISPLAY 4-1

American Registry of Radiologic Technology Standards of Ethics (*continued*)

11. Knowingly assisting, advising, or allowing a person without a current and appropriate state permit, license, registration, or an ARRT registered certificate to engage in the practice of radiologic technology, in a jurisdiction that mandates such requirements.

12. Delegating or accepting the delegation of a radiologic technology function or any other prescribed health care function when the delegation or acceptance could reasonably be expected to create an unnecessary danger to a patient's life, health, or safety. Actual injury to a patient need not be established under this clause.

13. Actual or potential inability to practice radiologic technology with reasonable skill and safety to patients by reason of illness; use of alcohol, drugs, chemicals, or any other material; or as a result of any mental or physical condition.

14. Adjudication as mentally incompetent, mentally ill, chemically dependent, or dangerous to the public, by a court of competent jurisdiction.

15. Improper management of patient records, including failure to maintain adequate patient records or to furnish a patient record or report required by law; or making, causing, or permitting anyone to make false, deceptive, or misleading entry in any patient record.

16. Revealing privileged communication from or relating to a former or current patient, except when otherwise required or permitted by law, or viewing, using, releasing, or otherwise failing to adequately protect the security or privacy of confidential patient information.

17. Knowingly providing false or misleading information that is directly related to the care of a former or current patient.

18. Violating a state or federal narcotics or controlled substance law, even if not charged or convicted of a violation of law.

19. Violating a rule adopted by a state or federal regulatory authority or certification board resulting in the individual's professional license, permit, registration, or certification being denied, revoked, suspended, placed on probation or a consent agreement or order, voluntarily surrendered, subjected to any conditions, or failing to report to ARRT any of the violations or actions identified in this rule.

20. Convictions, criminal proceedings, or military courts-martial:
    i. conviction of a crime, including a felony, a gross misdemeanor, or a misdemeanor, with the sole exception of speeding and parking violations. All alcohol- and/or drug-related violations must be reported; and/or
    ii. criminal proceeding where a finding or verdict of guilt is made or returned but the adjudication of guilt is withheld, deferred, or not entered or the sentence is suspended or stayed; or a criminal proceeding where the individual enters an Alford plea, a plea of guilty, or nolo contendere (no contest); or where the individual enters into a pretrial diversion activity; or
    iii. military courts-martial related to any offense identified in these Rules of Ethics.

21. Knowing of a violation or a probable violation of any Rule of Ethics by any Certificate Holder or Candidate and failing to promptly report in writing the same to ARRT.

22. Failing to immediately report to the Certificate Holder's or Candidate's supervisor information concerning an error made in connection with imaging, treating, or caring for a patient. For purposes of this rule, errors include any departure from the standard of care that reasonably may be considered to be potentially harmful, unethical, or improper (commission). Errors also include behavior that is negligent or should have occurred in connection with a patient's care, but did not (omission). The duty to report under this rule exists whether or not the patient suffered any injury.

Radiographers often find themselves in situations that present an ethical and legal issue. By following the *Scope of Practice* that is incorporated within the Practice Standards, and the Standards of Ethics, radiographers are less likely to choose an inappropriate course of action.

Reviewing these standards allows the student radiographer to reflect on possible issues that could arise and become a legal situation. Remembering the Code of Ethics may help one to always work inside the boundaries of the law. The two are closely tied together.

PATIENT RIGHTS

The radiographer has a legal responsibility to relate to colleagues, other members of the health care team, and the patient in a manner that is respectful of each person with whom interaction occurs and to adhere to *The Patient Care Partnership.* An abbreviated version of the actual bill can be found in Display 4-2. This bill, which replaced the Patient's Bill of Rights in 2003, delineates the rights of the patient as a consumer of health care. Because all health care workers are required to adhere to the provisions of this bill, they must be familiar with them. The radiographer must also be aware of the areas of practice in which health care workers may infringe upon the patient's rights and be held legally liable. Some examples follow:

- Acting in the role of a diagnostician and providing a patient with results, impressions, or diagnoses of **diagnostic imaging** examinations

- Failing to obtain appropriate consent from women of childbearing age before performing a diagnostic imaging procedure
- Failing to obtain a complete history from a patient before administering an iodinated contrast agent
- Failing to correctly identify a patient before performing an examination
- Failing to explain a diagnostic imaging procedure to a patient before the examination
- Failing to document technical factors used to facilitate dose calculations for a procedure
- Failing to maintain a patient's physical privacy during an examination
- Failing to maintain the highest quality of images with the lowest possible radiation dose for the patient

The radiographer must never assume the role of other medical personnel in the department. It is not within the scope of practice to read radiographic images or other diagnostic tests or to impart the results of these to the patient or the patient's family. This constitutes medical diagnosis and is the radiologist or physician's responsibility. If a patient is injured in the diagnostic imaging department in any manner, the radiographer must not dismiss the patient from the department until the patient has been examined by a physician and deemed safe for discharge.

Hospitals and clinics in which the radiography student may train may have a variation of this patient care statement, but all patients receive some type of assurance that the facility adheres to these standards.

CASE STUDY

Mary Ann is a 49-year-old outpatient woman who has an order for a routine chest radiograph. Donna, RT, is assigned to the dedicated chest room. Donna proceeds to call the patient back to the imaging room. During the introduction and patient identification phase, she recognizes Donna as a regular customer at the bank. Donna continues with the patient assessment, obtains the history, and is interrupted by Mary Ann. She politely asks Donna to let her know if there is still a spot on her right upper lung.

ISSUES TO CONSIDER

1. Could this be considered a violation of Health Insurance Portability and Accountability Act (HIPAA)?
2. How could this easily become an ethical violation?
3. How can Donna respond to Mary Ann and still remain professional?

DISPLAY 4-2

The Patient Care Partnership

The sections further explain some of the basics about how you can expect to be treated during your hospital stay. They also cover what we need from you to care for you better. If you have questions, please ask them. Your comfort and confidence in your care are important to us.

What to Expect During Your Hospital Stay:
- High-quality hospital care
- A clean and safe environment
- Involvement in your care to understand:
  - The benefit and risk involved
  - If your treatment is experimental or part of a research study
  - What you need to do after you leave the hospital
  - The financial consequences of using uncovered services or out-of-network providers
- Protection of your privacy
- Preparing you and your family for when you leave the hospital
- Help with your bill and filing insurance claims

Patient Responsibilities

Just as the radiographer has to abide by *The Patient Care Partnership*, the patient has responsibilities when presenting for health care. These responsibilities are as follows:

1. The patient has the responsibility to provide, as best as able, an accurate and complete health history.
2. The patient is responsible for keeping appointments and for notifying the responsible practitioner or the hospital when unable to do so for any reason.
3. The patient is responsible for all actions when refusing treatment or not following the practitioner's instructions.
4. The patient is responsible for fulfilling the financial obligations of any health care as promptly as possible.
5. The patient is responsible for following hospital rules and regulations, affecting patient care and conduct.
6. The patient is responsible for being considerate of the rights and property of others.

Not all patients may be able to follow these responsibilities and it is incumbent upon the radiographer to remain professional and ethical when encountering instances when the patient may not follow these conditions.

SYSTEMATIC ANALYSIS

Dealing with ethical challenges in an appropriate way is important for several reasons. One must assume that paying attention to ethical challenges involves paying attention to defining and improving the quality of patient care. Not paying attention to ethical challenges can be detrimental to patients, relatives, and health care professionals. It might challenge the patient's cooperation and diminish the quality of the decision-making processes. In order to avoid this, a systematic analysis of ethical problems must be undertaken. Although the process may seem lengthy, an analysis can be done in a few minutes.

When making an ethical decision, gather any facts of the situation and define the ethical issues that are involved. Next, determine the consequences of the actions that can be taken. If action A is put into place, what will happen? But, if action B is put into place, what will happen? Once the consequences are considered, professional obligations must be considered. Review the ethical principles list provided earlier to guide the decision-making process. Once the proper ethical action is decided on, the radiographer must be prepared to deal with the consequences of those actions; however, if this systematic approach is used, the best course of action is chosen.

Ethical Violations and Sanctions

Each person faced with an ethical dilemma and choosing a path has to be aware of the consequences of that action and be prepared to accept those consequences. The ARRT examination handbook (revised in 2022) and application requires each student to comply with the ARRT Standards of Ethics, including the Rules of

Ethics. All violations must be reported within 30 days its occurrence. The new handbook states:

> In addition, you must report applicants or R.T.s who don't comply. Applicants who don't follow these rules might become ineligible for certification and registration with ARRT. R.T.s who don't follow these rules might receive sanctions up to and including revocation of their ARRT credentials. (This is also stated as number 22 in the Rules of Ethics.)

The ARRT investigates every ethics infraction and decides if an ethical violation has occurred and if sanctions such as revocation are warranted. In 2020, only 1% of all investigations resulted in revocation. It is best to be up front with all situations and have the ARRT Ethics Committee review any issues.

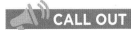

CALL OUT

It is strongly suggested that all radiography students download the *ARRT Primary Eligibility Pathway Handbook* and review it completely as soon as entering the program. Early application may keep the student on track for taking the examination on time.

As the scope of practice and professional responsibilities of radiologic technology grow, so do the ethical responsibilities of radiographers. Often with health care, an ethical decision involves a choice between two unsatisfactory solutions to a problem. If one conscientiously follows the professional code of ethics and ethical principles previously listed to make difficult decisions as they arise, one is able to resolve ethical dilemmas in a manner that allows knowing that the best solution was chosen.

ETHICAL DILEMMAS

All radiographers are expected to conduct themselves in a professional and ethical manner. They must be reliable and to report for work on time and complete the assigned share of the workload in a timely, competent, sensitive, and efficient manner. The radiographer is also expected to work as a cooperative member of the health care team. Speech must be articulate and free of vulgar expressions or inappropriate slang. All patients must be treated as persons of dignity and worth in a nondiscriminatory manner.

Individual and Societal Rights

Human rights (individual and society) are meant to guide the actions of the government. Ethics in health care broadly encompasses concerns for the actions of individuals and organizations. Human rights apply everywhere to everyone, regardless of country, culture, or status. There are five guiding principles (ethics) of human rights. They are:

- Universality of human rights applies to every member of the human race.
- Equality for the human race. Discrimination is a violation of human rights.
- Participation in the processes and decisions affecting one's own well-being and life
- Interdependence so that rights are interrelated. If one right is violated, another is also.
- Rule of law is the enforcement of all human rights.

In 2019, the world began a fight against coronavirus-19. This virus mutated several times, into the Delta and then the Omicron viruses. It was proven that the best way to prevent the spread of this virus was to maintain distance from other individuals and to wear a mask at all times. Eventually, a vaccine was developed that required two doses plus booster. However, many individuals believed that the vaccine contained products that would alter one's DNA or allow the government to track a person's location. Many other thoughts surrounded this vaccine, causing many individuals to refuse to take it. As the pandemic continued into a third year, many individuals began to rebel against wearing a mask. The federal government tried to enforce the use of masks and vaccine law, but many state governments fought against it, stating that individuals had the right over their own body to not take the vaccine or to not wear a mask if they desired. This is the epitome of individual and societal rights pushing up against the ethical issue of doing what is right to protect other members of society who have different views regarding the situation.

Cultural and Economic Considerations

One type of ethical behavior does not fit all individuals. Understanding of diversity and needs in other cultures may affect ethical decisions based on awareness of those needs. Chapter 7 explains culture diversity in detail, but for this limited scope of discussion, it must be made clear that individuals who may not believe in Western medicine or have religious beliefs that does not allow touching of the body must be treated with respect. Remember the first human right: that of universality. Respect the wishes of the patient, but every effort must be made to help the patient understand what is being done and the implications of refusing.

A patient's economic situation should not be a consideration in health care. However, that is often not the case. Pay for profit facilities and those that do not accept Medicaid or welfare often cause the patients without the ability to pay or be insured by an accepted agency to not be able to receive the care that is needed. This presents an ethical dilemma in that health care workers are to "do no harm." If a patient is denied treatment in a medical facility because that person is unable to pay, might that patient be harmed at some point?

Technology and Scarce Resources

Technologic changes have considerably affected health care practices. With these changes, ethical considerations must be made not only on the application of technology, but it should also focus on the problems and moral implications of this technology.

Addressing the pandemic once again, personal protective apparel was in extremely short supply in many health care facilities. The production of N95 masks could not keep up with the demand for them worldwide. Frontline health care workers were working around the clock to care for those individuals that became ill. Intensive care unit (ICU) beds and ventilators became a rare commodity, with some facilities erecting tents in the parking lots to house those patients that could not be accommodated in-house. The ethical dilemma here becomes, who should get the remaining hospital bed, the 5-year-old child that has appendicitis or the unvaccinated patient with COVID-19?

Access to Quality Health Care

Many people in the United States don't get the health care services they need. About 1 in 10 don't have health insurance, making them less likely to have a primary doctor. Chances are they are not able to afford the health care services and medication they need. Health disparities (health inequities) have received more attention from federal health agencies, physicians, and others since 2012. The American Hospital Association developed Path Forward in 2018 with a commitment for access to affordable health care. Despite this, people are unable to get the same quality of health care, especially in regions that are socially and economically disadvantaged.

Human Experimentation and Research

Bioethics discusses the ethics behind human research in areas such as stem cell. Human experimentation and research are performed to collect data and then analyze it to draw conclusions that may affect medicine in the future. Ethical principles that come into play when using humans in research are beneficence, nonmaleficence, fidelity, and trust. Others include dignity, autonomy, voluntary participation, and privacy. In 1981, the Department of Health and Human Services published regulations concerning the way in which biomedical research was to be performed. Some of the requirements are listed here.

- Minimal risk to the patient
- Equitable selection of participants
- Informed consent required and documented

These regulations help provide guidance to the ethical issues that arise.

Ethical Conduct of Research

Ethical considerations in research are a set of principles that guide the research design practices. The Patient Care Partnership assures the patient that research is not performed on the patient without the patient's knowledge and consent. When performing research on patients, ethical considerations must include protecting the right of the patient. The research must be voluntary and the patient must be informed. No research should be undertaken if it violates patient's rights.

Before beginning any research, the proposal must be submitted to an institutional review board where the design of the research is examined for ethical conduct. Once the board approves the design, data can be collected. As data are collected, the patient must remain anonymous. If the researcher knows the identity of a participant, it must be kept confidential when reporting the data.

Ethics Committee

For ethical dilemmas of some magnitude, most health care institutions have ethics committees that meet on a regular basis to solve problems and formulate policies that provide guidelines to facilitate decision-making. If an ethical dilemma is encountered in the workplace that cannot be readily resolved by following one's professional code of ethics, a person is obliged to present the problem to such a body.

A hospital ethics committee is comprised of individuals that have experience in ethical issues that may arise in a medical setting. Members of the committee come from various disciplines in the health care setting. People such as nurses, chaplains, physicians, social workers, and lawyers bring a different perspective to serve the patient in the best possible manner. The team should be diverse in terms of culture and skills as well as experience and knowledge. This team offers recommendations to the health care team, the patient, or the family to help make decisions in regard to care of the patients.

Structural Racism

Structural racism refers to disadvantages within society. It shapes and affects the lives of those individuals that fall into categories associated with structural racism. It exists in the social, economic, educational, and political systems in society. Racism is a form of structural inequity. The pandemic that began in 2019 escalated inequities. As an example, poverty rates are higher for African Americans and Pakistani groups because of being laid off with the closure of many businesses. People of color have higher death rates from the COVID-19 virus than others.

Social Justice

Social justice refers to the equal distribution of wealth, opportunities, and privileges within a society. It is fairness in health care, employment, housing, and more. It applies to all aspects of society including race and gender. Human rights and social justice are closely related. An example of social justice deals with health care. Everyone deserves equal rights and opportunities to good health. People of color are often unable to afford insurance, and therefore, they do not have access to care and other health resources. When they do find a source of care, they are often sicker and their costs are higher. All health care professionals must be aware of structural racism and social inequities and treat all patients and people with respect and dignity.

End-of-Life

Because advances in modern medical technology have prolonged life expectancies, end-of-life care has become increasingly difficult in terms of ethical considerations. Ethically speaking, the patient should make decisions regarding their end-of-life issues in consultation with the physician. However, if the patient is unable to make these decisions, it falls to family members who may be feeling sadness, fear, or anxiety. This could make it hard to make decisions that are most appropriate for the patient. Different family members may have different perspectives regarding decisions. Some may want everything that can be done to prolong life, whereas others may want to limit treatment and keep the patient as comfortable as possible. As explained in Chapter 2, advanced health care directives made by the patient let all individuals involved know the wishes of the ill patient, thus avoiding ethical dilemmas.

ETHICAL DILEMMAS IN MEDICAL IMAGING

With the advent of digital imaging, radiography has entered a new era of ethical dilemmas that were not an issue in the past. Prior to computerized images, the radiograph was produced and was either diagnostically acceptable or it had to be repeated. Technology has now allowed the radiographer to manipulate controls that may present unethical behavior on the part of the technologist.

Image Cropping or Masking

One of the most often used image manipulation tools is the cropping tool. Much like using the edit application on a cellular phone, unwanted anatomy can be "cropped" off of the image so that only the required anatomy is visible. Masking is another way to rid the image of anatomy that is not necessary for a diagnosis but in this instance, the anatomy is simply blackened out, and the image size remains the same. In either case, the patient was exposed to radiation to parts of the body that was not necessary to be irradiated. The ethical choice is to collimate so that the patient does not receive radiation to that part of the body at all. It is unethical to crop or mask off anatomy that should not be on the image. It is a myth that it is not possible to collimate with digital imaging. Not collimating causes a histogram analysis error.

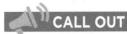 **CALL OUT**

Collimation is not the same as cropping with the postprocessing manipulation of digital equipment. Anything that is done after the exposure has not reduced the amount of radiation that the patient originally received. Collimate—do not crop!

Electronic Annotations

Annotating an image to add anatomic markers to indicate the patient's right or left side is not reliable in a court of law. Utilizing lead markers placed on the image receptor by the technologist at the time of the exposure is the only legally binding documentation of indicating anatomic sides. Other annotations that can be made on the image include supine, upright, inspiration, and expiration. Although annotating an image after exposure may seem preferable so as not to place a lead marker in an anatomic area of interest, malpractice cases have shown that the preferred method of identification on an image is with the lead markers placed before exposure.

Manipulation of Data

Another behavior that has been made possible with digital imaging is the manipulation of electronic data such as exposure indicators, processing algorithms, brightness, and contrast. It is possible to change the processing algorithm in order to "reprocess" the image under another anatomic part. For example, a pelvis image is underexposed. If the image is "reprocessed" under a lateral lumbar spine algorithm, the image has different numbers assigned to the radiation exposure to make it appear darker. It is also possible to then manipulate the brightness and contrast of the image to enhance the image. If the image is not diagnostically acceptable, one could say it has to be repeated. Others would argue that the patient is then receiving an additional dose of radiation. With digital imaging, the amount of radiation is much lower than with previous imaging techniques. The solution is not as clear-cut as the cropping of anatomy is. Is the extra amount of radiation worth seeing images that have not been manipulated that may or may not obscure pathology?

ALARA

The main premise of radiation protection for the patient has always been that radiation dose be kept As Low As Reasonably Achievable (ALARA). Digital imaging uses flat panel detectors that are extremely sensitive to radiation so that less radiation can be used and not compromise image quality. Ethical questions arise from the use of digital equipment, however, in the form of "dose creep." This is the gradual acceptance over time by radiographers to use higher exposure factors (and thus higher exposure to the patient) and then manipulate the exposure indicators to change the image to make it acceptable. Of course, this is not in keeping with ALARA. There needs to be an understanding of the relationship of exposure factors and image appearance to stop the practice of dose creep, which is an unethical practice of overexposure to the patient.

LEGAL ISSUES

Although ethics refers to a set of moral principles, law refers to rules of conduct as prescribed by an authority or group of legislators. Law can be defined as a "binding custom or practice of a community; a rule of conduct or action prescribed or formally recognized as binding or enforced by a controlling authority" (*Merriam-Webster*).

Many types of laws affect people in daily life; however, **statutory law** and **common law** are the most significant for the radiographer in professional practice. Statutory laws are derived from legislative enactments. Common law usually results from judicial decisions.

Two major classifications of the law are criminal law and civil law. An offense is regarded as criminal behavior and in the realm of criminal law if it is an offense against society or a member of society. If the accused party is found guilty, the person is punished.

Criminal law protects the entire community against certain acts. An example of this would be a terrorist bombing that results in the destruction of public property and the death of one or more persons. The crime is a crime against society and is a felony.

A misdemeanor is a crime of a less serious nature punishable by a fine or imprisonment for less than 1 year. In some instances, driving under the influence of drugs or alcohol may be a misdemeanor provided that no accident or injury has resulted.

Civil law has been broken if another person's private legal rights have been violated. The person who is found guilty of this type of offense is usually expected to pay a sum of money to repair the damage done. An example of a violation of civil law might be a suit by an individual against a physician for a misdiagnosis that results in injury. This injury is to one person and not to the entire society.

Tort law exists to protect the violator of a law from being sued for an act of vengeance, to determine fault, and to compensate the injured party. A tort involves personal injury or damage, resulting in civil action or litigation to obtain reparation for damages incurred. It is usually in this form of the law that a radiographer is found legally liable.

A tort may be committed intentionally or unintentionally. An intentional tort is a purposeful deed committed with the intention of producing the consequences of the deed. **Defaming** a colleague's character is an example of intentional tort. Other forms of intentional torts include assault and battery. Assault and battery are often linked together, meaning that a threat of harm existed before the actual contact; however, assault may be charged without any physical contact if the patient fears that this will occur. Battery may be charged by a patient to whom the radiographer has administered treatment against the patient's will. Other examples of intentional tort include the following:

- **Immobilizing** patients against their will (false imprisonment)
- Falsely stating that a patient has a socially unacceptable disease (defamation of character)
- Posting on social media about an interesting patient (violation of HIPAA)

An unintentional tort may be committed when a radiographer is negligent in the performance of patient care and the patient is injured as a result. The following are examples of unintentional torts:

- Improperly marking radiographic images, such as incorrectly labeling the side of the patient during a particular study for right and left, which could result in the surgeon removing the healthy kidney, leaving the diseased kidney
- Omitting to apply gonadal shielding on a female patient with a femur fracture who is subsequently discovered to be pregnant
- Improperly positioning a trauma patient for tibia and fibula projections so that the projections do not adequately demonstrate the entire lower leg, resulting in a fracture being "missed" by the orthopedic physician and the radiologists
- Handing the radiologist the incorrect syringe during a procedure, which results in the injection of Xylocaine (lidocaine) instead of the contrast media
- Leaving an unconscious patient on a gurney while the radiographer leaves the room, thus allowing the patient to jar the side rails and fall off the gurney because the safety belt was not secure
- Improperly positioning a footboard on an x-ray table that results in the patient sliding off the table when the table is placed in the upright position during an examination

• Not providing parents of pediatric patients with the proper protective attire when they are aiding in immobilizing their child, especially during fluoroscopic procedures

There are possibilities where a true "mistake" was made but the mistake can be proved to be an "intentional" tort. It is normal practice to call a patient from the waiting room to the imaging department by the first name. It is incumbent upon the radiographer to successfully prove the identity of the patient by asking for the last name and the date of birth. Failure to do so may result in the radiographer exposing the wrong patient to radiation. In legal discovery, it could be determined that the radiographer sincerely and honestly "forgot" to confirm the identity of the patient; however, in a court of law, this could be construed as an intentional act.

Radiographers are named in lawsuits now more than ever as the required education elevated the career to a profession. Radiographers most often have suits brought against them in cases of patient falls. Although the institution where the accident occurs (the employer) may be found **liable** for the actions of the radiographer (employee) under the principle of *respondeat superior* (let the master answer), technologists are responsible for their actions if named in a lawsuit. Another term that should be familiar to the radiographer is *res ipsa loquitur*, which is Latin for "the thing speaks for itself." This is a doctrine in the common law of torts that infers negligence from the nature of an accident or injury in the absence of direct evidence on how any defendant behaved.

Ethical and legal issues are frequently combined in the practice of imaging. The radiographer must be aware of this and take precautions to prevent situations that may lead to problems of this nature. Discrimination and **bias** shown toward a particular person constitute an example of this. It is unlawful to discriminate against any patient or coworker on the basis of race, color, creed, national origin, ancestry, gender, marital status, disability, religious affiliation, political affiliation, age, spoken language, or sexual orientation. Health care must be practiced in a totally nonjudgmental manner. No decisions must be made or any action taken on the basis of these issues.

LEGAL DOCTRINES AND STANDARDS

Legal Risk Reduction and Management

Managing risk in health care is evidenced in areas such as surgical cases. A "time out" is taken before the beginning of the surgery. This is when the patient is identified, the procedure that is being done is verified, and everyone present is aware of their roles in the procedure. This verification greatly reduces the potential risks of making mistakes during the procedure. The same should hold true in imaging, particularly in interventional radiography and computed tomography (CT). A quick time out to validate the patient, the procedure being done, the competence of the people performing the procedure, and, if appropriate, the documentation of consents can help individuals stay focused on the performance of the task at hand.

Risk management is everyone's job in the medical facility. Like risk reduction, managing the types of risks that can happen before they happen is pivotal in keeping everyone safe in health care. Annual training and evaluations are performed in all departments to ensure that employees know where the fire alarms are, or how to report a frayed cord on a mobile x-ray unit. Making every employee aware of the potential risks involved in the medical facility may prevent an injury from occurring.

Documentation in Health Records

Effective documentation is paramount in all areas of the health care profession. Students must not think that clerical work is beneath the profession of a radiographer or that it is not as important as other aspects of their duties.

In today's health care systems, computers are used for all functions within the imaging department. There are multiple computers placed in locations that make it easy for staff to check or document information about a patient. Patient records on computers may be called an e-chart (electronic) and holds information about the patient that is guarded by HIPAA. This makes using the computers in locations throughout the department a potential hazard if the chart is not closed and the technologist does not log off the computer when finished.

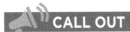 **CALL OUT**

To prevent possible unauthorized access to confidential information, all patient records must be closed and the technologist should log off the computer with each use.

Many imaging departments have their own form of documentation called a *radiology information management system* (RIMS). In some cases, the RIMS allows the technologist to access only specific information about the patient such as diagnostic imaging studies that have been performed in the past. Only managers and supervisors of the department may have authorization to access the patient's full chart, which provides appropriate confidentiality assurance. Other facilities allow full access to all staff. No matter what format a facility uses, an electronic log is kept each time a technologist logs into a computer and the length of time that a person has the patient's chart open. In the event something questionable occurs, there is documentation that can assist the facility and department in any legal matters that might arise.

Documenting information about the care the patient received while in the imaging department falls to the radiographer that provided that care, for example, administration of contrast media, medications given, and all treatment that may have been given to a patient while in the department. Consent forms and allergic history forms must be scanned into the e-chart. Documentation such as an incident report and all care that was given to the patient must be done as soon as it is safe to do so. Documentation may very well be the downfall or the supporting beam of a legal case. A phrase to remember is "if it isn't documented, it didn't happen." If the radiographer provided all the basics and more in the care of a patient that fell, but didn't document it, that care cannot be proved and, therefore, in the eyes of the law, did not occur.

All radiographic images are part of the patient's medical record and as such belong to the institution where they were taken. Because all images are covered under HIPAA, patients must sign a request to have their images sent to outside facilities. It is recommended that if the images cannot be transmitted virtually, then a CD be sent directly to the provider listed on the request.

Incident or Unusual Occurrence Reports

An injury to a patient or any error made by personnel in the **diagnostic imaging** department must be documented in an *incident report* as soon as it is safe to do so. By recording details immediately, the accuracy of the report is improved. The document may also be called an *unusual occurrence report* or an *accident notification report* (Display 4-3). An injury may seem slight and not worthy of such a report, but all injuries—whether to patients, visitors, students, or staff, or accidents involving

---

DISPLAY 4-3

Incident or Unusual Occurrence Reports—Sample Form

This is a confidential report.

Section 1

Name of the individual reporting the incident: _____

Institution where the incident occurred: _____

Date of incident: _____ Time of incident: _____ a.m. _____ p.m. _____

Exact location of incident: _____

Section 2

Incident occurred to: _____

❏ Staff ❏ Student   ❏ Patient-ID# _____   ❏ Equipment

Other. Explain: _____

_____

If staff, student, or patient is checked, see Sections 3 and 5.

If equipment is checked, see Sections 4 and 5.

Section 3

Occurrence: _____ Type of incident: _____

❏ Back injury from lifting patients   ❏ Reaction to foreign substances

❏ Miscellaneous back injury   ❏ Contagious disease

❏ Injury from a patient   ❏ Laceration

❏ Needlestick   ❏ Contusion

❏ Unsafe/defective equipment   ❏ Burn

❏ Improper use of equipment   ❏ Fracture

Incident or Unusual Occurrence Reports—Sample Form (*continued*)

❏ Patient contact   ❏ Sprain/strain
❏ Fall (attended)   ❏ Puncture
❏ Fall (unattended)   ❏ Other
❏ Fire
❏ Other
Did the injury require treatment by a physician?
Was the incident reported to the appropriate personnel?

Section 4
Type of equipment damaged: _____
How was equipment damaged: _____
Result of damage (e.g., equipment downtime for repair): _____

Section 5
Briefly describe the incident factually (what happened): _____
_____
_____

Name(s) of person(s) notified: _____
Name(s) of witness(es): _____
I certify that the above information is correct: _____/Title: _____
Home address: _____ Date of birth: _____ Telephone: _____
Signature of person filling out the form: _____ Date: _____
Witness Signature: _____ Date: _____

---

equipment regardless of severity—must be reported according to the department procedure. An error in medication administration, imaging the wrong patient, performing the wrong procedure, a patient falling, or any error in treatment or significant change in patient status must be documented in an incident report. The primary purpose is to uncover the circumstances and conditions that led to the event in order to prevent future incidents.

Every report should contain a minimum of the following:

- Type of incident (injury, property damage, theft)
- Location of incident
- Date and time of incident
- Name of the affected individual
- Narrative description of the incident, including the sequence of events and results of the incident
- Injuries and treatment required, if any

- Witness name(s) and statement(s)
- Other individuals involved

Many facilities have electronic report forms that can be attached to the patient's medical records, if that is the case. Regardless of how the form is presented, remember to state the facts and do not use phrases like "I believe" or "I feel that." State only facts that were seen and don't give opinions. Any patient injured in the imaging department must be examined by a physician before being allowed to leave the department. Injured health care workers or visitors must be examined according to the facility's policy. Because falls are the most common form of tort action in the imaging department, it cannot be stressed enough that documentation through the proper forms is warranted. Many times situations lead to litigation not because something was done incorrectly, but because there was no documentation that anything was done at all.

PATIENT CONSENT

There are procedures performed in diagnostic imaging departments that require special consent forms to be signed by the patient or, in the case of minor children or other special cases, by parents or legal representatives. The radiographer must be familiar with the procedures that require consent forms and not confuse these with the blanket consent forms, which are often signed when the patient enters the hospital, as these may not be valid for radiography procedures.

A consent is a contract wherein the patient voluntarily gives permission to someone (in this case, the imaging staff) to perform a procedure or service. The legal aspect of obtaining consent deals with the imaging staff's "duty to warn" and the ethic "do no harm." The medical aspect of consent hopes to establish rapport with the patient through communication to secure a successful outcome.

There are different levels of consents:

1. *Simple consent* is a matter of obtaining a patient's permission to perform a procedure without knowledge of that procedure. Simple consent is divided into express and implied consent.

    a. *Implied* consent is a form of consent that is inferred by the patient's actions or, in the case of an unconscious patient, would be given if the patient were able to do so. Implied may also be known as *implicit, deemed,* or *indirect* consent. An example would be a patient who has just had a heart attack and is unconscious. The emergency department gives medical treatment on the basis of implied consent assuming that the patient would, in fact, give consent for treatment to save their life.

    b. *Expressed* consent is clearly stated, although it does not have to be written. This may prove to be problematic if the patient denies that consent was given. Another type of expressed consent occurs when the patient does not stop the person from doing the study. An example would be a radiographer telling the patient that a chest x-ray is going to be taken and the patient does not stop the radiographer from doing it. Expressed consent is also known as *explicit* consent.

2. *Informed* consent is obtained after the patient has a clear understanding of what is being consented to, including the implications and future consequences. Informed consent is always in writing and is only legal if the patient is coherent, understands the language that the information was given in, and is of age to make decisions. Many informed consent forms require a witness to the signature of the patient. This type of consent is required for invasive radiographic procedures, procedures that require sedation or anesthesia, or any exam that may carry risk to the patient.

3. There is another type of consent that is known as *inadequate,* or *ignorant,* consent. This occurs when the patient has not been informed adequately to make a responsible decision. The patient can bring charges of negligence (an unintentional tort) when there has been an inadequate consent, particularly if the patient sustains injury (when consent is not obtained, battery may be charged).

Consent is not legal if the patient is not informed of all aspects of the procedure to be performed. These include the potential risks, benefits, and suggested alternatives. The patient must also be informed of the consequences if the suggested procedure is not completed. Because a patient usually consents or refuses a procedure on the basis of the information that the health care professional provides, the duty of obtaining the informed consent involves the patient's physician or radiologist and the radiographer.

Although special consent forms may be signed before the patient comes to the diagnostic imaging department, it is the duty of the radiographer to recheck the patient's medical records to be certain that this has been accomplished. The radiographer must also make sure that the patient understands what is going to be done and the essential nature of the choices available. If the patient, parent, or legal representative denies knowledge of the procedure or withdraws consent, the radiologist and/or the patient's physician should be notified of this. The procedure should be postponed until the matter is satisfactorily resolved. It is not the radiographer's responsibility to determine whether a procedure should be terminated. It is the radiographer's responsibility to bring the problem to the physician or supervisor in charge for resolution.

Obtaining informed consent helps to protect the health care worker from legal action. The radiographer must also understand that communicating effectively with the patient is essential to alleviate any anxiety as well as to improve outcomes from all procedures. Display 4-4 lists the criteria for valid informed consent.

Patients that have signed a consent form have the right to revoke that consent before the procedure takes place. However, it is incumbent upon the radiographer to alert the radiologist and the physician in charge of the patient of the patient's intent. Also, the patient must be made aware of the consequences of not having the x-ray or the procedure. The patient not only makes an informed consent but also an informed revocation of that consent.

DISPLAY 4-4

Types of Consent

Voluntary Consent

Valid consent must be freely given, without coercion.

Incompetent Patient

Legal definition: a patient who is unable to take a decision for themselves in relation to medical treatment because of an impairment of, or a disturbance in the functioning of, the mind or brain.

Informed Subject

Informed consent should be in writing. It should contain the following:

Explanation of the procedure and its risks

Description of benefits and alternatives

An offer to answer questions about the procedure

Instructions that the patient may withdraw consent

A statement informing the patient if the protocol differs from customary procedure

Patient Able to Comprehend

Information must be written and delivered in language understandable to the patient. Questions must be answered to facilitate comprehension if material is confusing.

CASE STUDY

During another busy afternoon at a community hospital in California, the emergency department was close to going on "Code Black" (a state of saturation where every bed and hallway gurney is full and patients are waiting for care without adequate resources to attend to them). A young, Spanish-speaking woman was being seen for low back pain. Because of the seriousness of other cases in the emergency department, the attending physician was unable to see the patient and the nurse sent the patient over to radiology for lumbar spine radiographs.

Upon arrival in the imaging department, the technologist correctly identified the patient, introduced herself, and explained that she was going to take x-rays of the back. The technologist was proficient enough in Spanish to communicate with the patient. While looking at the patient who appeared to be "chubby," the technologist thought that perhaps the patient might be pregnant, which might be the cause of the low back pain. The technologist questioned the patient about the possibility of "*el embarazo.*" The technologist patted her own abdominal area and asked the patient "*No niño esta acqui*?" The patient denied being pregnant in both cases and the technologist performed the spine study, which consisted of six images.

By the time the second image had been processed by the multiloader computed radiography (CR) reader, which was processing 12 to 15 images at the time, and seen by the supervisor, two more images were completed. It was at the time of viewing the second image that the supervisor was able to communicate with the radiographer that the patient was indeed pregnant with a well-developed fetus. (Note: this occurred before the advent of direct digital imaging.)

There are multiple legal ramifications that could present with this particular (true) case.

ISSUES TO CONSIDER

1. Should the radiographer do a study ordered by a nurse? (Presents an ethical as well as legal dilemma)

(*continued*)

2. Should the radiographer have used an interpreter to communicate with the patient? Why or why not?

3. Because the patient denied (to the technologist) any possibility of pregnancy, what responsibility rests with the patient?

4. Should the radiographer be held liable for exposing an unborn fetus to radiation? (It was determined that the woman was almost 7 months pregnant—should that matter to this case?)

5. What type of documentation should occur in this case?

This particular case presents a good demonstration of how ethics and the law can coincide but present different determinations.

Summary

1. Ethics is a set of moral principles that governs one's course of action. It is a combination of attributes of honesty, integrity, fairness, caring, respect, fidelity, competence, and accountability.

2. The origin of ethics goes back to Hippocrates and "to help and not to harm."
    a. Patients did not have many rights in the 1930s. They could be enrolled in experimentation without their knowledge.
    b. Patient Safety and Quality Improvement Act was enacted in 2005.
    c. The Institute for Healthcare Improvement and the National Patient Safety Foundation combined their efforts to promote better patient safety in the health care fields.

3. Ethical principles are derived from three ethical philosophies.
    a. The philosophies are:
        i. Utilitarianism (aka consequentialism). This advocates that the actions are correct if the greatest number of people are served by the decision made.
        ii. Deontology states that the rules matter above all else. Follow the rules at all times no matter the outcome.
        iii. Virtue focuses on using wisdom rather than emotional and intellectual problem solving. Holistic medicine uses this philosophy and incorporates certain principles of both utilitarianism and deontology.
    b. The principles are:
        i. Autonomy: people have the right to make decision without outside pressure.
        ii. Beneficence: act to attain a good result. What is beneficial for the patient?
        iii. Confidentiality: all patient information is to be kept confidential. This is a HIPAA requirement.
        iv. Justice: all people should be treated with fairness and equality.
        v. Nonmaleficence: do no harm.
        vi. Paternalism: an attitude of acting like a parent. This should not be done unless not acting would do more harm than acting.
        vii. Veracity: this is truthfulness and honesty.

4. Personal behavior standards are made up of a personal code of ethics that evolves from cultural and environmental background.
    a. Behaviors are also considered attributes and are important in the professional world.
    b. These include honesty, accountability, punctuality, technologic competence, and ethical behavior.

5. Professional attributes include demonstrating ethical behavior as well as competence and knowledge, respect, integrity, conscientiousness, appropriateness, emotional intelligence, and confidence.

6. Standards of Ethics in radiography are made up of two parts.
    a. The Code of Ethics is considered a guide.
    b. The Rules of Ethics are mandatory and must be followed. These Rules of Ethics are intended to promote the protection, safety, and comfort of patients. The Rules of Ethics are enforceable. Radiologic technologists are required to notify ARRT of any ethics violation, including state licensing issues and criminal charges and convictions, within 30 days of occurrence or during their annual renewal of certification and registration, whichever comes first.

7. Patient Care Partnership was previously known as the Patient's Bill of Rights. Every institution has some form of these procedures that are given to patients as they are admitted.
    a. Patient's rights can be infringed upon by the radiographer in the following ways:
        i. Making a diagnosis

    ii. Not obtaining a full allergic history prior to administering contrast

    iii. Not correctly identifying the correct patient or procedure

    iv. Failure to explain to the patient what is being done

    v. Not maintaining confidentiality or patient's physical privacy

    vi. Not providing high-quality images within the bounds of ALARA

8. Systemic analysis is the best way to approach an ethical challenge. By gathering all the facts about the issue, one is able to look at all actions that can be taken. Consequences of those actions have to be considered as well as professional obligations. However, the professional must be prepared to accept those consequences.

9. Sanctions can occur if a course of action is chosen that ended in a detrimental manner for the patient or others.

    a. Sanctions of ethical violations can include revocation of the certification to practice radiography.

10. Ethical dilemmas may include any of the following:

    a. Infraction on individual and/or societal rights

    b. Infraction on cultural or economic conditions

    c. Use of technology and scarce resources

    d. Access to quality health care

    e. Human experimentation and research

    f. Structural racism

    g. Social justice

    h. End-of-life issues

11. Ethical dilemmas in imaging may include any of the following:

    a. Masking or cropping off of anatomy instead of collimating

    b. Use of electronic annotation instead of lead markers placed prior to exposure

    c. Manipulation of data such as exposure indicators and processing algorithms

    d. Dose creep, which is the increase in technical factors and then manipulating the processing algorithms to obtain a satisfactory image

12. Legal issues are also governed by a set of rules of conduct as prescribed by an authority or groups of legislators.

    a. Two classifications of the law are criminal and civil law. Criminal law is against society, whereas civil law is against another person's rights.

    b. Civil law involves torts (either intentional or unintentional) and is normally what a radiographer can be sued under.

    c. Examples of intentional torts are immobilizing a patient against their will or violating HIPAA.

    d. Examples of unintentional torts (negligence) are mismarking an image with the letter markers indicating the correct side of the body, not protecting a patient from a fall, not shielding as appropriate.

13. Radiographers must reduce the risk of a mistake by taking the time to identify the patient, identify the procedure being performed, determine the status of pregnancy if appropriate, selecting appropriate technical factors for the procedure and patient body habitus, correctly collimating, and providing appropriate instructions.

14. Documentation is paramount in all areas of the health care profession.

    a. Patient records on computers are called an e-chart (electronic) and hold information about the patient that is guarded by HIPAA. This makes using the computers in locations throughout the department a potential hazard if the chart is not closed and the technologist does not log off the computer when finished.

    b. Many departments have their own form of documentation called an RIMS.

    c. Documenting patient care includes administration of contrast media, medications given, and all treatment. Consent forms and allergic history forms must be scanned into the e-chart. Documentation such as an incident report and all care that was given to the patient must be done as soon as it is safe to do so.

    d. Radiographic images are covered under HIPAA. Patients must sign a request to have their images sent to outside facilities.

    e. An injury to a patient must be documented in an *incident report* (aka *unusual occurrence report, accident notification report*)

        i. Every report should contain a minimum of the following:

            1. Type of incident (injury, property damage, theft)

            2. Location of incident

            3. Date and time of incident

            4. Name of the affected individual

            5. Narrative description of the incident, including the sequence of events and results of the incident

            6. Injuries and treatment required, if any

            7. Witness name(s) and statement(s)

            8. Other individuals involved

    f. Any patient injured should not be discharged without consent of the radiologist or physician in charge.

    g. Lack of documentation is detrimental to the radiography department in case of a lawsuit.

15. Patient consent must be made before certain types of procedures are performed, especially invasive procedures. There are different types of consent:

    a. Simple consent includes implied and expressed.

    b. Informed consent is only legal if the patient is coherent, the consent is in writing, the patient is old enough to make the decision and can sign it, and the patient understands.

    c. Inadequate or ignorant consents occur when the patient was not informed of everything or did not understand enough to make a responsible decision.

    d. Patients that have signed a consent have the right to rescind that consent and not allow the procedure to go forward. The radiographer must make certain that the patient understands the implications and consequences of such an action.

CHAPTER 4 REVIEW QUESTIONS

1. List three areas in which the radiographer may infringe upon patient rights.

2. What document represents the application of moral principles and moral values for radiologic technology?

3. Match the principle with the definition.

    a. Nonmaleficence   i. Right to make own decisions

    b. Autonomy   ii. Equal treatment and equal benefits

    c. Truthfulness   iii. Duty to refrain from inflicting harm

    d. Justice   iv. Honesty to patients

4. The radiographer who mistakenly administers an incorrect drug to a patient may be guilty of:

    a. Intentional tort
    b. Negligence
    c. Crime
    d. Battery

5. As a radiographer, you refuse to work with a patient because you do not care for persons of the patient's religion. You are guilty of violating:

    a. The Standards of Practice
    b. The Code of Ethics
    c. You own moral values
    d. Both a and b

6. What documentation should a radiographer provide when a patient falls from a table?

7. Professional ethics may be defined as:

    a. A set of principles that govern a course of action
    b. Standards of any professional person
    c. The same as not violating the law
    d. A set of rules and regulations made up by the department in which you work

8. If you are unable to solve a professional ethical dilemma after discussing it with your supervisor, you must present the problem to:

    a. Your attorney
    b. The ethics committee of the institution for which you work
    c. Your colleagues
    d. Your peers

9. Assault occurs when a person feels that there is a danger of bodily harm by another person.

    a. True
    b. False

10. An unconscious child is brought to the emergency suite in your hospital for a diagnostic radiograph. There is no parent or legal guardian with the child. You proceed with the procedure and are functioning under the rule of implied consent.

    a. True
    b. False

11. When a medical professional makes a decision for a patient that the professional believes is in the patient's best interest, the medical professional is engaging in:

    a. Paternalism
    b. Patient advocacy
    c. Self-determination
    d. Veracity

12. Which of the following ethical principles guides health care providers?

    a. Ethical and moral responsibility
    b. Beneficence and nonmaleficence
    c. Humanity and compassion
    d. Trust and respect

13. Which of the following is the principle of truth telling?

    a. Nonmaleficence
    b. Beneficence
    c. Justice
    d. Veracity

14. Law is divided into which two broad categories?

    a. Civil and tort
    b. Criminal and statutory
    c. Tort and malpractice
    d. Criminal and civil

15. Which of the following is mandatory and enforceable?

    a. ARRT Code of Ethics
    b. ARRT Rules of Ethics
    c. ARRT Ethics Committee
    d. ARRT Standards of Practice

PART II

PATIENT INTERACTIONS AND MANAGEMENT

Safety, Patient Care, and Transfer

5

OBJECTIVES

After studying this chapter, the student will be able to:

1. Describe environmental, occupational, and patient safety techniques.

2. Describe methods to evaluate patient physical status.

3. Demonstrate correct principles of body mechanics applicable to patient care.

4. Demonstrate techniques for specific types of patient transfer.

5. Discuss the legal ramifications for failing to safely move a patient.

6. Demonstrate select procedures to turn patient who has various health conditions.

7. Describe specific patient safety measures and concerns.

8. Describe immobilization techniques for various types of procedures and patient conditions.

KEY TERMS

Ambulatory: Walking or able to walk

Atrophy: Decrease in the size of the organ, tissue, or muscle

Decubitus ulcer: A pressure sore

Dyspnea: Labored or difficult breathing

High-Fowler position: Patient semi-sits with head raised 45° to 90°. This position is used to alleviate respiratory distress.

Immobilizer: Any device that is used to limit or prevent movement of a patient that might cause injury to self or others

Ischemia: Deficiency of blood in a body part because of functional constriction or actual obstruction of a blood vessel

Lateral recumbent (side-lying): Patient is on the right or left side with both knees slightly flexed.

Semi-Fowler position: Patient's head is raised at an angle of 15° to 30°.

Sims position: Patient lays on left side with top knee bent and slightly forward. The body is rolled forward as well. This position is used for diagnostic studies of the lower gastrointestinal (GI) tract.

Supine position: Patient is flat on the back.

Tissue necrosis: Localized death of tissue because of injury or lack of oxygen

Trendelenburg position: Patient's head is lowered, or the feet and legs are raised to promote venous return in patients with inadequate peripheral perfusion.

Ulceration: An area of tissue necrosis that penetrates below the epidermis; excavation of the surface of any body organ

INTRODUCTION

Ensuring environmental safety is part of the scope of practice of any health care worker. Reporting fire and electrical hazards may avert a catastrophic incident in the future. Occupational Safety and Health Administration (OSHA) and the Environmental Protection Agency (EPA) have set standards that must be followed so as to keep personnel and the environment safe.

Radiographers are responsible for protecting themselves and the patient from injury in every way possible. Health care workers are often injured while moving and lifting patients, but almost all these injuries are preventable if the correct body mechanics and rules of safety are used. Patients are also victims of injuries caused by being improperly moved or lifted. Most of these injuries can also be prevented. It is imperative that each situation be assessed and enough help is obtained to prevent injury.

Moving a patient from the radiographic table to a gurney or wheelchair, or from a hospital bed to a gurney or wheelchair, requires some forethought regarding the safety of the patient as well as to the body mechanics used. Special care with the ancillary equipment must be taken when moving it with a patient during transport. A patient's integumentary system must be protected from damage. This is of particular concern when the patient is unable to assist in a move.

Patient care extended to ensuring that their belongings are safe and secure. Assisting patients to change into patient gowns or changing soiled gowns may be required by the radiographer in order to protect the patient's skin and well-being.

Occasionally, a patient may have to be immobilized for safety reasons during a radiographic procedure. Not only must the institution-specific rules concerning immobilizers be learned, but the correct use of these devices must also be carefully learned to protect the patient from harm.

SAFETY

Prevention of patient and personnel injury is the responsibility of all health care workers. It is the responsibility of the radiographer to practice safety in all aspects of work. This includes fire and electrical safety, prevention of patient or staff falls, prevention of poisoning, and safe disposal of hazardous waste and toxic chemicals. Facilities are required to test their employees over on safety areas on a yearly basis. This annual testing helps refresh employees on the use and location of equipment and the procedures necessary for keeping themselves and the patients safe.

Environmental Safety

Institutional, local, state, and federal agencies regulate safety in health care institutions, and there are safety committees in all The Joint Commission (TJC)-accredited health care agencies. Fire departments in all cities routinely evaluate the fire safety of health care and community institutions. Poison control centers advise health care institutions if poisoning is possible. The Nuclear Regulatory Commission enforces radiation safety and nuclear medicine standards, and the EPA establishes guidelines for the disposal of radioactive waste. OSHA requires employers to protect all persons employed in the imaging department from exposure to ionizing radiation sources that are not regulated by the Nuclear Regulatory Commission or other federal agencies.

Fire Safety

The radiographer has an obligation to learn fire containment guidelines in any institution where employed. All departments within a facility are required to comply with the following in order to gain or keep accreditation:

1. The telephone number of the institution for reporting a fire; the number must be posted in a clearly visible location next to the telephone.
2. The agency's fire drill and fire evacuation plan.
3. The location of the fire alarms.
4. The routes of evacuation in case of fire.
5. The locations of fire extinguishers and the correct type of extinguisher for each type of fire.
   Carbon dioxide extinguisher: grease or electrical fire
   Soda and acid water extinguisher: paper and wood fire
   Dry chemical extinguisher: rubbish or wood fire
   Antifreeze or water: rubbish, wood, grease, or anesthetic fire
6. A fire must be reported before an attempt is made to extinguish it, regardless of the size.
7. Hallways must be kept free of unnecessary equipment and furniture.
8. Fire hoses must be kept clear at all times.
9. Fire extinguishers must be inspected at regular intervals. Fire drills must be regularly scheduled for agency personnel.
10. Warning signs must be posted stating that, in case of fire, elevators are not to be used and stairways must be used instead.

If fire occurs, the correct procedure for patient safety must be followed, including the following:

1. Persons in imminent danger are to be moved out of the area first.
2. Windows and doors are to be closed.
3. If oxygen is in use, it must be turned off.
4. Patient and staff evacuation procedures must be followed.

General rules for the prevention of accidents involving electrical equipment should include the following:

1. Use only grounded electrical plugs (three pronged) inserted into a ground outlet.

2. Do not use electrical equipment when the hands or the feet are wet or when standing in water because water conducts electricity.

3. When removing an electrical plug from an outlet, grasp the plug at its base. Do not pull on the electrical cord.

4. Electrical cords must not be kinked or frayed; if they are, don't use them.

5. Any electrical equipment must be in sound working order to be used for patient care. If it is not, the equipment must be returned to the area designated for repair service.

6. All electrical equipment must be tested before it is used for patient care.

7. Report any shock experienced; do not use equipment if a patient reports that it gives a tingling feeling or a shock.

8. Do not use a piece of electrical equipment that has not been explained.

9. To prevent falls, do not use extension cords that are not rounded and secured to the floor with electric tape.

Technologists are not responsible for maintaining facility equipment maintenance, but they are responsible for reporting equipment that is not in proper working condition. Each facility has its own forms for reporting this, and it is the responsibility of the student to make sure that they have been adequately orientated and trained in all procedures listed earlier.

Magnetic Resonance Safety

Magnetic resonance (MR) is a form of medical imaging that measures the response of the atomic nuclei of the body when placed in a strong magnetic field. The radio waves cause the nuclei to "spin" and then slow and return to normal. This allows images of the internal organs to be produced. It is noninvasive and utilizes no radiation to create three-dimensional images. Magnetic resonance imaging (MRI) is discussed in a later chapter; however, students must be aware of the potential danger while performing clinical rotations in this area.

The American College of Radiology has published a manual on MR safety that is intended as a guide for facilities with MRI when developing policies and procedures for safety. Metallic objects can become a projectile and cause a fatal injury to the patient or others; or it might fly into the machine itself, damaging the equipment and causing costly repairs. Because the radio waves cause the nuclei in the body to spin, the body's temperature can increase and may cause burns if metal objects are within the magnetic field.

Careful screening of people and objects entering the MR environment is critical to ensure that nothing can become a projectile. There are zones within the MR area that are restricted for safety purposes.

Zone I is freely accessible to the general public as the field poses no hazard.

Zone II requires supervision. This area usually includes the reception area, dressing rooms, and screening areas for patients.

Zone III is access restricted. Only approved MR personnel and patients that have undergone screening are allowed within this area. This is where the control room is located.

Zone IV is where the magnet is located. Only those individuals that have been thoroughly screened and have had all metal removed are allowed within this area.

There are many issues in MR safety that must be considered when a student radiographer is within the confines of the magnetic field. As such, a qualified MR individual should assess all students for the ability to enter into Zone III. Students should be supervised at all times while in the MR area.

Poisoning and Disposition of Hazardous Waste Materials

The number of the nearest Poison Control Center must be posted near department telephones. As the radiographer, the following must be understood and adhered to:

1. Any toxic chemical or agent that may poison patients or staff must be clearly labeled as such.

2. These substances must be stored in a safe area as designated.

3. Emergency instructions to be followed in case of poisoning must be conspicuously posted in the diagnostic imaging department.

4. Chemicals must remain in their own containers and marked as toxic substances.

5. Chemical and toxic substances must be disposed of according to federal mandates and institutional policy.

6. Restrictions for disposal of hazardous materials must be posted in a conspicuous area and followed by all in the department.

7. Contrast media and other drugs must be kept in a safe storage area where access to them is not available to anyone not designated to use them.

8. All containers of hazardous substances must be clearly marked with the name of the substance, a hazard warning, and the name and address of the manufacturer.

9. Hazardous substances may be labeled with a color code that designates the hazard category, for instance, health, flammability, or reactivity.

The radiographer must read and fully understand all hazard warnings before using any product, and follow the guidelines as stated on the label. If there is no label, or if the label is unclear, the product should not be used and properly discarded.

If an accidental spill of a hazardous substance occurs, first aid guidelines are as follows:

- *Eye contact*: Flush eyes with water for 15 minutes or until irritation subsides. Consult a physician immediately.
- *Skin contact*: Remove any affected clothing; wash skin thoroughly with gentle soap and water.
- *Inhalation*: Remove from exposure; if breathing has stopped, begin cardiopulmonary resuscitation; call emergency number and a physician.
- *Ingestion*: Do not induce vomiting; call emergency number and Poison Control Center.

Diagnostic imaging personnel must understand the potential hazards of these materials. Every imaging department should have Material Safety Data Sheets (MSDSs) in an accessible location. These sheets contain information that employees need to know about the hazards of materials being handled. Display 5-1 shows a sample MSDS.

DISPLAY 5-1

Sample MSDS

Issuing Date _____ Revision Date _____ Revision Number _____

1. Identification of the Substance/Preparation and of the Company/Undertaking
   Product identifier
   Other means of identification
   Recommended use of the chemical and restrictions on use
   Details of the supplier of the safety data sheet
   Emergency telephone number

2. Hazards Identification
   Classification
   Globally Harmonized System (GHS) label elements, including precautionary statements
   Emergency overview
   Signal word
   Hazard statements
   Precautionary statements—prevention
   Precautionary statements—response
   Precautionary statements—storage
   Precautionary statements—disposal
   Hazards Not Otherwise Classified (HNOC)

3. Composition/Information on Ingredients
   Unknown toxicity
   Other information
   Interactions with other chemicals

4. First Aid Measures
   Most important symptoms and effects, both acute and delayed
   Indication of any immediate medical attention and special treatment needed

5. Firefighting Measures
   Suitable extinguishing media
   Unsuitable extinguishing media
   Specific hazards arising from the chemical
   Explosion data
   Protective equipment and precautions for firefighters

6. Accidental Release Measures
   Personal precautions, protective equipment, and emergency procedures
   Environmental precautions
   Methods and material for containment and cleaning up
   Precautions for safe handling
   Conditions for safe storage, including any incompatibilities

DISPLAY 5-1

Sample MSDS (*continued*)

7. Exposure Controls/Personal Protection
   Control parameters
   Appropriate engineering controls
   Individual protection measures, such as personal protective equipment

8. Physical and Chemical Properties
   Appearance
   Odor
   pH
   Melting/freezing point
   Flash point
   Evaporation rate

9. Stability and Reactivity
   Reactivity
   Chemical stability
   Possibility of hazardous reactions
   Conditions to avoid
   Incompatible materials
   Hazardous decomposition products

10. Toxicologic Information
    Information on likely routes of exposure
    Information on toxicologic effects
    Delayed and immediate effects as well as chronic effects from short- and long-term exposure
    Numerical measures of toxicity—product information

11. Ecological Information
    Ecotoxicity
    Persistence and degradability
    Bioaccumulation
    Other adverse effects

12. Disposal Considerations
    Disposal methods
    Contaminated packaging

13. Transport Information
    Department of Transportation (DOT)
    Transport of Dangerous Goods (TDG)
    International Civil Aviation Organization (ICAO)
    International Air Travel Association (IATA)
    International Maritime Dangerous Goods (IMDG)
    International Maritime Organization (IMO)

14. Regulatory Information
    Chemical inventories
    U.S. state regulations
    International regulations

15. Other Information
    National Fire Protection Association (NFPA)
    Hazardous Materials Identification System (HMIS)
    General disclaimer

End of Safety Data Sheet

EVALUATING PATIENT NEEDS

Evaluating patient needs includes understanding the social determinants of health (poor socioeconomic areas have less access to health care) and using critical thinking skills to assess patient status. It is the systematic approach to ensuring that the patient is receiving what is needed to diagnose and treat what is wrong. This requires the understanding of what is involved, the time necessary to undertake the assessment, and then using the critical thinking skills learned to plan what is necessary for the best interest of the patient.

Social Determinants of Health

Social determinants of health are conditions in places where people live, learn, work, and play that affect a wide range of health and quality-of-life risks and outcomes. Resources that enhance quality of life can influence health outcomes. These resources include safe and affordable housing, access to education, public safety, and local emergency/health services. Differences in health are significant in communities with poor social determinants. Low income and substandard education are major limiting factors. These determinants should be taken into account when evaluating the needs of the patient for radiography services.

Assessing Patient Status

Every patient and every diagnostic procedure may present problems ranging from simple to complex. When the radiography student obtains a patient for imaging, it must be decided how to perform the assignment quickly, efficiently, and as comfortably as possible for the patient. This requires going through the problem-solving process before beginning the exam. Critical thinking is necessary to achieve a satisfactory outcome. The radiographer should consult the clinical information that is available by reviewing the patient's history in the e-chart and consulting with the staff associated with the patient as appropriate. Combining this knowledge with the patient assessment done by the radiographer helps determine the best and safest method to transfer a patient. Patient assessment can be successfully performed by following these steps:

- Data collection
- Data analysis
- Planning
- Implementation
- Evaluation

Although it may seem unrealistic to the beginning student to go through this process, once skills have been practiced and competence is gained, the entire process takes less than a few minutes to complete. Critical thinking skills are practiced every day and eventually become a habit. Going through this process to evaluate patients' needs becomes the same.

Data Collection and Analysis

There are two types of data, subjective and objective. Subjective data include anything that the patient or family member who accompanies the patient might say that is pertinent to the patient care. The patient is the subject; therefore, the data are subjective. Objective data include anything that the radiographer sees, hears, smells, feels, or reads on the patient's chart reported by other health care workers that may affect the patient or the procedure to be performed.

Analysis of the data integrates all segments of critical thinking. The radiographer mentally reviews both subjective and objective data to make a decision as to what data are relevant to the assignment. A decision is then made as to what data are relevant to the assignment and consider any problems and potential problems.

Planning and Implementation

A goal is set for successful completion of the procedure and a plan for achieving the goal is made. Patient involvement in goal setting and formulating a plan to achieve the goal is essential. A patient who is not made part of the care planning is not able to cooperate in achieving the desired goal. Collaborating with patients in planning their care instills in the patient a feeling of responsibility for a successful outcome.

Implementation of the plan depends on the patient's problems and the need for assistance to achieve the desired goal safely. Patient safety and comfort during the implementation of the plan must always be the priority. The radiographer must consider what instructions need to be given to the patient as well as any assistance that may be needed.

Evaluation

After the plan has been implemented, the outcome must be evaluated. Image quality is certainly the goal; however, if the patent's safety was jeopardized or if the patient was subjected to a great amount of pain as the plan was implemented, the outcome of the procedure was less than perfect. Honest inquiry is the key to evaluation.

- Were the patient's needs met while maintaining safety?
- Did unanticipated problems arise? If so, what might have been done differently?

Pain Assessment

All accredited health care facilities must have a pain assessment tool to rate the degree of pain the patient is feeling. This tool may differ according to the patient's age, cultural background, and medical condition so that each patient can easily understand it. The scales used are either numbers from 1 to 10 or facial expressions showing a face with tears to a smiling face. Figure 5-1 shows a tool that contains both a numeric scale and expressions including English and Spanish directions.

Gender plays a role in pain assessment. Males typically need stronger or higher doses of pain medication than women. Age should be a consideration in pain assessment. The young patient may overreact for the benefit of the parent; however, the pain may be real. The elderly may have lost some pain-sensing mechanisms and may not be aware of some injuries that could inflict pain. Culture is also a determinant. There are those who believe "mind over matter" controls or even removes the cause of the pain. There are also religious beliefs that prayer heals without the benefit of medical care, and patients with this belief may not show the true amount of pain being experienced. Anxiety and stress make pain worse no matter what the age, gender, or culture. Fatigue can make pain worse as well. With so many factors involved, the technologist should always believe the patient and treat the patient with the care necessary to prevent further injury and pain.

The radiographer most often interviews the patient to determine any level of pain that might be occurring. This is most important if the exam that is to be completed is to determine the cause of the pain. Examples of this might be a kidney, ureter, and bladder (KUB) x-ray for abdominal pain or chest images for chest pain with associated shortness of breath. A complete description of the pain must be obtained and documented for the radiologist. The location of the pain should be accurate and include the intensity and duration of the pain being experienced. Documentation should also include what factors cause the pain to be worse (aggravating factors) or when the pain might be lessened (alleviating factors).

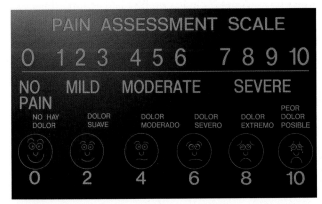

FIGURE 5-1 Pain assessment tool found in an Emergency Department. This combines facial expressions, number scales, and written description, which is excellent for all age groups.

BODY MECHANICS

Although safety should be the top priority for all health care workers, it is easy to take shortcuts and try to save time when performing a transfer. Constant abuse of the spine from moving and lifting patients is the leading cause of injury to health care personnel in all health care institutions. Forty-five percent of all musculoskeletal disorders in health care are due to injury from improper patient lifting. Following the correct rules of body mechanics reduces the amount of fatigue and chance of injury. Rules of body mechanics are based on the laws of gravity.

Gravity is the force that pulls objects toward the center of the earth. Any movement requires an expenditure of energy to overcome the force of gravity. When an object is balanced, it is firm and stable. If it is off-balance, it falls because of the pull of gravity. The center of gravity is a hypothetical point at which the mass of any body is centered. When a person is standing, the center of gravity is at the center of the pelvis near the sacrum.

Safe body mechanics require good posture. Good posture means that the body is in alignment with all the parts in balance. This permits the musculoskeletal system to work at maximal efficiency with minimal amount of strain on joints, tendons, ligaments, and muscles. Good posture also aids other body systems to work efficiently. For instance, if the chest is held up and out, then the lungs can work at maximal efficiency.

Correct upright posture is accomplished by

- Holding the chest up and slightly forward with the waist extended. This allows the lungs to expand properly and fill to capacity;
- Holding the head erect with the chin held in. This puts the spine in proper alignment, with a normal curve in the neck;
- Standing with the feet parallel and at right angles to the lower legs. The feet should be 4 to 8 inches apart. Keep body weight equally distributed on both feet;
- Keeping the knees slightly bent. They act as shock absorbers for the body;
- Keeping the buttocks in and the abdomen up and in. This prevents strain on the back and abdominal muscles.

The forces of weight and friction must be overcome when moving and lifting objects. Keep the heaviest part of the object close to the body. If this is not possible, additional help should be obtained to assist with moving or lifting the load. To avoid self-injury when moving heavy objects, remember to keep the body's line of balance closest to the center of the load.

Friction opposes movement. Reduce the surface area to be moved. Pulling rather than pushing also reduces friction when moving a heavy object or person.

To avoid self-injury when moving heavy objects, remember to keep the body's line of balance closest to the center of the load. Keep the following rules in mind when lifting or moving heavy objects:

- When picking up an object from a low table or the floor, bend the knees (Fig. 5-2A1) and lower the body. Do not bend from the waist (Fig. 5-2A2). The biceps are the strongest arm muscles and are effective when pulling; therefore, pull heavy items or patients rather than push them.
- Always protect the spine. Rather than twisting the body to move a load, change the foot position instead (Fig. 5-2B1 and B2). Always keep the body balanced over the feet, which should be spread to provide a firm base of support.
- Keep the heaviest part of the load close to the body (Fig. 5-2C1). Having the object farther from the body (Fig. 5-2C2) causes strain on the back.
- When assisting a patient to move, balance the weight over both feet and keep one foot slightly ahead of the other. Stand close to the patient, flex the gluteal muscles, and bend the knees to support the load. Use arm and leg muscles to assist in the move.
- Make certain that the floor area is clear of all objects.

Proper body mechanics alone do not prevent injury; it only decreases the chance of injury. It must be remembered

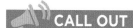
CALL OUT

Keep the body balanced over the feet to provide a broad base of support.

Correct Body Mechanics	Incorrect Body Mechanics
Figure 5-2A1	Figure 5-2A2
Figure 5-2B1	Figure 5-2B2
Figure 5-2C1	Figure 5-2C2

CALL OUT

To prevent lower back injury, always keep the center of gravity, with the knees flexed and the weight over both feet. Do not bend at the waist or twist with the body.

that body mechanics only focus on the lower back when doing lateral transfers and not on the other parts of the body such as the shoulders and lower neck muscles that are injured from boosting and repositioning a patient. As our body ages, the chance of injury to the back increases. More care must be taken by obtaining more assistance to prevent injury to both the worker and the patient.

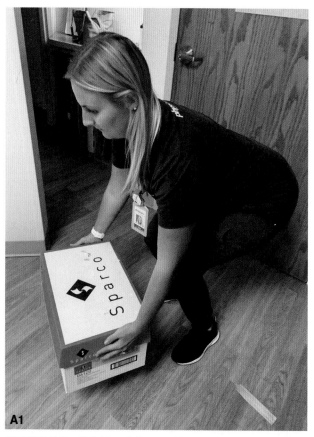

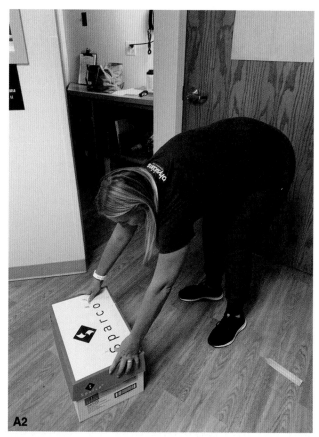

FIGURE 5-2 (A1) Kneel down with the back straight. **(A2)** Don't bend at the waist as this strains the back.

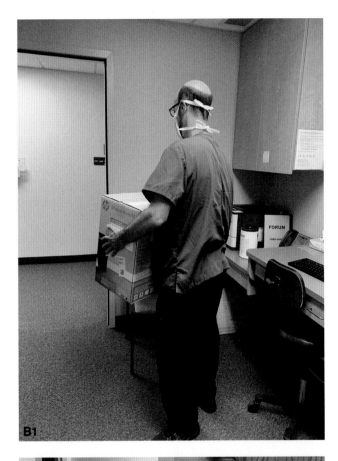

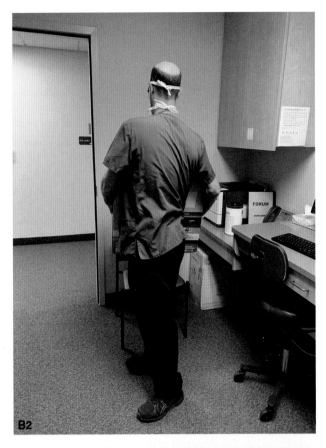

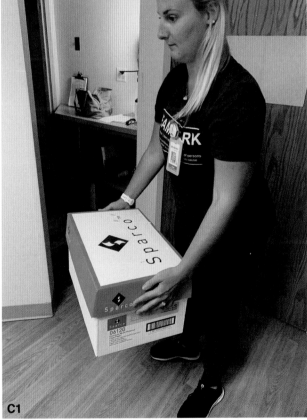

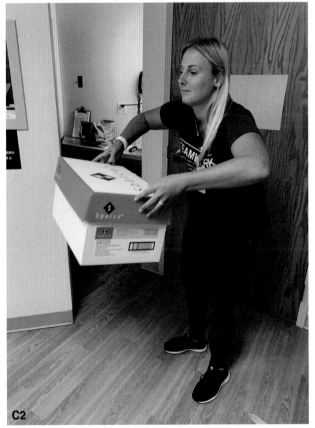

FIGURE 5-2 *(continued)* **(B1)** Move the feet in a new direction. **(B2)** Don't twist at the waist. **(C1)** Keep a heavy object close to the body. **(C2)** Don't reach out to lift when the object is far from the body.

PATIENT TRANSFER AND MOVEMENT

The radiographer may be called upon to transfer or assist in transferring a patient from a hospital room to the diagnostic imaging department. Involving patients in the transfer when being moved provides them with a positive sense of being part of their care. Speaking with the patients and reviewing their capability regarding the transfer and mobility tasks greatly reduces the risk of injury from mistakes.

Assessing Patient Mobility

Before moving the patient, the radiographer must assess the ability of the patient for pain and mobility. Patients in pain are less likely to be mobile and willing to help in the transfer. Ask the patient about any limitations that may hinder the move. If the patient responds positively, the radiographer must use critical thinking skills developed to determine the best method to safely move the patient. However, if the patient responds there are no limitations, the radiographer must still make plan for the transfer as many patients may think they can do something and are not aware that they are weaker than they think. Whether getting an outpatient from the waiting room or transferring a patient from the floor, look for the following during patient assessment:

- *Deviations from correct body alignment.* Deviations in formal physiologic body alignment of the patient may result from poor posture, trauma, muscle damage, dysfunction of the nervous system, malnutrition, fatigue, or emotional disturbance. Positioning sponges or pillows must be available to make the patient comfortable.
- *Immobility or limitations in range of joint motion.* Any stiffness, instability, swelling, inflammation, pain, limitations of movement, or **atrophy** of muscle mass surrounding each joint must be noted and considered in the plan of transfer and care.
- *The ability to walk.* Gait includes rhythm, speed, cadence, and any characteristic of walking that may result in a problem with balance, posture, or independence of movement. Before beginning the move, the amount of assistance needed to safely complete the move and procedure must be planned.
- *Respiratory, cardiovascular, metabolic, and musculoskeletal problems.* Obvious respiratory or cardiovascular symptoms that impair circulation and signal potential problems in positioning must be planned for. (Symptoms and care of patients with medical problems are discussed in Chapter 9.)
- *The patient's general condition.* What is the range of motion and weight-bearing ability of the patient? Evaluate the patient for strength and endurance, and balance.

- *The patient's ability to understand what is expected during the transfer.* Is the patient responsive and alert? Has the patient received a sedative, hypnotic, or other psychoactive drug in the past 2 or 3 hours? Will any medication that has been taken affect the ability to move safely?
- *The patient's acceptance of the move.* Does the patient fear or resent the transfer? Will the transfer increase any pain? Does the patient feel that the move is unnecessary, or perhaps the procedure itself?

Before going to the patient, a consultation with the staff in charge of the patient is recommended so that the patient's condition and limitations can be understood. If assistants are needed, they must be on hand or readily available for the radiographer. A patient must never be moved without adequate assistance because doing so may cause injury to the patient or the radiographer. The radiographer must decide how the patient can be transferred safely and comfortably, whether by gurney or by wheelchair. In some cases, the radiology request states that the patient can travel by wheelchair, but upon accurate assessment and consultation, the radiographer discovers that the patient is unable to sit in a wheelchair and must be transported by gurney. Hospital patients should never be allowed to walk to and from the imaging department for safety reasons.

Rules for Safe Patient Transfer

Several precautions must be taken when moving a patient from the hospital room to the imaging department. The following rules should be observed during a move:

1. Establish the correct identity of the patient.
2. Request pertinent information concerning the patient's ability to comply with the physical demands of the procedure, ability to ambulate, or any restrictions or precautions to be taken concerning the patient's mobility.
3. Use correct body mechanics to protect the mover's back.
4. Use devices that are designed to transfer patients safely.
5. Lock all wheels on beds, gurneys, and wheelchairs before the move begins. At the same time, remove anything that might be in the way or might be a tripping hazard.
6. Give only the assistance that the patient needs for comfort and safety.
7. Always transfer a patient across the shortest distance.
8. Generally, it is better to move a patient toward the stronger side while assisting on the patient's weaker side.
9. The patient should wear shoes or hospital socks for standing transfers, not personal socks, which may be slippery. Hospitals do provide transfer socks that have

gripping soles to prevent the patient from slipping on the tile floors of the hospital as seen in Figure 5-3.

10. Inform the patient of the plan for moving and encourage any help.

11. Give the patient short, simple commands and help the patient to accomplish the move.

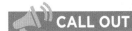
CALL OUT

Never move a patient without first ensuring the patient's identity matches the requested order!

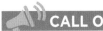
CALL OUT

Never move a patient without enough assistance to prevent injury to you and/or the patient.

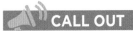
CALL OUT

Never move a patient without assessing the patient's ability to assist.

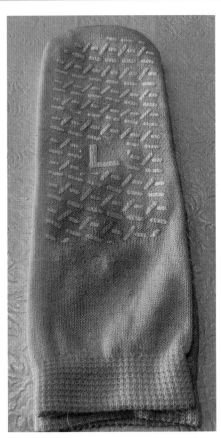

FIGURE 5-3 All inpatients are given a pair of these nonskid socks upon admission to help prevent falls.

When the imaging procedure is completed, return the patient to the hospital room using the following procedures:

1. Stop at the appropriate station and inform the unit personnel that the patient is being returned to the room. Request help if it is needed at this time.

2. Return the patient to the room, help the patient get into bed, and ensure comfort and safety. Place the patient's bed in the position that is closest to the floor with the side rails raised and the call button within reach in case the patient needs assistance.

 WARNING!

To prevent possible patient injury, always lower the bed to the lowest position and secure the rails in the upright position when a patient is returned to bed.

If the patient is from the outpatient waiting area, walk the patient back to the waiting room and thank them. Communication with the patient at the end of the study is just as important as performing the study itself. Walking the patient to the waiting area where the interaction began is courteous and should be part of the completion of the examination.

METHODS OF MOVING PATIENTS

There are essentially three ways of transferring patients: by gurney, by wheelchair, and by **ambulation**. Walking a patient from a room within the hospital to the imaging department is not advisable for safety reasons. Patients that are in the outpatient waiting area should also be assessed before deciding on the ability to walk into the examining room. Be sure to determine what is allowable and appropriate in the facility.

Gurney

When a patient is moved from a gurney to a radiographic table, or the reverse, great care must be taken to prevent injury. If the patient is unconscious or unable to cooperate in the move, the patient's spine, head, and extremities must be well supported. Convenient and safe ways to do this are using a sheet or a sliding board to move the patient from one surface to another. Refer to the "Procedure" sections for information on how to use a sheet or sliding board to transfer a patient.

Wheelchair

Although it may seem that a patient in a wheelchair is more capable of assisting with a transfer, such is not always the case. Always be by the patient's side to assist in any manner that is needed. The patient being moved from a room on the floor may not have been out of bed for a period of time and may be light-headed and less strong than was anticipated. This, combined with the motion of the wheelchair as it moves quickly down the hall to the radiology department, may be enough to cause the patient to become dizzy and fall. Using proper body mechanics helps prevent an injury to the technologist as well as to the patient in situations that may arise because of unsteadiness.

For patients who are able to transfer themselves, the radiographer must provide instructions and provide standby assistance. Place the wheelchair at a 45° angle with the patient's strongest side closest to the radiographic table. The radiographer must secure the wheelchair locks and lift the footrests so that the patient does not trip over them. In this type of standby assistance, the radiographer must not leave the patient alone to get out of the wheelchair and get onto the table. Doing so invites disaster in the form of a fall, which is the most common patient injury in an imaging department.

Use the following flowchart to assess the patient's need for assistance. Once the assessment has been made, refer to the "Procedure" section and watch the video clip to ensure complete knowledge of the transfer.

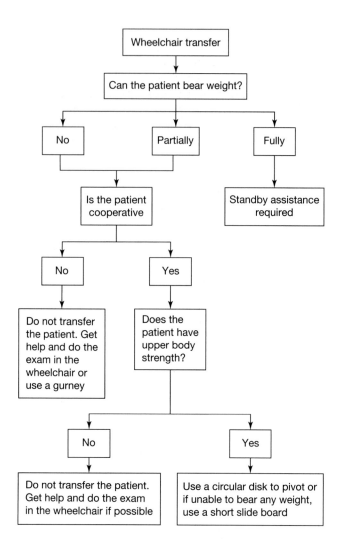

PROCEDURE

Sheet Transfer

To place a sheet under a patient:

1. Obtain a heavy draw sheet or a full bed-sheet that is folded in half. Have one person stand on each side of the table or bed at the patient's side.

2. Turn the patient onto the side that is opposite to the side or direction that the patient is being moved to.

3. Place the sheet on the table or bed with the fold against the patient's back (Fig. 5-4A).

4. Roll the top half of the sheet as close to the patient's back as possible (Fig. 5-4B). Inform the patient to roll onto the back and over the rolled sheet.

5. Finally, turn the patient to the other side and off the roll of the sheet. The assistant should straighten the sheet, making it flat for the patient to be laid on (Fig. 5-4C). Return the patient to a supine position, and the transfer may begin.

To transfer the patient after placing the sheet:

If the patient is an adult, three or four people should participate in the maneuver. One person stands at the patient's head to guide and support it during the move, with another at the side to which the patient is moved, and a third person at the side where the patient is lying. If there are four people, two may stand at each side. The force of friction opposes movement. When moving or transferring a patient, reduce friction to the minimum to facilitate movement. This can be done by reducing the surface area to be moved or, in the case of a patient, using some of the patient's own strength to assist with the move, if possible. If the patient is unable to assist, reduce friction by placing the patient's arms across the chest to reduce the surface area. The surface over which the patient must be moved must be dry and smooth. Pulling rather than pushing also reduces friction when moving a heavy

object or person. A sliding board or pull sheet placed under an immobile patient also reduces friction. Directions for use of these items are presented later in this chapter.

The sheet is rolled at the side of the patient so that it can easily be grasped, close to the patient's body. In unison (usually on the count of three), the team transfers the patient to the other surface. Extra care over the radiographic table's metal edges should be taken as well as ensuring that the x-ray tube housing is positioned out of the way.

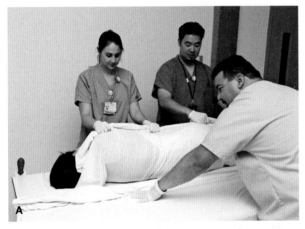
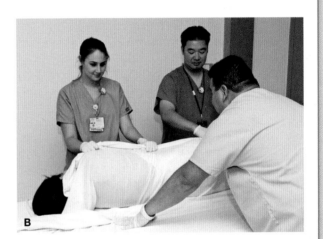
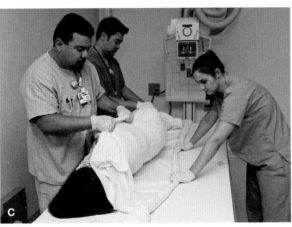

FIGURE 5-4 **(A)** Place the sheet on the table with the fold against the patient's back. **(B)** Take the top half of the sheet and roll it against the patient. **(C)** After the patient is rolled to the opposite side, the rolled half of the sheet is straightened out.

PROCEDURE

Log Roll

In the event a trauma patient must be moved and there is no sheet or other means to transfer the patient, a procedure known as a log roll must be used. The objective of the log roll procedure is to maintain correct anatomic alignment in order to prevent the possibility of further, catastrophic neurologic injury and the prevention of pressure sores.

At least three people are required to assist in the log roll procedure:

1. One person must hold the patient's head.

2. Two people must support the chest, abdomen, and lower limbs on either side of the patient. If the patient is obese, tall, or has lower limb injuries, a fourth person on the patient's side may be necessary.

3. Explain the procedure and ask the patient to lie still and to not move.

4. Make sure that urinary catheters, intravenous (IV) tubing, and so on are repositioned to prevent overextension and dislodgement during movement. Make sure that the patient is anatomically aligned before rolling.

5. The patient's arm away from the side of intended turn must be extended along the thorax and abdomen or bent over the chest if appropriate.

6. Place a pillow between the patient's legs.

7. One assistant on the side of the patient supports the patient's upper body by placing one hand on the shoulders and the other hand around the patient's thighs.

8. The other assistant supports the patient's abdomen and lower limbs by overlapping with the first assistant's arm to place one hand under the patient's lower back and the other hand over the patient's lower legs.

9. The technologist holding the patient's head directs the turn. Upon direction, the patient is turned in anatomic alignment in one smooth action.

10. Once a sheet or smooth mover is placed under the patient to assist in the move, the patient is returned to the supine position to be moved as stated earlier.

 WARNING!

The patient who is suspected of spinal injury must be kept in correct anatomic alignment at all times.

PROCEDURE

Lateral Transfer

The lateral transfer is best accomplished with the use of a sliding board (also called a smooth mover or a "smoothie"). There are two lengths of this glossy, plasticized board that are used in different situations. The long board is approximately 5 ft 10 inches in length and about 2 ft 6 inches wide. This length is used to transfer a supine patient from one flat surface to another. There is also a short board that is approximately 3 ft long and 2.5 ft wide and is used for transfer from

a sitting position to another surface. The sliding board usually requires fewer personnel to make the move than the sheet transfer because it creates a firm bridge between the two surfaces over which the patient can be easily moved. The sliding board transfer procedure is as follows:

1. After assessing whether the patient is able to assist in the move, and the patient's approximate size, a determination

of the number of assistants necessary can be made. Use the long board and two to four assistants. A Hoyer lift (Fig. 5-5) may be necessary if moving a bariatric patient. All individuals using this device to transfer patients must be trained in its functions.

2. Obtain the transfer board and spray it with antistatic spray if necessary. Moving a patient on this board may create static electricity and cause the technologist to be shocked when touching the metal edges of the table or gurney.

3. Move the patient to the edge of the gurney. One person should hold the sheet that the patient is lying on over the top of the patient to keep the patient from possibly rolling off the gurney.

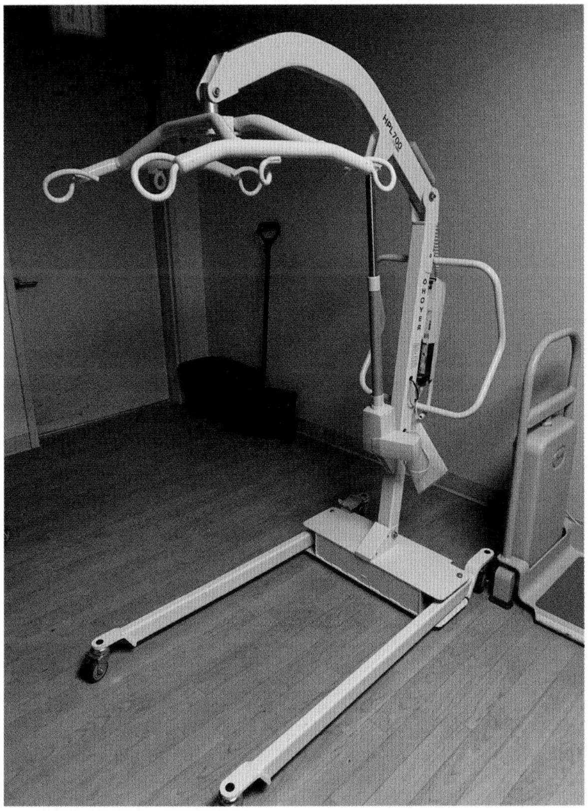

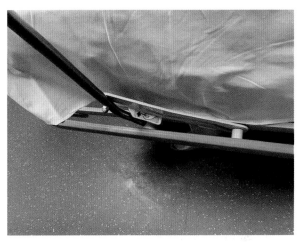

FIGURE 5-5 The frame of a Hoyer lift used to lift large patients or those that are unable to move. A hammock style seat wraps around the patient and hooks to the top of the lift.

4. Lower the side rails by releasing the lock at the bottom of the rail (Fig. 5-6) and move the gurney to the table so that there is no gap between them. Lock the wheels of the gurney. Brakes on the gurney are color coded. When the red side is down, the brakes are locked as seen in Figure 5-7. The patient's strongest side should be against the radiographic table.

5. Assist the patient to turn onto the side, away from the radiographic table, and place the sliding board under the sheet upon which the patient was lying.

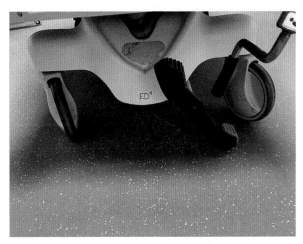

FIGURE 5-6 A toggle lock releases the side rails of the gurney so that they can be raised or lowered.

FIGURE 5-7 By stepping on the red side of the foot brake, the gurney is in the locked position.

(continued)

6. Create a bridge with the board between the edge of the radiographic table and the edge of the gurney (Fig. 5-8A).

7. Place the sheet over the board, and allow the patient to roll back onto the board.

8. With one person at the side of the radiographic table and the other at the side of the gurney, slide the patient over the board and onto the radiographic table. Make sure that the patient's lower extremities are moved in unison with the body to prevent injury to them (Fig. 5-8B).

9. Assist the patient to continue the roll away from the side that the gurney was on, keeping the patient secure by holding onto the sheet. The person standing on the side of the gurney should remove the sliding board from under the patient (Fig. 5-8C).

10. One person removes the gurney, whereas the other assistant remains to ensure the patient's safety. Perform the radiographic procedure.

11. When the procedure is completed, the patient can be transferred back to the gurney by repeating the steps earlier.

12. Once back on the gurney, place a pillow under the patient's head, if this is permitted, and put the side rails of the gurney up. Be sure to cover the patient with a blanket and place a soft immobilizer over the waist. The patient may then be transferred.

13. When the move is complete, discard the soiled linen that was used on the radiographic table, and clean the sliding board and the table with a disinfectant spray.

14. After washing hands, place clean linen on the table.

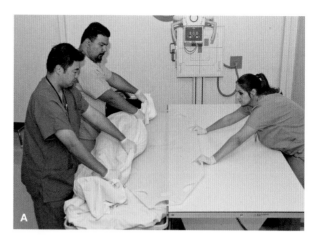

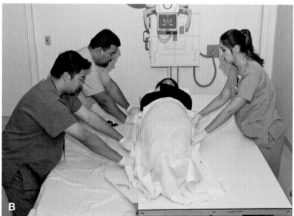

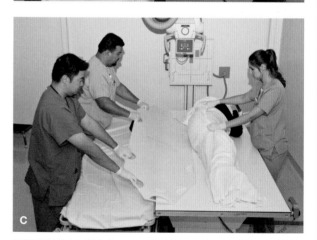

FIGURE 5-8 **(A)** Create a bridge with the board between the table and the gurney. **(B)** Roll the sheet close to the patient and slide the patient onto the table. **(C)** Remove the sliding board while safely securing the patient.

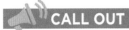 **CALL OUT**

Always obtain enough assistance to move a patient, even with a sliding board. This is for the safety of both the patient and the radiographer.

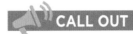 **CALL OUT**

Patients who have suffered a stroke or who have varying levels of paralysis should be transferred with certain safety concerns in mind.

CALL OUT

When moving a patient from a gurney, be sure to lower the side rails so that a back injury is less likely.

 PROCEDURE

Wheelchair Transfer

A patient that is able to get in and out of a wheelchair still needs standby assistance. To help a patient out of the wheelchair and onto the table, the following procedures should be followed:

1. Lower the table or place a step stool with a handle next to the table.

2. Push the wheelchair to the edge of the table at a 45° angle (Fig. 5-9A), lock the brakes, and raise the footrests (Fig. 5-9B and C).

3. Stand by the patient's elbow to provide stabilizing assistance if needed (Fig. 5-9D).

4. Instruct the patient to stand and sit on the edge of the table (Fig. 5-9E).

5. Once the patient is seated on the table, remove the wheelchair so that the procedure can begin.

To help a patient off the radiographic table and into a wheelchair, the following procedures should be followed:

1. Place the wheelchair at an angle next to the table before sitting the patient up, lock the brakes, and put the footrests up. Do not lower the table if the patient requires help to sit up. Lowering the table may cause injury to the radiographer's back.

2. If the patient requires help to a sitting position, have the patient turn to the side with knees flexed; stand in front of the patient with one arm under the shoulder and the other across the knees (Fig. 5-9F).

3. The patient can assist by pushing up with the arm when told to do so (Fig. 5-9G).

4. On the count of three, move or help the patient to a sitting position at the edge of the table. Allow the patient to sit for a moment and regain a sense of balance. While the patient is "dangling," place nonskid slippers on the patient's feet. Lower the table if appropriate (Fig. 5-9H).

5. If the patient needs minimal assistance to get off the table, stand at the patient's side and take the patient's arm to help (Fig. 5-9I).

6. If the radiographic table is high, never allow a patient to step down without providing a secure stepping stool. Always stay at the patient's side to assist. A telescoping radiographic table must be placed in the lower position before a patient is assisted to move off it.

7. The wheelchair must be close enough so that the patient can be seated in the chair with one pivot. The use of a circular disk for the patient to stand on allows a pivot

(continued)

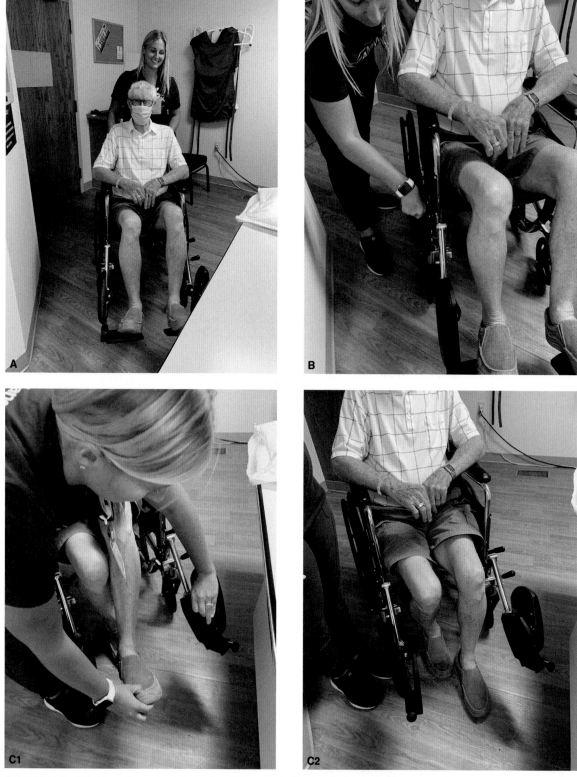

FIGURE 5-9 **(A)** Place the wheelchair at a 45° angle to the table. Lock the brakes and raise the footrests. **(B)** Always lock the brakes of the wheelchair on both sides of the chair. **(C1)** Remember to raise the footrests up before allowing the patient to stand up. **(C2)** Both feet should be squarely on the floor.

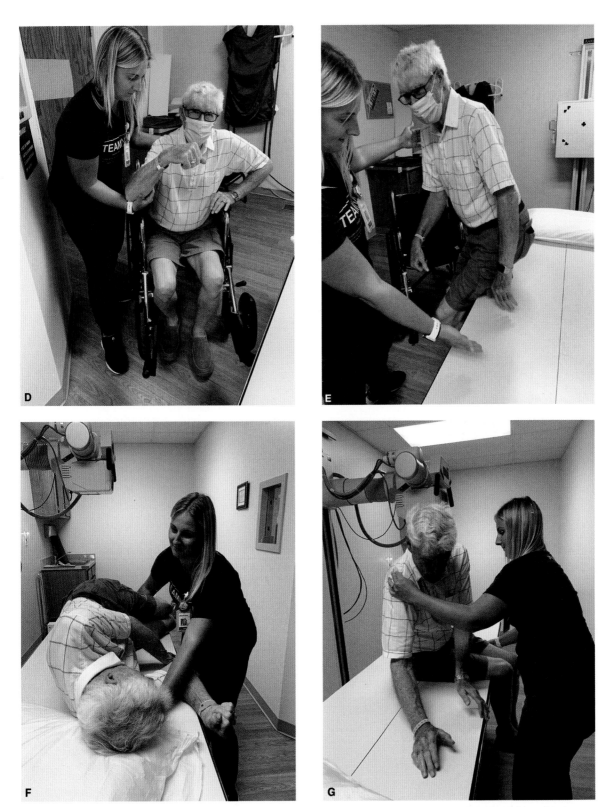

FIGURE 5-9 (*continued*) **(D)** Stand by the patient's elbow to provide assistance as needed. **(E)** Stand in front of the patient and indicate where the patient is to sit on the table before lying down. **(F)** Stand in front of the patient and place an arm under shoulders and over knees. Assist to a sitting position. **(G)** Have the patient assist by pushing with the arm that is down.

(*continued*)

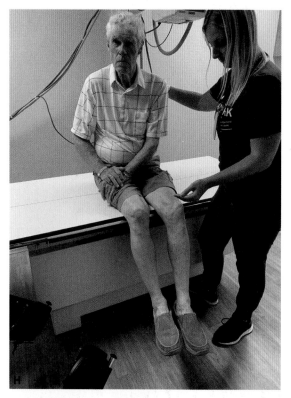

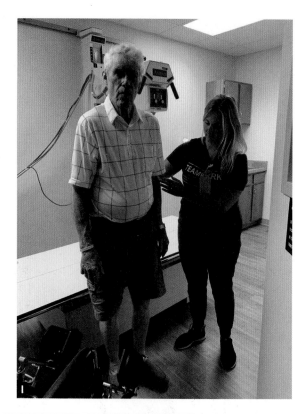

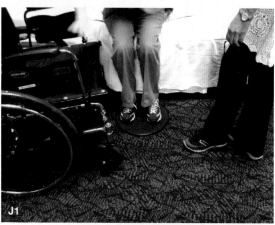

J1

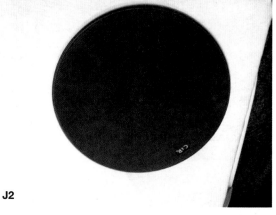

J2

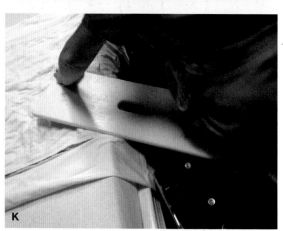

K

FIGURE 5-9 (*continued*) **(H)** Allow the patient to "dangle" for a few moments while the table is lowered. Do not leave the patient's side. Note how the technologist rests her hand on the patient's shoulder for reassurance. **(I)** Provide assistance back to the wheelchair by holding the patient's elbow for stability. Do not leave any patient's side, no matter the age of the patient. **(J1)** A circular disk placed on the floor between the table and the wheelchair allows the patient to pivot with minimal movement and help from the radiographer. **(J2)** The disk is approximately 12 inches in diameter and allows a complete circular movement. **(K)** The short board is placed under the patient's hips and bridges the distance to the radiographic table, allowing the patient to slide from the chair to the table.

action with minimal help from the radiographer (Fig. 5-9J1 and J2).

8. The footrests on the wheelchair should then be put down and the wheels unlocked. A safety belt should be put across an unsteady patient. Once the patient is in the wheelchair, cover the patient with a sheet or blanket to protect privacy and dignity during the transport within the building.

Another method of moving a patient in a wheelchair, who is able to assist but unable to bear weight, is to use the short board described in the lateral transfer procedure. This is accomplished by the following steps:

1. Remove the arm rail on the side of the chair that is to be placed alongside the radiographic table that has been completely lowered. Make sure that the brakes have been set on both sides.

2. Have the patient raise the thigh on the side next to the table and place the short board under that hip and bridge the gap between the table and the chair as seen in Figure 5-9K.

3. The patient then is able to slide across the board to the radiographic table. The technologist must stand next to the patient to provide assistance and ensure the patient's safety.

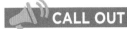

CALL OUT

When moving a patient from a hospital bed to a wheelchair, always place nonskid slippers on the patient's feet, provide assistance to prevent falls, and secure the seatbelt on the wheelchair.

WARNING!

Before allowing a patient to get out of a wheelchair, raise the foot supports out of the way. Many patients step on these, causing the wheelchair to flip over, which causes injury to the patient!

WARNING!

A patient who has received a narcotic, hypnotic, or other type of psychoactive medication; a confused, disoriented, unconscious, or head-injured person; or a child must never be left alone on a radiographic table or gurney. If the patient's behavior cannot be predicted or if the patient is in a wheelchair, careful observation is a must. A soft immobilizer belt should be placed over any patient on a gurney or in a wheelchair. The side rails of the gurney must always be up.

LEGALITIES OF AN INCORRECT TRANSFER

As stated earlier, assistants must be available for help when moving a patient from a gurney or wheelchair to the x-ray table and back. The radiographer must never assume that the patient fully understands the ability to move from one area to another. It is the radiographer who is responsible for making the decision to request help. Not obtaining the help or resources available may end in severe consequences for both the patient and the radiographer.

The following case study is a true story. Although the student might think that no one would do something like this, it only takes a moment of poor judgment to assume that nothing happens and lives are changed forever. The technologist's strongest ally is critical thinking in terms of action and consequences. Every action has a consequence. The most important one is the one that has a good outcome.

POSITIONING FOR SAFETY, COMFORT, OR EXAMS

When the patient must spend a long period in the imaging department, it is the radiographer's duty to assist the patient to maintain normal body alignment for comfort and to maintain normal physiologic functioning. Proper long-term positioning should allow the patient to interact with those around them and accommodate their needs. Long-term positioning methods must be used to reduce pressure on bony prominences so as not to create a pressure ulcer.

CASE STUDY

The late afternoon shift was just beginning at a well-known medical center in one of the largest cities in the United States. A patient, who was 1-day postoperative brain surgery, was in the department for radiographic studies. The technologist explained the move from the gurney to the examining table to the patient. She assured the technologist that she was able to move. After locking the brakes on the gurney, the technologist went around the table to pull the patient onto the table. However, the patient was only able to move her upper body from the gurney to the table and not her lower body. Every time she pushed with her heels to try and move her hips over, the gurney moved slightly away from the table. The technologist held onto the patient's arm, but was unable to keep her from falling between the gurney and the table, causing her to strike her head against the corner as she fell.

Through the legal discoveries in this court case, it was determined that there were other technologists readily available outside the room. There was also a smooth transfer board hanging on the wall in the radiographic room.

ISSUES TO CONSIDER

1. What did the technologist do correctly? What went wrong with the gurney?
2. Once it became apparent that the patient was unable to accomplish the move as directed, what should have occurred?
3. Do you believe that the patient "was at fault" for informing the technologist that she could, in fact, move on her own? Why or why not?
4. Explain how this entire event could have been prevented if the technologist had used critical thinking skills. What are several ways that the study could have been performed without injury to the patient or the technologist?

There are several protective positions that allow for comfort. Patients in respiratory distress must not be left in a recumbent position for long. Place the patient in a **high-Fowler position** (Fig. 5-10A) in which the head is raised to an angle of 45° to 90° to avoid the patient becoming **dyspneic**. If this is not possible, a **semi-Fowler position** (Fig. 5-10B) may help alleviate respiratory distress. In this position, the patient's head is raised 15° to 30°.

Patients that may experience hypotension (low blood pressure) may need to have their head lowered so that their feet are higher. Known as the **Trendelenburg position** (Fig. 5-10C), it promotes venous return to the heart. If the table does not tilt down, a modified Trendelenburg position may be used by placing pillows or blocks under the patient's legs and feet. If a patient feels nauseated and may vomit, the patient should be placed in a recovery position, which is a modified lateral recumbent position with the top knee bent and forward to stop the patient from rolling onto the stomach. The recovery position (Fig. 5-10D) keeps patients from aspirating foreign material if they should vomit. Although this might seem like a **Sims position** used in lower GI procedures, the patient is not rolled slightly forward but is completely on the side. A Sims position requires the patient to be on the left side and rolled slightly forward, with both legs slightly bent but the top leg is forward of the bottom leg.

In the **supine position**, the patient's knees and hips should be slightly flexed. This takes the pressure off the patient's lower back. With the patient in a **lateral recumbent (side-lying)** position, consider the safety of the patient. Is it possible that the patient might roll off the radiographic table? If the patient must be left alone in this position for any reason, a gurney can be placed alongside the table, or a compression band can be used to keep the patient safe.

Skin Care

The radiographer is responsible for the care of the patient's skin or integumentary system while in the diagnostic imaging department. Skin breakdown can occur within a brief period (1 to 2 hours) and result in an ulcer that may take weeks or months to heal. Mechanical factors that may predispose the skin to break down are immobility, pressure, and shearing force.

Immobilizing a patient in one position for an extended period creates pressure on the skin that bears the patient's

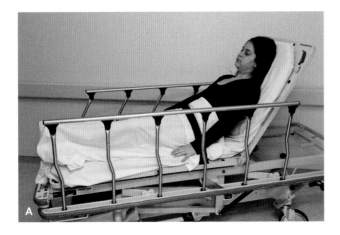
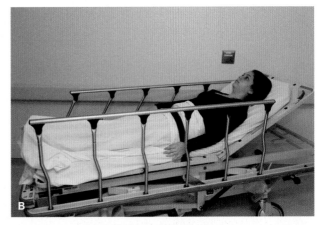
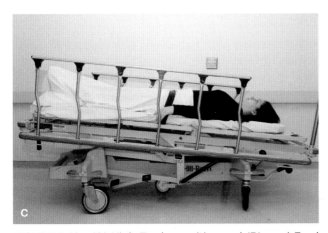
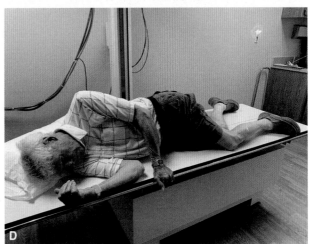

FIGURE 5-10 **(A)** High-Fowler position and **(B)** semi-Fowler position are both used to relieve respiratory distress. **(C)** Trendelenburg position is used when a patient's blood pressure drops. **(D)** Recovery position keeps a patient from aspirating vomitous.

weight. This, in turn, restricts capillary blood flow to that area and can result in **tissue necrosis**.

Moving a patient to or from an imaging table too rapidly or without adequately protecting the patient's skin may damage the external skin or underlying tissues because they are pulled over each other, creating a shearing force. This, too, may lead to tissue necrosis.

Another factor that contributes to skin breakdown is friction caused by movement back and forth on a rough or uneven surface, such as a wrinkled bedsheet. Allowing a patient to lie on a damp sheet or remain in a wet gown may lead to skin damage. Similarly, urine and fecal material that remain on the skin act as an irritant and are damaging to the skin.

Early signs that indicate imminent skin breakdown are blanching and a feeling of coldness over pressure areas. This condition is called **ischemia**. Ischemia is followed by heat and redness in the area because the blood rushes to the traumatized spot in an attempt to provide nourishment to the skin. This process is called *reactive hyperemia*. If, at the time of reactive hyperemia, the pressure on the threatened area is not relieved, the

tissues begin to necrose, and a small **ulceration** soon becomes visible. Ischemia and reactive hyperemia are difficult to observe in patients who are dark skinned. In these cases, the skin must be felt to assess any threat of damage. A shearing injury to the skin may cause it to appear bluish and bruised. If such an area is not cared for, necrosis and ulceration occur.

Persons who are most prone to skin breakdown are the malnourished, the elderly, and the chronically ill. A patient who is elderly and in poor health may have dehydrated skin, an accumulation of fluid in the tissues (edema), increased or decreased skin temperature, or a loss of subcutaneous fat that acts to protect the skin. Any of these factors can contribute to skin breakdown, and the radiographer must be particularly cautious when moving or caring for this type of patient.

Preventing Decubitus Ulcers

Protection against **decubitus ulcers** must always be a consideration when caring for patients in the diagnostic imaging department. The tables on which the patients must be placed for care are hard, and often the surface is unprotected. Areas most susceptible to decubitus ulcers are the scapulae, the sacrum, the trochanters, the knees, and the heels of the feet.

Although a patient is not likely to be kept on a radiographic table for long periods of time, the patient should be allowed to change position occasionally to keep pressure off the hips, knees, and heels. This can be done by placing a pillow or soft blanket under the patient or by turning the patient to a different position whenever possible. This is done in the usual hospital situation every 2 hours. If the patient is lying on a hard surface, such as the radiographic table, it should be done every 30 minutes. If a patient is perspiring profusely or is incontinent of urine or feces, make certain that the area is kept clean and dry, and take precautions when moving the patient to prevent skin abrasions.

Special precautions should be taken to protect the patient's feet and lower legs during a position change or transfer, particularly with an elderly patient because the skin is often extremely thin and easily torn. Shoes should protect the feet, and care should be taken to prevent bruising while the move is made. Circulatory impairment in the lower extremities is common, and the slightest bump may be the beginning of ulceration.

FALL PREVENTION

Patient falls are one of the most common hospital accidents. Patient rooms now have environmental devices such as cordless sensors that are found in the patient's bed. These sensors promptly alert caregivers when a patient tries to leave a bed. When getting a patient from a hospital bed into a wheelchair or onto a gurney, these alarms must be disconnected. The radiographer must always be on guard to prevent falls. No patient should be allowed to get out of a wheelchair or off a gurney or radiographic table without assistance from the radiographer or other health care worker.

Patients most prone to falls are the frail, the elderly, persons with neurologic deficits, persons who are weak and debilitated because of prolonged illness or lengthy preparations for procedures, persons with head trauma, persons with sensory deprivations, persons who have been medicated with sedating or psychoactive drugs, and confused patients. Adhere to the following rules to prevent falls:

1. Learn the condition of the patient and determine whether safety can be maintained while entering, remaining in, or leaving the diagnostic imaging department without assistance.
2. Keep floors clear of objects that may obstruct pathways.
3. Keep equipment such as gurneys, mobile radiographic machines, and wheelchairs in areas where they do not obstruct passageways.
4. Side rails must always be up when a patient is on a gurney.

5. A wheelchair must be locked if a patient is in it; a soft restraint may be needed if the patient is not reliable and may try to get up without assistance.
6. Patients returned to their hospital room must have the bed lowered and side rails up.

If it is decided that the patient is unable to walk safely into the radiography room, the technologist must assist the patient. Once the procedure is over, the patient must be assisted back to a waiting room, emergency department (ED), or other origination area. Never leave these patients alone. The risk of fall is high, and the technologist is held legally responsible under a tort.

CARE OF THE OUTPATIENT

A patient who comes to the radiology department as an outpatient is frequently required to remove all or some items of clothing and to put on a patient gown before a procedure or treatment can be performed. It is usually the radiographer who receives the patient and determines which items of clothing are to be removed. The patient's discomfort or embarrassment can be decreased if the situation is approached in a courteous and professional manner.

After the patient is taken to the specific dressing area, clearly explain how to put on the examining gown and point out where to go for the examination once prepared. Remember that not everyone knows that some types of examining gowns open at the back rather than at the front; this information should be part of the explanation. Doing this takes only a few moments, and it makes the patient feel more comfortable and eliminate any embarrassment when told to turn the gown around.

If it is permissible to leave clothing in the dressing room, explain this to the patient. Dressing room doors or cubicles should have hooks provided for the patient to hang up clothes. If the patient cannot leave the clothing in the dressing cubicle, make this part of the explanation. Many departments provide plastic bags with handles that are large enough to hold all clothes, shoes, and even purses. These bags allow patients to take their items with them. It is important that purses, jewelry, and other valuables should be treated with special care so that they are not lost or stolen.

Many female patients wear jewelry and/or carry a purse to the radiology department. The dressing rooms in most departments are not safe places to leave these items, and the patient may feel justifiably uneasy about leaving them there. Again, consider the patient's concern and explain what must be done with personal items to keep them safe.

Metal items, such as necklaces, rings, and watches, are not to be worn for particular diagnostic procedures and must be removed before beginning the procedure. An envelope or other container large enough to accommodate all such items should be offered to the patient. In the event that the items must be removed from the room, identifying information should be written down, and all items should be tagged and placed in the designated safety area. This procedure prevents losses that may result in inconvenience and expense to both the patient and the department. If the patient is allowed to wear the items into the radiography room for a short procedure (such as chest images), the patient should be allowed to hold the jewelry if possible. If this is not possible, place the jewelry in a cup, basin, or envelope and place the container in an area where the patient can see it.

Patients may have body piercings that are not visible. It is important to ask the patient if there is any jewelry or body piercings. If so, ask the patient to remove the jewelry (if possible) so that it is not visible on the radiographic image. If the patient refuses to do so, which may be likely for body piercings, especially if they are new, this must be noted on the request so that the radiologist can make this known in the report to the referring clinician.

Do not place a personal value on a patient's belongings. An item that may seem insignificant to others may be the patient's most treasured belonging. Every article of clothing or jewelry and the personal effects that a patient brings to the diagnostic imaging department should be treated with care.

Assisting the Patient to Dress and Undress

The patient may arrive in the diagnostic imaging department alone if coming from outside the hospital. The patient may need assistance in removing clothing. This may be necessary if the patient has an injured extremity, or is in a weakened condition. The patient may have a contracture of an extremity or poor eyesight. Whatever the problem, if the radiographer senses that the patient has difficulty undressing if left alone, then assistance should be offered and given as needed.

If a trauma patient is brought to the diagnostic imaging department from the ED, removing the clothing in the conventional manner may cause further injury or pain. It may be necessary to cut away garments that interfere with acceptable radiographs; however, clothing must not be cut without the patient's consent except in extreme emergencies. If the patient is unable to give consent, a family member should do so in writing. Most often, the clothing will have been removed in the ED before arriving in the imaging department.

A young patient accompanied by a family adult may be more relaxed if the adult helps with the dressing process. Explain to the adult how the child should be dressed for the procedure, arrange a meeting place, and leave them alone.

If a patient with a disability of the lower extremities must have assistance, do so in the following manner:

1. Remove the clothing from the upper body first. Place a long examining gown on the patient. Instruct the patient to loosen belt buckles, buttons, or hooks around the waist and slip the trousers over the hips. If the patient cannot do this, explain that you are going to help and then reach under the gown and pull the trousers down over the hips.
2. Have the patient sit down. Squat down in front of the patient and gently pull the clothing over the legs and feet to remove it. If the patient is not able to help, call for an assistant.

Some dresses may be removed in the same way. If this method is not practical, however, and the dress must be pulled over the woman's head, proceed as follows:

1. After removing the dress, have the patient sit down.
2. Place a draw sheet over the patient and then help her to remove her slip and brassiere.
3. Help her to put on an examining gown and then remove the draw sheet.

The following are steps to redress a patient with an injury to a lower extremity:

1. Slide the clothing (pants or skirt) over the feet and legs as far as the hips while the patient is sitting and still wearing an examining gown.
2. Have the patient stand and pull the clothing over the hips if it can be tolerated.
3. If the patient is not able to pull the clothing over the hips alone, have an assistant raise the patient off the chair so that you may slip the clothing over the hips and waist.
4. Remove the patient's arms from the sleeves of the gown and hold it over the chest. Carefully pull the shirt over the head, or put it on one sleeve at a time.
5. When the outside items of clothing are on the patient, remove the gown from under the clothes.

When changing the gown of a patient who has an injury or is paralyzed on one side, remove the gown from the unaffected side first. Then, with the patient covered by the soiled gown, place the clean gown first on the affected side and then on the unaffected side, pulling the soiled gown from under the clean one.

Always make sure that the patient is covered during the process as seen in Figure 5-11.

CALL OUT

When changing a disabled patient's gown, allow enough material to work with by removing the unaffected side first or by placing the gown on the affected side first.

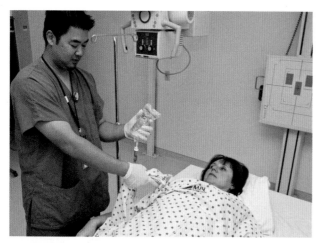

FIGURE 5-11 Make sure to keep the patient covered while placing a new gown on the patient.

USE OF IMMOBILIZERS

Immobilizers are defined as any physical or mechanical device, material, or equipment attached or adjacent to the person's body that the person cannot remove easily and that restricts freedom of movement or normal access to one's body. In radiography, the need for immobilization most often arises when radiographing pediatric patients. The most effective method of avoiding the need to inhibit movement of an adult patient is the use of communication. If a patient seems fearful or is striking out or moving in an unsafe manner, assure the patient that the procedure will be carried out as quickly and as comfortably as possible. If this does not reassure the patient, other less restrictive devices, such as soft, Velcro straps (Fig. 5-12A), sandbags (Fig. 5-12B and C), and sponges, may be used to remind the patient to refrain from moving. If immobilizers are to be used, be certain that they are being used to protect the patient's safety and that their use is the only alternative. TJC states that immobilizers should be used only after less restrictive measures have been attempted and have proved ineffective in protecting the patient. Immobilizers are used only when patients' behavior presents a danger to self or others and should never be used as a convenience for the staff.

There are various types of immobilizing devices that may be used for adult patients:

1. Ankle or wrist immobilizers (Fig. 5-13)
2. Immobilizing vest for keeping a patient in a wheelchair

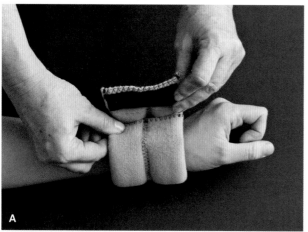

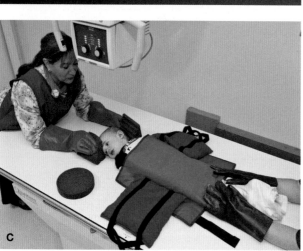

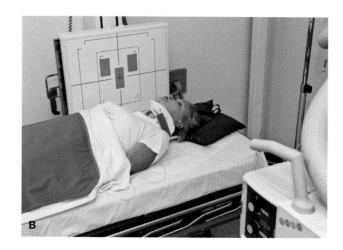

FIGURE 5-12 **(A)** A Velcro strap being placed snuggly but not tightly. **(B)** Sandbags help remind the adult patient to remain still. **(C)** Sandbags also assist in immobilizing the infant while holding the shield in place.

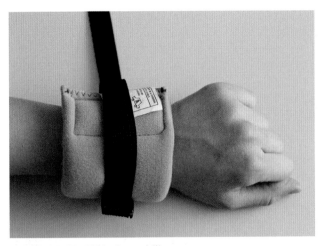

FIGURE 5-13 Wrist immobilizer.

3. Waist immobilizer, which keeps the patient safe on an examining table or in a bed, but allows the patient to change position

Reasons for application of immobilizers in the care of an adult patient include the following:

1. To control movement of an extremity when an IV infusion or diagnostic catheter is in place
2. To remind a patient who is sedated and having difficulty remembering to remain in a particular position
3. To prevent a patient who is unconscious, delirious, cognitively impaired, or confused from falling from a radiographic table or a gurney; from removing a tube or dressing that may be life sustaining; or from injury by impact with diagnostic imaging equipment.

When caring for someone who has been immobilized, explain the reason for using immobilizers to the patient and to anyone who may accompany the patient. After immobilizers are applied, do not leave the patient unattended. Remind the patient of the reason for the straps, and explain that the immobilizers are only temporary. As soon as the procedure is finished, the immobilizer is removed. A calm, reassuring manner often soothes an agitated or confused patient who has been immobilized. A patient in this state needs repeated orientation as well as a quiet and quick explanation to complete the procedure. Always apply immobilizers carefully and in the manner prescribed by the manufacturer of the device. The type of immobilizer to be used is dictated by need. All radiographers must document any application of immobilizers.

Remember this and use critical thinking skills to avoid the use of immobilizers if at all possible.

The following are rules for application of immobilizers:

1. The patient must be allowed as much mobility as is safely possible.

2. The areas of the body where immobilizers are applied must be padded to prevent injury to the skin beneath the device.
3. Normal anatomic position must be maintained.
4. Knots that do not become tighter with movement must be used (a half-knot is recommended; Fig. 5-14).
5. The immobilizer must be easy to remove quickly, if this is necessary.
6. Neither circulation nor respiration must be impaired by the immobilizer.
7. If leg immobilizers are necessary, wrist immobilizers must also be applied to prevent the patient from either unfastening the device or, in an attempt to leave the radiographic table or gurney, accidentally becoming entangled.

For young patients such as toddlers, tape or Velcro straps are an option to hold the hand of a child flat while sitting in a parent's lap. The use of tape comes with precautions, however. Try not to place the sticky surface of the tape directly onto the skin. Instead, fold the tape in half lengthwise as seen in Figure 5-15A and B, then twist it so the tape can be adhered to a solid surface (Fig. 5-15C). Remember that adhesive tape hurts when removed from skin. Stockinettes are an excellent means of securing the arms of a pediatric patient above the head. Because stockinettes are stretchable and come in a roll, they can be cut to any length.

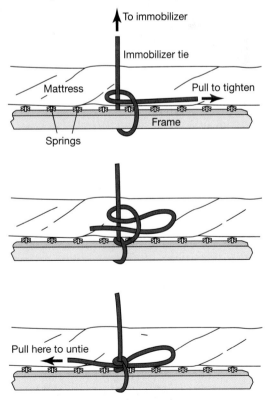

FIGURE 5-14 Following this sequence results in tying a half-bow knot. The knot remains secure until the free end is pulled.

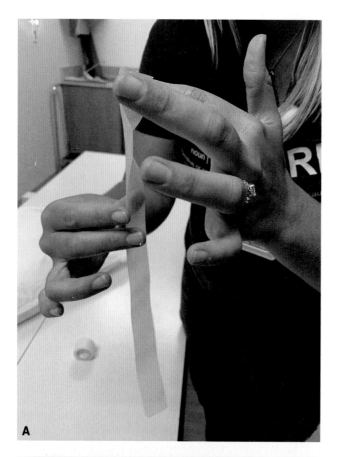

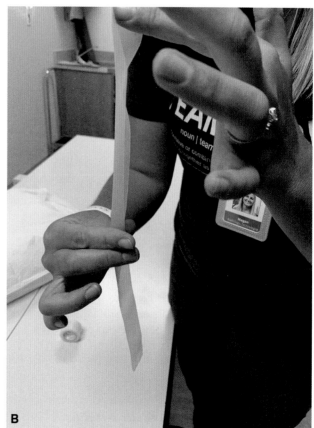

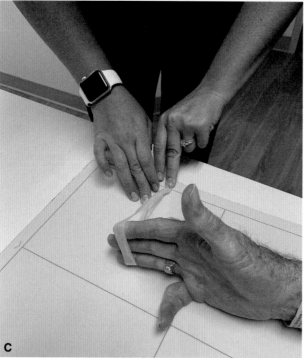

FIGURE 5-15 (A, B) When using tape to secure a body part, be sure to put the sticky sides of the tape together so that it does not adhere to the skin. **(C)** The tape can now be twisted to adhere it to the table or the image receptor (IR).

Summary

1. Safety in the imaging department is critical for the patient as well as the employee.
   a. Areas to consider are environmental safety through OSHA, EPA, and the National Commission on Radiation (NCR).
   b. The radiographer is responsible for reporting frayed cords and other items that present a fire hazard.
      i. Know the locations of fire extinguishers, how to evacuate patients, and phone numbers to report a fire.
   c. The MR department has safety zones that must be adhered to in order to prevent injury from flying metal objects.
   d. Hazardous materials must be stored and disposed of in a manner indicated on the MSDSs.
2. Evaluating patient needs includes understanding the social determinants of health (poor socioeconomic areas have less access to health care) and using critical thinking skills to assess patient status.
   a. Patient assessment can be performed by data collection and analysis; planning and implementing the plan; and then evaluating the outcome
      i. Subjective data come from the patient and objective data are what is seen, heard, or felt by the health care worker.
   b. Pain assessment in the radiography department is done by questioning and interviewing the patient as to location, duration, and alleviating or aggravating factors.
3. Correct body mechanics must always be used to prevent injury to the radiographer.
   a. When moving or lifting, keep the weight close to the body and maintain a firm base of body support.
      i. This is accomplished by having the feet slightly spread out and knees flexed.
      ii. Never twist or bend the body at the waist when lifting a heavy load.
      iii. Weight should be pulled, not pushed. Use arm and leg muscles, not the spine for lifting.
4. When moving and lifting a patient, assess the patient and resolve potential problems before beginning the transfer.
   a. After identifying the patient with two identifiers, explain the move to the patient and notify the ward personnel when taking a patient to or from a hospital room.
   b. The use of enough assistants and equipment such as a smooth mover facilitates the move and protects personnel and the patient from possible injury.
   c. When a patient is on the radiographic table or on a gurney in the diagnostic imaging department, the body must be in good alignment. If the patient is moved to a particular position for an examination, restore correct body alignment as soon as possible.
5. Three ways of moving patients are by gurney, by wheelchair, or by ambulation.
   a. Never walk a patient from a hospital room to the radiology department for safety reasons.
   b. Make sure all equipment is in working order and lock the brakes before beginning the transfer.
   c. Provide for the patient's safety by using safety belts on both the gurney and the wheelchair.
   d. Always move the patient toward the strongest side.
   e. When moving by gurney, use adequate assistance and transfer equipment to aid in the move for safety reasons to protect both the radiographer and the patient.
6. Take care to prevent the patient's skin from being damaged through immobility, pressure, shearing force, or friction.
   a. Patients most susceptible to skin breakdown are the malnourished, the elderly, and the chronically ill. Injury may result in a decubitus ulcer that can take months to heal.
   b. Patients must be kept clean and dry. It is the radiographer's duty to change the disabled patient's gown and covering if they become wet or soiled.
7. When an outpatient arrives in the diagnostic imaging department, it is often necessary for that patient to undress entirely or partially for the diagnostic examination or treatment. Always show the patient where and how to do so in a sensitive manner to spare the patient embarrassment.
8. It is the responsibility of the radiographer to provide the patient with a safe place for personal belongings. Remember that the patient may treasure an article of clothing or jewelry that may not seem valuable.
9. The use of immobilizers must be done only as a last resort.
   a. Most often, it is the pediatric patient which needs immobilization; however, there are times when immobilizers must be used for the safety of the adult patient.
   b. When immobilizers are required, apply them according to the manufacturer's directions and the policy of the institution.
   c. Do not immobilize a patient without an order by a physician. A patient that is immobilized should be attended to at all times and the immobilizer released at least every 2 hours.
   d. Follow the correct manner of documenting immobilization use.

CHAPTER 5 REVIEW QUESTIONS

1. Written instructions for handling hazardous material, safe use of the product, and cleanup and disposal directions are called:
   a. Package inserts
   b. HIPAA
   c. MSDS
   d. Hazardous warning systems

2. Patient transfers from gurney to x-ray table and back to gurney should be performed:
   a. By the radiographer only if the patient thinks they can move
   b. By two or more radiographers to ensure patient and radiographer safety
   c. By the radiographer only if the department is short staffed
   d. By the radiographer only so as not to frighten the patient

3. The most effective means of reducing friction when moving a patient is by:
   a. Placing the patient's arms across the chest and using a pull sheet
   b. Pushing rather than pulling the patient
   c. Rolling the patient to a prone position
   d. Asking the patient to cooperate by moving alone

4. Toxic chemicals may be:
   a. Poured down the sink in the restroom
   b. Poured down any sink as long as it doesn't go into the ground
   c. Disposed of only as specified by the MSDS
   d. Capped in a container and thrown in the trash

5. A patient explains to the radiographer what type of pain is being experienced, which is known as:
   a. Objective data
   b. Subjective data
   c. Data analysis
   d. Plan implementation

6. Pain control is not within the radiographer's scope of practice and should not be a concern.
   a. True
   b. False

7. Patients most prone to falls are: (Circle all that apply)
   a. The frail or elderly
   b. The person who is confused
   c. Persons who have been given a psychoactive drug
   d. Persons with sensory deficits

8. The leading cause of work-related injuries in the field of health care is:
   a. Bumping into misplaced equipment
   b. Overexposure to radiation
   c. Infection owing to poor handwashing techniques
   d. Abuse of the spine when moving and lifting patients

9. When transporting a patient back to the hospital room, some *safety* measures to be used are: (Circle all that apply)
   a. Place the side rails up, the bed in the low position, and call bell at hand.
   b. Inform the nursing staff that the patient has been returned to the room.
   c. Give the patient something to eat or drink.
   d. Be sure that the TV is in place for the patient's viewing.

10. Correct body mechanics include: (Circle all that apply)
    a. Abdomen sucked in
    b. Buttocks normal and low
    c. Chest up
    d. Head up and chin out
    e. Feet apart with equal weight distribution
    f. Knees slightly bent

11. The radiographer can leave a patient who is getting out of a wheelchair.
    a. True
    b. False

12. TJC says it is acceptable to use immobilizers if all other alternatives have been exhausted.
    a. True
    b. False

Vital Signs, Laboratory Tests, and Oxygen Administration

6

OBJECTIVES

After studying this chapter, the student will be able to:

1. Define vital signs and explain when assessment should be done.

2. List the rates of temperature, pulse, pulse oximetry, respiration, and blood pressure that are considered to be within normal limits for a child and an adult, male and female.

3. Describe any interfering factors that affect the normal values of vital signs.

4. Identify sites and methods available for measuring body temperature.

5. Identify the most common types of oxygen administration equipment and explain any potential hazards.

6. Describe all equipment used to monitor blood pressure, take temperature, and administer oxygen.

7. Accurately monitor pulse rate, respiration, and blood pressure.

8. Explain the purpose of basic laboratory values such as blood urea nitrogen, creatinine, and glomerular filtration rate.

KEY TERMS

Bradycardia: A slow heart rate of less than 60 beats per minute

Chronic obstructive pulmonary disease (COPD): Disease of the lungs in which inspiratory and expiratory lung capacity is diminished

Cyanosis: A condition in which the blood does not supply enough oxygen to the body, causing a bluish tone to the lips and fingertips

Dehydration: Excessive loss of fluids from the body causing effects such as headaches and constipation

Diastolic: The blood pressure reading that occurs during the relaxation of the ventricles (the lowest number of the reading)

Dyspnea: Difficult breathing resulting from insufficient airflow to the lungs

Hypercapnia: Carbon dioxide being retained in the arterial blood

Hypertension: High blood pressure in which long-term pressure against artery walls may eventually cause heart problems

Hypotension: Low blood pressure that may cause dizziness or fatigue

Hypothalamus: The ventral and medial region of the diencephalon of the brain

Hypoxemia: Low levels of oxygen in the blood

Korotkoff sounds: Extraneous sounds heard during the taking of blood pressure and may be a tapping, knocking, or swishing sound

Orthostatic hypotension: A form of low blood pressure that occurs when the blood pressure quickly

drops upon standing from sitting or recumbent positions. It is also known as postural hypotension.

Sphygmomanometer: A blood pressure cuff

Systolic: The blood pressure reading taken during the contraction of the ventricles while the blood is in the arteries (the highest number of the reading)

Tachycardia: A fast heart rate of more than 100 beats per minute

Tympanic: Bell-like; resonance pertaining to tympanum

Vital signs: Assessment of the patient's blood pressure, temperature, pulse, pulse oximetry, and respiration

Volatile: Easily vaporized or evaporated; unstable or explosive in nature

INTRODUCTION

Many imaging departments in large facilities employ radiology nurses and do not rely on radiologic technologists to perform routine monitoring of patient's vital signs. However, there are still some hospitals that do not have the luxury of nursing staff to perform these routine assessments of the patient or to operate ancillary equipment. All technologists and student technologists must have the knowledge and understanding of how to monitor and record vital signs. Recording vital sign information in the patient's medical record or on the radiology requisition is an important part of the care of the patient.

Technologists must have an understanding of how to operate the oxygen administration equipment and what the oxygen flow rate should be for the different conditions the patient might have. Because oxygen is a potentially toxic and **volatile** substance, the radiographer needs to understand the precautions that are to be taken when assisting with oxygen administration.

A physician's order is not required for vital signs to be measured. Unless a registered nurse is present to do so, vital signs should be taken by the radiographer when a patient is brought into the diagnostic imaging department for any invasive diagnostic procedure or treatment, before and after the patient receives medication, any time the patient's general condition suddenly changes, or if the patient reports nonspecific symptoms of physical distress, such as simply not feeling well or feeling "different."

MEASURING VITAL SIGNS

Taking a patient's **vital signs** is an important part of a physical assessment and includes measurement of body temperature, pulse, pulse oximetry, respiration, and blood pressure. In the event of an emergency situation, the technologist must be prepared by knowing how to measure each of the vital signs and know what those readings mean. It is also important to learn what the patient's vital signs are under normal circumstances as everyone has some variation from what is considered normal for a particular age group. After the baseline vital signs for a patient have been established, it is easy to determine whether the patient's current vital signs are deviating from that of the baseline. Vital signs must be measured if the patient comes to the diagnostic imaging department for an extensive procedure. Changes in vital signs can be an indication of a problem or a potential problem. As a part of the assessment of vital signs, the technologist should be aware of the patient as a whole; the color and temperature of the skin (cool or clammy), the level of consciousness and anxiety, and the patient's communication provide additional information prior to a procedure.

It is the responsibility of the radiographer to ensure that there is a functioning sphygmomanometer, a stethoscope, and the equipment necessary to administer oxygen in each diagnostic imaging room at the beginning of each shift. Emergencies requiring these items arise, and that is not the time to look for this equipment.

Body Temperature

Body temperature is the physiologic balance between the heat produced in body tissues and heat lost to the environment. It must remain stable if the body's cellular and enzymatic activities are to function efficiently. Changes in the body's physiology occur when the body temperature fluctuates even 2 to 3° F (1.2 to 1.8° C). Body temperature is controlled by a small structure in the basal region of the diencephalon of the brain called the **hypothalamus**, sometimes referred to as the body's thermostat.

Chemical processes that result from metabolic activity produce body heat. When the body's metabolism increases, more heat is produced. When it decreases, less heat is produced. Both normal and abnormal conditions in the body can produce changes in body temperature. The environment, time of day, gender, age, weight, hormone levels, emotions, physical exercise, digestion of food, disease, and injury are some factors that influence body temperature. The body's cellular functions and cardiopulmonary demands change in proportion to temperature variations outside of normal limits.

A patient whose body temperature is elevated above normal limits is said to have fever or *pyrexia*. Fever indicates a disturbance in the heat-regulating centers of the body, usually as a result of a disease process. As the body temperature increases, the body's demand for oxygen increases. Symptoms of fever are increased pulse and respiratory rate, general discomfort or aching, flushed dry skin that feels hot to the touch, chills (occasionally), and loss of appetite. Fevers that are allowed to remain very high for a prolonged period can cause irreparable damage to the central nervous system (CNS).

The normal body temperature remains almost constant; however, a variation of 0.5 to 1° F (0.3 to 0.6° C) above or below the average is within normal limits. The normal body temperature of infants and children up to 13 years of age varies somewhat from these readings. Average body temperatures for each group of individuals are found in Display 6-1.

A person with a body temperature below normal limits is said to have *hypothermia*, which may be indicative of a pathologic process. Hypothermia may also be induced medically to reduce a patient's need for oxygen. It is rare for a person to survive with a body temperature between 105.8° F (41° C) and 111.2° F (44° C) or below 93.2° F (34° C).

DISPLAY 6-1

Normal Vital Sign Ranges for Groups of Individuals

Temperature

Adult	97.8-99° F
Child (5-13 years)	97.8-98.6° F
Infant (3 months to 3 years)	99-99.7° F

Pulse

Adult	60-90 beats per minute
Child (4-10 years)	90-100 beats per minute
Infant	12 beats per minute

Respiration

Adult	15-20 breaths per minute
Infant	30-60 breaths per minute

Blood pressure

Adult	90-120 systolic over 50-70 diastolic
Adolescents	85-130 systolic over 45-85 diastolic

Measuring Body Temperature

There were four areas of the body in which temperature was commonly measured: the oral site, the tympanic site, the rectal site, and the axillary site. With changing technology, the oral and rectal sites are not as common and have been replaced by the temporal site. The site selected for measuring body temperature must be chosen with care depending on the patient's age, state of mind, and ability to cooperate in the procedure. Because the reading might vary depending on where it is measured, be sure to specify the site used when reporting the reading. Temperature readings are reported in most health care facilities as follows:

- An oral temperature of 98.6° F is written 98.6 O.
- A tympanic temperature of 97.6° F is written 97.6 T.
- A temporal temperature of 97.6° F is written 97.6 Tm.
- An axillary temperature of 97.6° F is written 97.6 Ax.
- A rectal temperature of 99.6° F is written 99.6 R.

Whatever method of measuring body temperature is chosen, the radiographer must assemble the necessary equipment and abide by medically aseptic technique (such as washing the hands and wearing gloves if there is a possibility of coming in contact with blood or other body fluids).

Oral Temperature Oral digital thermometers use heat sensors to measure body temperature. It is the most effective method to get an accurate reading on adults and for children over the age of 4 if they are able to keep their mouth closed around the thermometer. The average temperature reading is 98.6° F (37° C). The thermometer consists of a probe that is placed under the patient's tongue and held in place until the instrument signals that it has registered a temperature (Fig. 6-1). The temperature of the mouth may change the temperature registered on the thermometer.

Tympanic Temperature The **tympanic** membrane thermometer (also called an *aural thermometer*) is a small, handheld device that measures the temperature of the blood vessels in the tympanic membrane of the ear (Fig. 6-2). This provides a reading close to the core body temperature if correctly placed. The patient may be sitting upright or may be in a supine position. In the clinical setting, this is a fast and easy method to obtain an accurate temperature reading of the patient in the diagnostic imaging department.

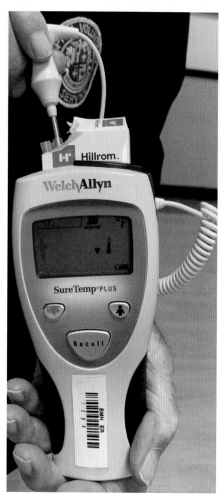

FIGURE 6-1 Digital oral thermometer.

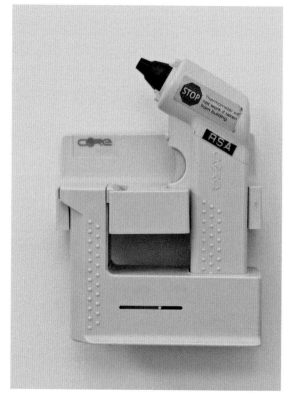

FIGURE 6-2 Tympanic membrane thermometer.

Axillary Temperature Use of the axillary site is the safest method of measuring body temperature because it is noninvasive. It is particularly useful when measuring an infant's temperature. Unfortunately, the time and precision of placement needed to obtain an accurate reading make this method somewhat unreliable. When it is necessary to measure temperature using the axillary site, an electronic or disposable thermometer may be used. The average axillary temperature is 97.6 to 98° F (36.4 to 36.7° C).

Rectal Temperature Rectal temperature is taken at the anal opening to the rectum. The average rectal temperature is 99.6° F (37.5° C). The rectal site is considered to provide the most reliable measurement of body temperature because factors that can alter the results are minimized. It is also in close proximity to the pelvic viscera or "core" temperature of the body. Body temperature should not be measured rectally if the patient is restless or has rectal pathology such as tumors or hemorrhoids. Normally, a rectal temperature is only taken on infant patients and not on adults.

Temporal Temperature There are two methods of taking a temporal temperature: (1) scanner (Fig. 6-3) and (2) touchless (Fig. 6-4). The scanner method is more accurate than the touchless method, but both types are noninvasive, fast, and easy methods of obtaining a body temperature.

The scanner works through a process of measuring the balance between tissues warmed by arterial blood (from behind the ear) and tissues that are cooled as a result of heat loss (from the forehead). Temporal temperatures are accurate to within 1° F of the oral method.

Contactless Temperature Recognition The contactless scanners are mounted on kiosks and automatically read normal versus abnormal body temperature in seconds (Fig. 6-5A). These thermometers are most often used in institutions where the patient walks up to the scanner, placing the face within the boundaries indicated on the scanner (Fig. 6-5B). Within seconds, the thermal detection technology scans the internal body temperature, identifying and recording abnormal temperatures. During times when temperatures must be taken on every individual entering a facility, this is the best and most accurate method of obtaining normal or abnormal results. These scanners do not give an actual temperature reading but rather an indication of normal or abnormal.

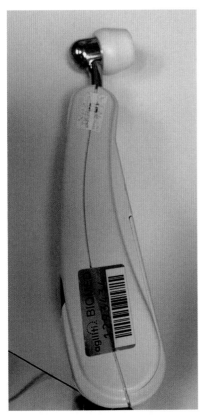

FIGURE 6-3 Temporal thermometer that scans the forehead to detect the patient's temperature.

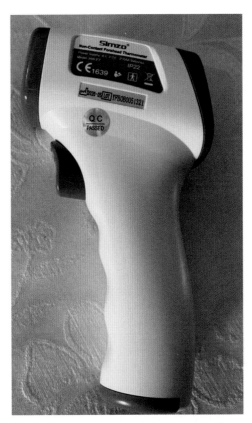

FIGURE 6-4 Temporal thermometer is contactless and does not touch the patient's head.

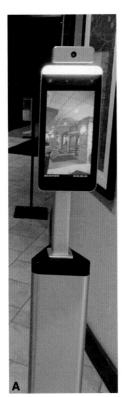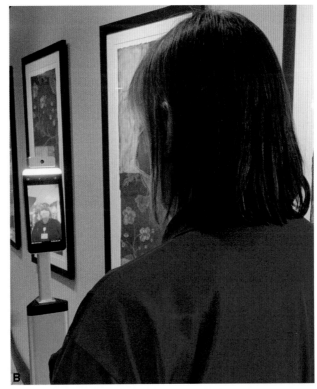

FIGURE 6-5 **(A)** Contactless temperature recognition scanner. **(B)** The patient aligns their face within the monitor of the scanner, which then detects the body temperature as normal or abnormal.

PROCEDURE

Taking a Tympanic Temperature

1. Place a clean sheath or cone on the probe that is to be inserted into the external auditory canal.

2. Place the probe into the external auditory canal and hold it firmly in place (Fig. 6-6) until the temperature registers automatically on the meter held in the nondominant hand.

3. Remove the probe and read the indicator.

4. Remove the probe's cover and dispose it correctly. Remove any gloves and wash hands.

5. Record the reading. Immediately report any abnormal temperature to the radiologist in charge of the procedure.

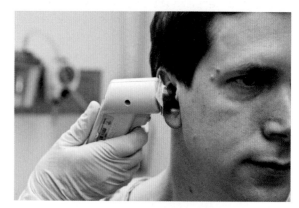

FIGURE 6-6 Measuring temperature with a tympanic thermometer. The probe is placed inside the external auditory canal.

PROCEDURE

Taking a Temporal Temperature

1. Obtain the instrument to be used. If it is a scanner-type thermometer, place a protective cap on the probe as appropriate.

2. Place the scanner thermometer in the center of the forehead and slide it to either the right or left in a straight line toward the ear (Fig. 6-7).

3. Gently touch the thermometer behind the ear closest to the thermometer until the instrument beeps indicating it has reached a measurement.

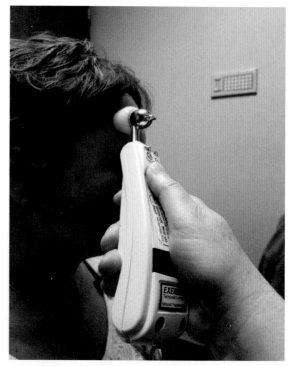

FIGURE 6-7 Measuring temperature with a scanning-style temporal thermometer. If a cap is not used to protect the scanning head, it must be cleaned after use.

4. With a contactless thermometer, hold the instrument close to the center of the forehead and press the start button. The thermometer reads the temperature being emitted by the patient's forehead (Fig. 6-8).

5. Remove the scanner and read the temperature.

6. Record the reading.

7. Dispose of the protective cap as appropriate.

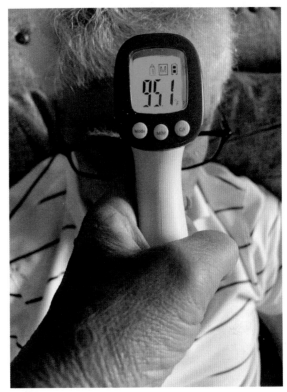

FIGURE 6-8 Measuring temperature with a contactless style temporal thermometer. The temperature is digitally displayed on the front.

Pulse

As the heart beats, blood is pumped in a pulsating fashion into the arteries. This results in a throb, or pulsation, of the artery. At areas of the body in which arteries are superficial, the pulse can be felt by gently pushing the artery lying beneath the skin against a solid surface such as bone. The pulse can be detected most easily in the following areas of the body:

- *Apical pulse*: over the apex of the heart (heard with a stethoscope) (Fig. 6-9A)
- *Radial pulse*: over the radial artery at the wrists at the base of the thumb (Fig. 6-9B)
- *Carotid pulse*: over the carotid artery at the front of the neck (Fig. 6-9C)
- *Femoral pulse*: over the femoral artery in the groin (Fig. 6-9D)
- *Popliteal pulse*: at the posterior surface of the knee (Fig. 6-9E)
- *Temporal pulse*: over the temporal artery in front of the ear (Fig. 6-9F)
- *Dorsalis pedis pulse* (*pedal*): at the top of the feet in line with the groove between the extensor tendons of the great and the second toe (may be congenitally absent) (Fig. 6-9G)

- *Posterior tibial pulse*: on the inner side of the ankles (Fig. 6-9H)
- *Brachial pulse*: in the groove between the biceps and the triceps muscles above the elbow at the antecubital fossa (Fig. 6-9I)

The pulse rate is usually the same as the heart rate. The pulse rate is rapid if the blood pressure is low and slower if the blood pressure is high. The patient who is losing blood has an unusually rapid pulse rate and a very low blood pressure. This occurs because the body knows that it is not getting enough blood to the body's organs. Therefore, the heart pumps harder to get more blood out to the body. The normal average pulse rate in an adult man or woman in a resting state is between 60 and 90 beats per minute. The normal average pulse rate for an infant is 120 beats per minute. A child from 4 to 10 years of age has a normal average pulse rate of 90 to 100 beats per minute. For the normal values for each group of patients, refer to Display 6-1.

Assessment of the Pulse

The pulse rate is a rapid and relatively efficient means of assessing cardiovascular function. **Tachycardia** is an abnormally rapid heart rate (over 100 beats per minute), and **bradycardia** is an abnormally slow heart rate (below

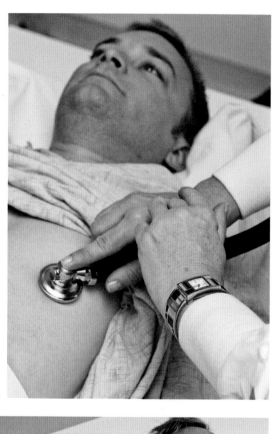

A

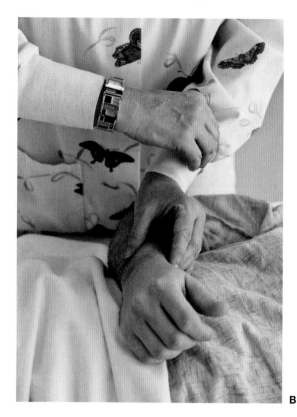

B

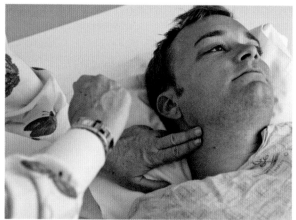

C

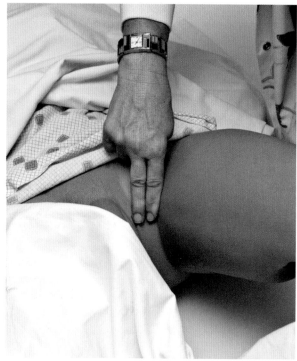

D

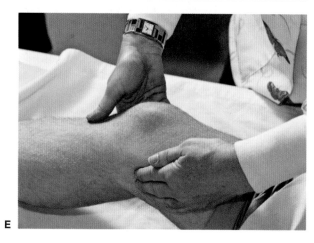

E

FIGURE 6-9 **(A)** Apical pulse. **(B)** Radial pulse.
(C) Carotid pulse. **(D)** Femoral pulse. **(E)** Popliteal pulse.

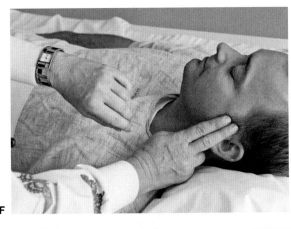
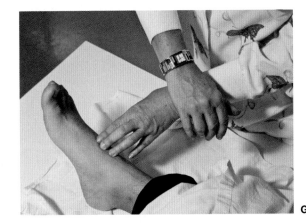
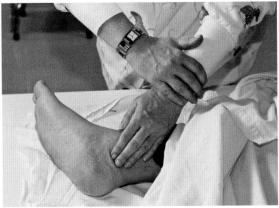
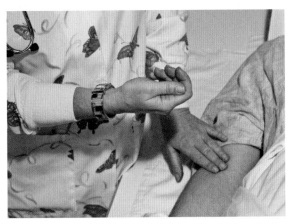

FIGURE 6-9 *(Continued)* **(F)** Temporal pulse. **(G)** Dorsalis pedis pulse (pedal). **(H)** Posterior tibial pulse. **(I)** Brachial pulse.

60 beats per minute). All technologists and students should be prepared to make this assessment before beginning any invasive diagnostic imaging procedure in order to establish a baseline reading. It must be reassessed frequently until the procedure is complete and the patient leaves the department. The radial pulse is usually the most accessible and can be taken conveniently on an adult patient. It should be counted for one full minute. If there is any irregularity in the radial pulse rate, take the apical pulse. The carotid pulse is also monitored if the patient's radial pulse is inaccessible.

For infants and children, the apical pulse is the most accurate for cardiovascular assessment. The femoral, popliteal, and pedal pulses are assessed bilaterally if peripheral blood flow is to be assessed.

When assessing pulse rate, report the strength and regularity of the beat as well as the number of beats per minute. The normal rhythm of the pulse beat is regular, with equal time intervals between beats. The pressure of the fingers should not obliterate the pulse. When even the slightest pressure of the fingers causes this to happen, report the pulse as weak or thready. If the beat is irregular, unusually rapid, unusually slow, or unusually weak, immediately report this to the physician in charge of the patient. Changes in pulse rate during a procedure must also be reported.

Equipment needed to assess the pulse includes a watch with a second hand and a pad and pencil to record the findings. For monitoring the apical pulse, a stethoscope that has been cleaned is needed.

PROCEDURE

Assessing Pulses

1. After completing the necessary hand washing, place the index finger and middle finger flat over the artery chosen for assessment.

2. When the throbbing of the artery is felt, count the throbs for 1 minute.

(continued)

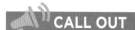

CALL OUT

Be careful not to press too hard with the finger or the pulse will be compressed and not felt.

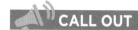

CALL OUT

Do not use the thumb to count the pulse because it has its own pulse.

PROCEDURE

Taking an Apical Pulse

1. Clean the earpieces and the bladder of the stethoscope with alcohol wipes and then wash hands.

2. Place the patient in a semi-Fowler or supine position.

3. Drape the patient so that the lower chest area is exposed.

4. Place the bladder of the stethoscope at the fifth intercostal space 5 cm from the left sternal margin (the nipple of a man's breast can be used as a landmark for 5 cm).

5. If the beat cannot be heard, move the stethoscope slightly in every direction until it can be heard.

6. Count the beats for 1 minute and assess for regular rate and rhythm.

7. Remove the stethoscope and cover the patient. Clean the earpieces and bladder again with alcohol.

8. After completing a 30-second hand wash, record the pulse rate and report any irregularities.

The pedal, popliteal, and femoral pulses are often monitored during special diagnostic imaging procedures to ascertain that the patient's circulatory status in the lower extremities is satisfactory. When this is done, the pulses are not always counted. Instead, they are palpated and assessed as present and strong, weak, regular, or irregular. Mark the areas on the body with a marking pen where the pedal and popliteal pulses are palpated so that they may be rechecked as necessary.

When recording pulse rate, use the abbreviation P for pulse and AP for apical pulse. For example, P 80 equals a pulse rate of 80 beats per minute. AP 88 equals an apical pulse rate of 88 beats per minute. Record any abnormalities and immediately report these to the patient's physician.

Respiration

The function of the respiratory system is to exchange oxygen and carbon dioxide between the external environment and the blood circulating in the body. Oxygen is taken into the lungs during inspiration. It passes through the bronchi, into the bronchioles, and then into the alveoli, which are the gas exchange units of the lungs. Oxygen is transported to the body tissues by the arterial blood. Deoxygenated blood is returned to the right side of the heart through the venous system. It is then pumped into the right and left pulmonary arteries and reoxygenated by passing through the capillary network on the alveolar surfaces. The blood is then returned to the left side of the heart through the pulmonary veins for recirculation. During this process, carbon dioxide is also deposited in the alveoli and exhaled from the lungs during expiration.

The average rate of respiration (one inspiration and one expiration) for an adult man or woman is 15 to 20 breaths per minute, and for an infant it is 30 to 60 breaths per minute. Respiration of fewer than 10 breaths per minute for an adult may result in **cyanosis**, apprehension, restlessness, and a change in the level of consciousness because the supply of oxygen is inadequate to meet the needs of the body.

Normal respirations are quiet, effortless, and uniform. Medication, illness, exercise, or age may increase or decrease respirations, depending on the metabolic need for oxygen in the body. When patients are using more than the normal effort to breathe, they can be described as dyspneic or as having **dyspnea**.

Assessment of Respiration

As with other vital signs, it is important to establish a baseline respiratory rate because changes in respiration are often an early sign of a threatened physiologic state. Remember, however, that the rate of respiration increases with physical exercise or emotion. Respiration is also quicker in newborns and infants. When assessing respiration, observe the rate, depth, quality, and pattern.

When recording respiration, use the abbreviation "R." R 20 equals 20 rises and falls of the chest wall. Any abnormalities or deviations from the baseline should be reported to the physician in charge of the patient and recorded; for example, *R 28, shallow and labored.*

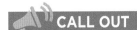

CALL OUT

Patients who are aware of respiration assessment may alter their normal pattern of breathing.

PROCEDURE

Assessing Respiration

1. *Keep the patient in a seated or supine position.* The patient should be in a quiet state and be unaware that the breathing pattern is being observed. The most convenient time to count respirations is immediately after the pulse count. This gives the appearance of continuing to count the pulse rate and helps to keep the patient unaware of the respiratory movement. Patients who become aware that respiration is being assessed may consciously or unconsciously alter the pattern.

2. *Observe the chest wall for symmetry of movement.* There should be an even rise and fall of the chest with no involvement of muscles other than the diaphragm. In the adult patient, abdominal, intercostal, or neck muscle involvement in breathing is a sign of respiratory distress and should be noted. Other signs of respiratory distress in an adult patient include the need to assume a sitting position or the need to lean forward and place the arms over the back of a chair or on the knees in order to breathe easily.

3. *Observe skin color.* Cyanosis, or bluish discoloration, is easily observed around the mouth, in the gums, in nail beds, or in the earlobes. Cyanosis may be a sign of respiratory distress.

4. *Count the number of times the patient's chest rises and falls for 1 full minute.* An easy way to count respirations is to cross the patient's arm across the chest and count the rise and fall of the arm.

Blood Pressure

In general terms, pressure is defined as the product of flow times resistance. Blood pressure is the amount of blood flow ejected from the left ventricle of the heart during systole and the amount of resistance the blood meets because of systemic vascular resistance. Maintenance of blood pressure depends on peripheral resistance, pumping action of the heart, blood volume, blood viscosity, and the elasticity of the vessel walls.

If the volume of blood decreases because of hemorrhage or dehydration, the blood pressure falls because of a diminished amount of fluid in the arteries. Fluid or blood replacement reverses the problem.

The number of red blood cells (RBCs) in the blood plasma determines the viscosity of the blood. With an increased number, the blood thickens or becomes more viscous and, subsequently, increases the blood pressure.

The arteries are normally elastic in nature; however, age or buildup of atherosclerotic plaque reduces the flexibility of the arteries and increases blood pressure.

The peripheral blood vessels distribute blood ejected into the circulatory system to the various body organs. When the peripheral blood vessels are in normal physiologic state, they are partially contracted. If this normal physiologic state is changed because of changes in environmental factors such as heat or cold, medication, disease, or other obstructive conditions, peripheral blood vessel resistance may increase. This increase causes an increase in blood pressure. Conversely, if the peripheral blood vessel resistance declines, this causes a decrease in blood pressure.

Blood pressure normally varies with age, gender, physical development, body position, time of day, and health status. As a person ages, the blood pressure usually increases as the body systems that control blood pressure deteriorate.

Physiologic factors that may increase blood pressure are increased cardiac output, increased peripheral vascular resistance, increased blood volume, increased blood viscosity, and decreased arterial elasticity. Physiologic factors that decrease blood pressure are decreased cardiac output, decreased peripheral vascular resistance, decreased blood volumes, decreased blood viscosity, and increased arterial elasticity.

Blood pressure is usually lower in the morning after a night of sleep than later in the day after activity. Blood pressure increases after a large intake of food. Emotions and strenuous activity usually cause systolic blood pressure to increase.

Men usually have higher blood pressure than women. Infants generally have higher blood pressure than adults, and adolescents have the lowest overall blood pressure. Because the range of blood pressure varies in these age groups, measurements for infants and children should be taken in series.

The instrument used to measure blood pressure is called a **sphygmomanometer**. Two numbers, read in millimeters of mercury (mm Hg), are recorded when reporting blood pressure: systolic pressure and diastolic pressure. The **systolic** reading is the highest point reached during contraction of the left ventricle of the heart as it pumps blood into the aorta. The **diastolic** pressure is the lowest point to which the pressure drops during relaxation of the ventricles and indicates the minimal pressure exerted against the arterial walls continuously.

According to the National Heart, Lung, and Blood Institute, for men and women, normal blood pressure is anything below 120 mm Hg for systolic pressure and 80 mm Hg for diastolic pressure. Adolescent patients' blood pressure ranges from 85 to 130 mm Hg systolic and 45 to 85 mm Hg diastolic. Adult patients who fall

into a **hypertensive** stage 1 have a blood pressure of 130 to 139 mm Hg/80 to 89 mm Hg. Hypertensive stage 2 reading is 140/90 or higher. Patients in crisis have blood pressures over 180/120. If a radiographer encounters a patient with these readings, help must be sought immediately. A patient is considered **hypotensive** if the systolic reading is consistently less than 90 mm Hg. These numbers are only a guide, and concern should not be extreme if a measurement falls outside this guide for a single episode.

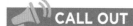
CALL OUT

Radiographers must be aware of a condition known as orthostatic hypotension that occurs when a patient has been recumbent for a lengthy period of time, causing the blood pressure to be low, and the patient may faint upon standing.

Pulse pressure is the difference between the systolic and the diastolic blood pressure and is an indicator of the stroke volume of the heart (the amount of blood ejected by the left ventricle during contraction). Pulse pressure decreases when a patient is in a state of hypovolemic shock.

Equipment Needed to Measure Blood Pressure

There are two types of sphygmomanometers: a mercury manometer and an aneroid manometer (Fig. 6-10A, B). Each has a cloth cuff, which comes in a variety of sizes.

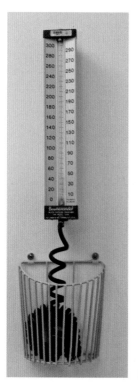
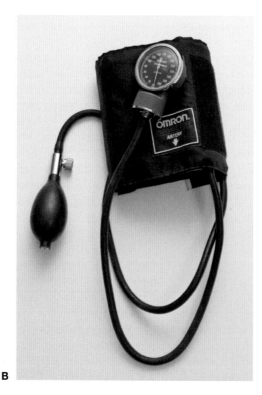

A   **B**

FIGURE 6-10   (A) A mercury manometer.
(B) An aneroid manometer.

Within the cuff is an inflatable bladder, which should be nearly long enough to encircle the arm. Each also has a pressure manometer, a thumbscrew valve to maintain or release the pressure, a pressure bulb to inflate the bladder, and a rubber tubing that leads to the gauge and to the pressure bulb. The bulb and the tubing must be free of leaks.

The mercury manometer is the more accurate of the two, but because of environmental concerns, it is being gradually phased out of use. The aneroid manometer needle should point to zero before the bladder of the cuff is inflated. Its calibration should be checked for accuracy and recalibrated by means of a perfectly accurate mercury manometer at least once each year.

The blood pressure cuffs should be selected according to patient size. A cuff that is too large or too small for the patient's arm gives an incorrect reading.

A good-quality stethoscope (Fig. 6-11) has a bladder and a bell, strong plastic or rubber tubing 12 to 19 inches (30 to 40 cm) in length that leads to firm but flexible binaural tubes (the metal tubing leading to the earpieces), and earpieces that fit snugly and securely into the ears. The bladder or the bell of the stethoscope can be used for assessing blood pressure. The bell transmits low sound and should be held lightly against the skin; the bladder transmits high-pitched sound and is held firmly against the skin. When holding the bladder, place your finger around the base of the bell, rather than holding the bell with your thumb. This allows you to have an even pressure on the bladder to hold it snugly against the patient's arm.

An automated vital sign monitor (Fig. 6-12) is used during special diagnostic imaging procedures when it is necessary to know the patient's circulatory status at all times. The pulse, blood pressure, and mean arterial pressure are measured with this instrument. Many types of Doppler and electronic blood pressure monitoring devices are used in clinical practice. Although these automated monitors may be available in the imaging

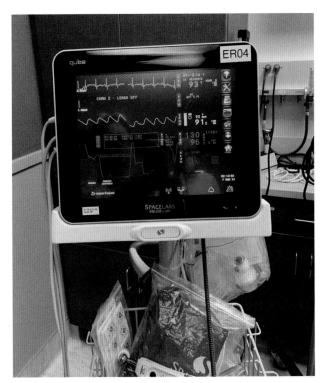

FIGURE 6-12 Automated equipment is used in many CT departments to monitor vital signs.

departments, it is important that technologists know how to perform manual blood pressure and a monitor may not be available on a moment's notice if a patient has a crisis.

Measuring Blood Pressure

Have the patient sit in a chair with the left arm supported or recline in a supine position. Although pressure can be taken while the patient is standing, it is not recommended. Most often, the patient will be recumbent when it becomes necessary for the radiographer to perform a blood pressure reading.

The room should be as quiet as possible to facilitate hearing the pulsations. Make sure that no clothing is between the blood pressure cuff and the skin. If the sleeve of the patient's shirt or blouse is too tight when rolled up, the garment should be removed before taking the blood pressure. The brachial artery of the left arm should be used as it is a direct line from the patient's heart and gives the truest indication of blood pressure. The bladder and bell of the stethoscope and the earpieces should be cleansed with alcohol sponges before and after each use to prevent passing infection indirectly from one person to another.

When the diastolic pressure is heard, there may be a change in the intensity of the sound before the sound is completely muffled. Note the point at which the softer sound is heard, and then note the point at which

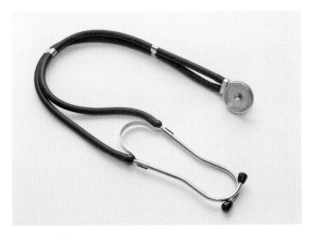

FIGURE 6-11 A stethoscope.

the pulsations are completely absent. This reading is a more accurate indication of intra-arterial diastolic pressure. Record both readings, but record the softer sound first. There are times when extraneous sounds such as tapping, knocking, or swishing may be heard. These are known as **Korotkoff sounds**, and they must be recorded as well.

If the systolic reading is 120 and the diastolic reading is 80, the blood pressure is recorded as BP 120/80 and is read "one twenty over eighty." If the diastolic reading is soft at 80 and then completely muffled at 60, it should be written BP 120/80/60 (the 60 reading being the Korotkoff sound).

Blood pressure measurement for infants and small children is a more complex procedure and requires a smaller sphygmomanometer cuff and less pressure exerted upon inflation. A physician or nurse educated in this skill should perform this assessment. Usually, a nurse is on hand to monitor when invasive diagnostic imaging procedures are to be done for patients in this age group.

 WARNING!

Do NOT perform a B/P measurement on the same side if a patient has an arteriovenous fistula for dialysis, an IV in the antecubital fossa, has had breast surgery on one side, edema in the arm, or paralysis from a stroke on one side.

PROCEDURE

Measuring Blood Pressure

1. Roll up the patient's sleeve, if necessary. The brachial artery must be free of clothing.

2. Place the deflated sphygmomanometer cuff evenly around the patient's upper arm above the elbow; secure it so that it does not work loose. Make sure that the cuff is facing the correct direction and that the arrow indicating the artery is placed appropriately (Fig. 6-13).

3. Place the gauge of the sphygmomanometer on a flat surface or attach it to the top edge of the cuff so that it can be easily read.

4. Place the bladder or bell of the stethoscope over the brachial artery. This artery is located at the center of the anterior elbow and may be identified by feeling its pulsations. Place the instrument flat against the brachial artery. Do not allow the stethoscope or the tubing to touch the patient's clothing because it creates sounds that may confuse the reading.

5. After positioning the stethoscope, tighten the thumbscrew of the pressure bulb and pump the bulb until the indicator or mercury reaches 180 mm Hg or until the pulse beat is no longer heard (Fig. 6-14).

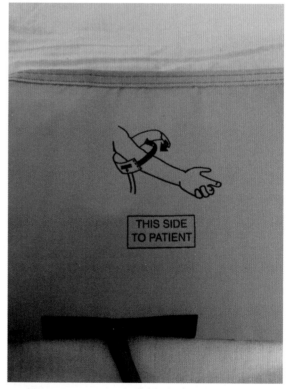

FIGURE 6-13 The cuff explains which side should be placed next to the patient.

6. Open the valve by slowly loosening the thumbscrew. Allow the indicator to fall at a moderate pace and listen for the first audible pulse beat. Listen carefully for the

pulse beat to begin and take the reading on the gauge where it is first heard. *This first reading is the systolic pressure.*

7. Continue to listen to the pulsations until they become soft or the sound changes from loud to very soft or is inaudible. Note where the sound changes or is no longer heard. *This is the diastolic reading.*

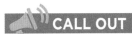

CALL OUT

Blood pressure should be taken on the left arm above the brachial artery.

CALL OUT

Clothing must be removed from the area before placing the cuff of the sphygmomanometer on the arm so that the sounds will not be obscured.

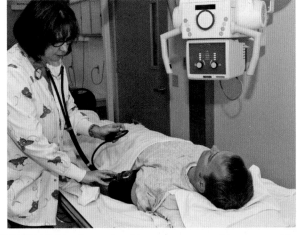

FIGURE 6-14 Assessing blood pressure with an aneroid sphygmomanometer.

WARNING!

The technologist must practice how to release the blood pressure cuff accurately. A cuff that is deflated too slowly gives false high readings. A cuff that is deflated too quickly gives false low readings.

OXYGEN ADMINISTRATION

Oxygen is an essential physiologic need for survival. The human brain cannot function for longer than 4 to 5 minutes without an adequate oxygen supply. Because oxygen cannot be stored in the body, the supply from the external environment must be constant. When a human being's oxygen supply is suddenly interrupted or interfered within any manner, it is an emergency that must be dealt with immediately to prevent a life-threatening situation. This type of emergency may occur in the diagnostic imaging department, thus making the radiographer performing the procedure the first person to observe such a problem. It is the technologist's responsibility to ensure that the equipment needed to administer oxygen is available at all times and is in functioning condition in the work area. It is also the radiographer's responsibility to assist with oxygen administration in emergency situations. Therefore, understanding the methods of oxygen administration that may be encountered in the care of the patient is critical.

The lungs supply oxygen and remove carbon dioxide from the body. Oxygen and carbon dioxide are carried to and from the various body systems in the blood. Only small amounts of oxygen are carried in solution in the blood. The major supply of oxygen is carried in chemical combination with hemoglobin. The oxygen capacity of the blood is expressed as a percentage of the volume. The amount of oxygen in either air or blood is called the oxygen tension (partial pressure) and is written Po_2. Carbon dioxide is described similarly as Pco_2.

Carbon dioxide diffuses into the plasma of systemic capillary blood, but the major part enters the RBCs. Carbon dioxide is also carried in combination with hemoglobin, which assists with its removal from the body. When there is an excessive buildup of carbon dioxide in the bloodstream, the pH (acidity or alkalinity) of the blood changes, often with dire physiologic effects. Prevention of excessive acidity of the blood is achieved through the presence of a bicarbonate (HCO_3) buffer in the bloodstream.

The effectiveness of pulmonary function (the lungs' ability to exchange oxygen and carbon dioxide efficiently) is most accurately measured by laboratory testing of arterial blood for the concentrations of oxygen, carbon dioxide, HCO_3, acidity, and the saturation of hemoglobin with oxygen (SaO_2). Laboratory values (called *arterial blood gases*) considered within normal limits are:

pH: 7.35 to 7.45
$PaCO_2$: 32 to 45 mm Hg
PaO_2: 80 to 100 mm Hg
HCO_3: 20 to 26 mEq/L
SaO_2: 97%

When pulmonary function is disturbed, the level of oxygen in the arterial blood becomes inadequate to meet the patient's physiologic needs. This condition is referred to as **hypoxemia**. Carbon dioxide may be retained in the arterial blood, which results in a condition called **hypercapnia**. When the PaO_2 is below 60 mm Hg or the hemoglobin saturation is less than 90%, it can be assumed that adequate oxygenation of the blood is not taking place. Physical symptoms of this problem, discussed in Chapter 9, are a good indicator that hypoxemia is occurring.

Pulse Oximetry

The purpose of pulse oximetry is to check how well the heart is pumping oxygen through the body. It may be used to monitor the health of individuals with any type of condition that can affect blood oxygen levels. These conditions include:

- chronic obstructive pulmonary disease (COPD)
- asthma
- pneumonia
- lung cancer
- anemia
- heart attack or heart failure
- congenital heart defects

There are a number of different reasons for performing pulse oximetry, including:

- to assess how well a lung medication is working
- to evaluate whether a patient needs help breathing
- to evaluate how helpful a ventilator is
- to monitor oxygen levels during or after procedures that require sedation
- to determine how effective supplemental oxygen therapy is, especially when treatment is new
- to assess a patient's ability to tolerate increased physical activity

During a pulse oximetry (abbreviated SaO_2) reading, a small clamp-like device is placed on a finger, earlobe, or toe. Small beams of light pass through the blood in the finger, measuring the amount of oxygen. It does this by measuring changes in light absorption in oxygenated or deoxygenated blood. The meter reports oxygen saturation levels and heart rate (Figs. 6-15 and 6-16).

Typically, more than 89% of the blood should be carrying oxygen (known as oxygen saturation). This is a minimum level needed to keep the body's cells healthy. Normal rates in a healthy adult patient are between 95% and 100%, indicating the amount of oxygen levels found in the blood. High-quality equipment found in most medical offices or hospitals consistently provide results within a 2% difference either way of what it really is. There are several factors that can affect the accuracy of the readings. A level that is consistently lower than 92% indicates potential hypoxemia. Patient movement, nail polish on a finger where the probe is placed, or poor placement of the probe itself are all possible causes for the reading to be inaccurate. These must be checked and remedied before accepting a low reading and falsely stating the condition of hypoxemia.

Hazards of Oxygen Administration

Oxygen is considered to be a medication and, like all other forms of medical therapy, must be prescribed by

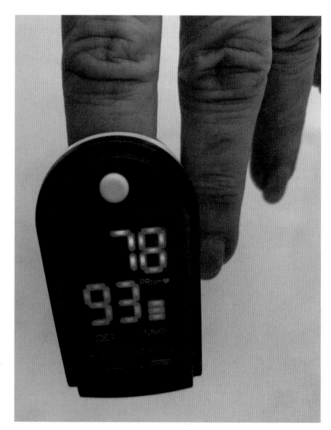

FIGURE 6-15 Portable pulse oximeter can be used when the oxygen level needs to be checked quickly.

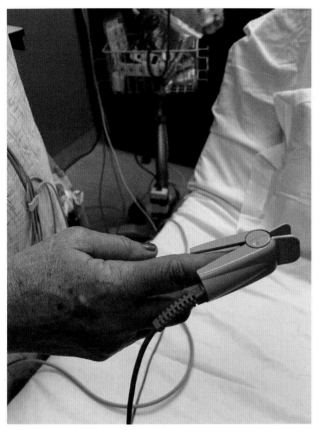

FIGURE 6-16 A pulse oximeter attached to the automated equipment shown in Figure 6-12.

WARNING!

High flow rates of oxygen are dangerous to patients who have COPD because their respiration is controlled by higher levels of carbon dioxide in the blood.

Infection and bacteria thrive in oxygenated environments. Therefore, the equipment used to deliver oxygen is a potential source of infection to the patient. Be certain that the tubing, cannulas, and masks for oxygen delivery are used for one patient only and then discarded. Oxygen supports combustion; therefore, take care to prevent sparks or flames from occurring where oxygen is being administered. Smoking is prohibited where oxygen is in use, and anything that may produce sparks or flames must be used with extreme caution. Take precautions when mobile radiographic equipment is used in the presence of pure oxygen to be certain that it does not produce sparks.

WARNING!

Oxygen is part of the triad of a fire, so great care must be taken to prevent sparks from occurring while imaging a patient with the mobile unit.

Oxygen Delivery Systems

Oxygen is administered by artificial means when the patient is unable to obtain adequate amounts from the atmosphere to supply the needs of the body. If the patient requires supplementary oxygen, it is delivered to the respiratory tract under pressure. When the flow rate is high, the oxygen is humidified to prevent excessive drying of the mucous membranes. Passing the oxygen through distilled water can do this as oxygen is only slightly soluble in water. The procedure for moisturizing oxygen varies somewhat from one institution to another, but often, the receptacle for distilled water is attached at the wall outlet, and the oxygen passes through the water and then into the delivery system.

In most hospitals, oxygen is piped into patient rooms, post-anesthesia areas, emergency suites, and the diagnostic imaging department. Wall outlets make it readily available. Oxygen supplied in this fashion comes through pipes from a central source at 60 to 80 pounds of pressure per square inch. A flow meter is attached to each wall outlet to regulate flow.

If oxygen is not piped in through wall outlets, it is available compressed and dispensed in tanks of varying sizes (Fig. 6-17). A large, full tank contains 2,000 lbs of pressure per square inch. These tanks have two regulator

a physician. Excessive amounts of oxygen may produce toxic effects on the lungs and CNS or may depress ventilation.

Varying degrees of oxygen toxicity may result from inhalation of high concentrations of oxygen for more than a brief period. Mild oxygen toxicity may produce reversible tracheobronchitis. Severe oxygen toxicity may cause irreversible parenchymal lung injury. Because of the potential for adverse effects from excessive amounts of oxygen, oxygen should be administered as prescribed and in the lowest possible amount to achieve adequate oxygenation.

Special care is necessary when oxygen is administered to patients who have **chronic obstructive pulmonary disease (COPD)**. Excessive oxygen in the blood of the patient who has COPD may depress the respiratory drive, and the patient may stop breathing. This occurs because patients with a chronic lung disease have chemoreceptors that no longer respond to the stimulus of CO_2 to breathe, as occurs in a healthy person. They must rely on hypoxemia as a respiratory stimulus. If they receive an excessive amount of oxygen, hypoxia is no longer present and respiration ceases.

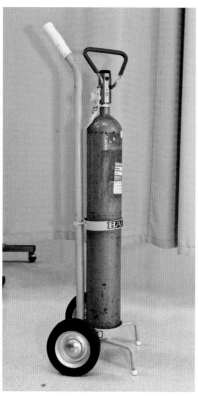

FIGURE 6-17 A small oxygen tank used to transport patient from one area to another.

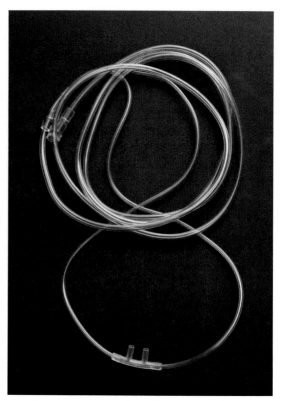

FIGURE 6-18 Nasal cannula.

valves: one valve indicates how much oxygen is in the tank and the other valve measures the rate of oxygen flow through the delivery tubing. If this type of system is used, take care not to allow the tank to fall or the regulator to become cracked. If this were to happen, the buildup of pressure within the tank may cause the regulator to act as a dangerous projectile.

Twenty-one percent of the air we breathe is normally composed of oxygen, often abbreviated as F_{IO_2}. This percentage of oxygen may need to be increased if a patient is in respiratory distress and unable to inspire enough room air to fulfill the body's oxygen needs.

There are many types of oxygen delivery systems that transport oxygen from wall outlets or tanks. The more complex systems deliver a controlled amount of premixed room air and oxygen. The simpler systems deliver a prescribed amount of oxygen mixed with room air, but the concentration varies as the patient's rate of respiration varies because they are not closed systems. The physician determines the amount of oxygen that the patient needs and the type of delivery device needed. The flow rate of oxygen is measured in liters per minute (LPM). The systems that the radiographer will see most often deliver low-to-moderate concentrations of oxygen.

Nasal Cannula

The nasal cannula is a disposable plastic device with two hollow prongs that deliver oxygen into the nostrils

(Fig. 6-18). The other end of the cannula is attached to the oxygen supply, which may or may not pass through a humidifier. The cannula is held in place by looping the tubing over the patient's ears. This device is the most commonly seen delivery system in the diagnostic imaging department. Patients on long-term oxygen delivery have a nasal cannula because of the comfort and convenience of the cannula.

The concentration of oxygen delivered by nasal cannula varies from 21% to 60%, according to the amount of room air inspired by the patient. Oxygen delivery by nasal cannula is indicated for patients whose breathing range and depth are normal and even. With this method, 1 to 4 LPM of oxygen is usually prescribed for adults. For children, the rate is much lower (1/4 to 1/2 LPM). Rates at higher levels dry the nasal mucosa because of the position of the tubes against the skin of the nostrils.

The oxygen should be turned on and flowing at the desired rate before placing any low-flow device on a patient. This prevents a sudden burst of oxygen into the patient's nostrils when the regulator is first turned on. The nasal prongs must be kept in place in both nostrils.

Nasal Catheter

A nasal catheter is another means of low-flow delivery of oxygen. Although this method of oxygen delivery is not routinely used, it warrants description in the event that the radiographer may come in contact with it. In this system, a French-tipped catheter is inserted into one nostril until it reaches the oral pharynx. This type of catheter is used to deliver a moderate-to-high concentration of oxygen. As with the nasal cannula, the other end of the French-tipped catheter is attached to the oxygen supply with a flow meter attached. The prescribed flow rate for this method of delivery is usually 1 to 5 LPM. Oxygen delivered by this method does have associated hazards. For example, oxygen may be misdirected into the stomach, causing gastric distention, or the mucous membranes may become dry, causing a sore throat.

Face Mask

A face mask is used to deliver oxygen for short periods (Fig. 6-19). It is attached to an oxygen supply and a flow meter. The mask is placed over the nose and mouth and attached over the ears and behind the head with an elastic band (Fig. 6-20). Wearing a mask for long periods is uncomfortable because the patient is unable to eat, drink, or talk with it in place. Moreover, the percentage of oxygen is so variable with the face mask that it is not the method of choice for long periods. Because the mask

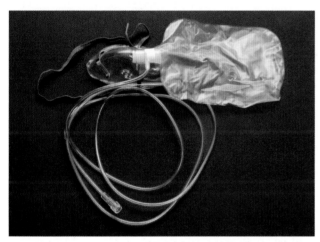

FIGURE 6-19 Face mask with rebreather mask attached.

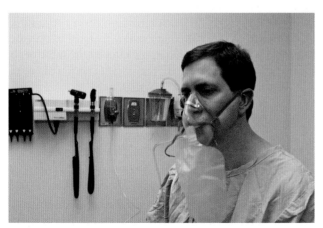

FIGURE 6-20 The face mask is secured over the head with an elastic strap.

does not fit tightly against the face, the concentration of oxygen delivered varies from 30% to 50%.

When the face mask is used, it should be run at no less than 5 LPM. This rate is needed to flush the CO_2 from the mask. Other face masks are usually used to administer more precise concentrations of oxygen. Several types of face mask delivery systems are available at present, and the physician prescribes the one best suited to the patient's needs.

The different types of masks include a *non-rebreathing mask*, which, if correctly used, may supply 100% oxygen. This high-flow system has a reservoir bag attached. The bag fills with oxygen to provide a constant supply of oxygen. A valve prevents the exhaled gases from entering the reservoir bag and prevents rebreathing of exhaled gases. A *partial rebreathing mask* (Fig. 6-19), which delivers 60% to 90% oxygen, operates similarly to the non-rebreather mask. The rebreather mask does not have a valve between the mask and the bag; therefore, exhaled air flows into the reservoir bag and allows the patient to breathe a mixture of oxygen and carbon dioxide. Two other types of face mask delivery systems include a *Venturi mask*, which mixes the oxygen flow with ambient air to achieve the desired oxygen concentrations between 0.24 and 0.6, and an *aerosol mask*, which is used when oxygen concentration needs of the patient change and provides 60% to 80% oxygen mixed with particles of water.

Other Oxygen Delivery Systems

Persons who must have continuous oxygen therapy for long periods may have a *transtracheal delivery system*. This system has a catheter that is inserted into the trachea and tubing that is connected to a portable tank.

Patients in acute respiratory failure are often placed on *mechanical ventilators* (also known as respirators), which control or partially control inspiration and expiration and FIO_2. The radiographer usually encounters these patients in the critical care units of the hospital while performing mobile radiography. These patients are generally unable to breathe on their own accord. The rate of oxygen flow is determined by many factors and is regulated by the equipment. Because the ventilator tubing is generally over the patient during the performance of the procedure, adequate help must be obtained before moving the patient and placing the image receptor. The nursing personnel in charge of the patient in the critical care unit who is on high-flow oxygen therapy or a mechanical ventilator must be consulted so that the patient's care is not jeopardized.

Home Oxygen Delivery Systems

There are agencies that hire radiographers to take radiographs in the home of a patient who is unable to be transported to a health care facility. These patients often use oxygen, and the oxygen may be delivered as compressed gas, as a liquid, or by means of an oxygen concentrator.

Compressed oxygen comes in tanks, which are usually smaller than the tanks used in the hospital; however, the principles of delivery are similar. Pure oxygen may be delivered by this method.

Liquid oxygen is a liquefied gas that concentrates oxygen into a lightweight container the size of a thermos bottle. It is conveniently portable and lasts longer than other forms of oxygen; therefore, people who must take oxygen with them use this method when they leave home. This is an expensive method, chiefly because the oxygen evaporates quickly.

The oxygen concentrator is economical and is an excellent source of oxygen. Oxygen is concentrated by means of an electric machine that removes the nitrogen, water vapor, and hydrocarbons from room air. Oxygen is delivered at 90% by this means.

Oxygen Delivery Equipment for the Imaging Department

The following is a list of equipment that must be on hand for oxygen administration in the diagnostic imaging department:

1. An oxygen source, either a piped-in source or a tank. If the source of oxygen is a tank, the tank must be checked daily to make certain that it is filled. Tanks should be stored on their side and not in the upright position if standard carriers are not available. This is to avoid accidental falling of the tank, which may cause an explosion.
2. A sterile nasal cannula or simple face mask that is packaged and has not been used. These are disposable items.
3. Connecting tubing and an adapter to fit into a wall unit or tank.
4. A humidifier, if indicated. Humidifiers are not always used for short-term oxygen administration.
5. A flow meter.
6. A "no-smoking" sign.

RADIOGRAPHIC EXAMINATIONS OF THE CHEST

Normal lung tissue is radiolucent; therefore, pathologic conditions that produce opacities may be detected by radiographic imaging techniques (Fig. 6-21). Posterior/anterior and lateral radiographic images are frequently ordered to diagnose pulmonary pathology and to determine placement of endotracheal tubes and hemodynamic devices. These radiographic images are frequently taken at the patient's bedside because they are too ill to be moved. If this is the case, the patient may have difficulty complying with

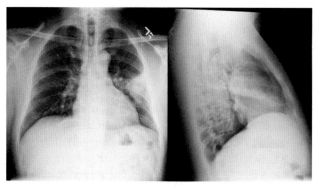

FIGURE 6-21 Posteroanterior (PA) and lateral chest image showing pneumonia.

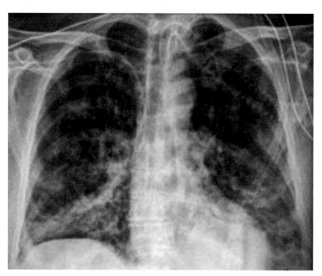

FIGURE 6-22 Anteroposterior (AP) mobile chest radiograph with the ventilator tube across the lung on the patient's left side.

directions for positioning and breathing. Critical thinking and problem-solving skills need to be employed in order to obtain a diagnostically acceptable image.

Before the image is taken, the oxygen delivery system, the oxygen monitoring equipment, and the placement of associated tubing must be assessed to prevent repeating the exposure (Fig. 6-22). Transporting patients or moving patients from a wheelchair or stretcher to the table or to the upright position can pull on oxygen tubes and cause pain to the patient.

LABORATORY DATA USED IN PATIENT ASSESSMENT

Although diagnostic radiographers are not normally required to monitor laboratory results such as blood urea nitrogen (BUN) and creatinine, basic knowledge of these values and what they mean can help determine a course of patient care. Patients undergoing procedures involving contrast media are most often required to have certain laboratory tests performed prior to the contrast procedure. Normal tests and values are listed in Display 6-2.

Kidney Function Assessments

Kidneys maintain the pH of the blood and as such are critical to life. Different laboratory assessments can be measured to determine whether the kidneys are functioning properly and whether a contrast media injection might prove harmful to the patient. The BUN, creatinine, and glomerular filtration rate (GFR) are three laboratory values that the radiographer must be familiar with.

The kidneys maintain the blood creatinine in a normal range. Creatinine is a waste product created by metabolism in the muscle. It has been found to be a fairly reliable indicator of kidney function as the waste material is eliminated from the body through urine. Elevated creatinine level signifies impaired kidney function or kidney disease.

As the kidneys become impaired for any reason, the creatinine level in the blood rises because of poor clearance of creatinine by the kidneys. Abnormally high levels of creatinine warn of possible malfunction or failure of the kidneys. It is for this reason that standard blood tests routinely check the amount of creatinine in the blood.

A more precise measure of the kidney function can be estimated by calculating how much creatinine is cleared from the body by the kidneys. This is referred to as creatinine clearance, and it estimates the rate of filtration by kidneys (GFR). The creatinine clearance can be measured in two ways. It can be calculated (estimated) by a formula using serum (blood) creatinine level, patient's weight, and age. Although the radiographer does not need to know how to figure the level, it is important that the levels are

known and what they mean. Normal creatinine clearance for healthy women is 0.6 to 1.2 mg/dL with males having a slightly higher rate. A person with only one kidney may have a normal level of about 1.8 or 1.9. Creatinine levels that reach 2.0 or more in babies and 5.0 or more in adults may indicate severe kidney impairment.

The need for a dialysis machine to remove wastes from the blood is based on several considerations, including the BUN, creatinine level, potassium level, and how much fluid the patient is retaining.

BUN level is another indicator of kidney function. Urea nitrogen is a normal waste product that the body creates after eating. The liver breaks down the proteins in food, which creates BUN. This substance is released by the liver into the blood and eventually ends up in the kidneys. When the kidneys are healthy, the BUN is removed, leaving only a small amount of it in the blood. This is then excreted out of the body through urine. The BUN-to-creatinine ratio generally provides more precise information about kidney function and its possible underlying cause compared with creatinine level alone. BUN also increases with **dehydration**. Normal range for BUN is 7 to 20 mg/dL. If values are off the normal range, it could mean that either the liver or kidneys are not working properly.

The GFR test measures how the kidneys are carrying out their filtration function. Diabetics are more at risk for kidney disease, and this test is particularly important as early kidney disease often has no symptoms. Any rate higher than 60 is considered normal. When the GFR falls to 15 or lower, it can be a sign that you have kidney failure.

GFR measurements vary by age. For most adults, over 90 is considered normal, but age causes the GFR to decrease. Once a patient reaches 60, the GFR is still normal at a rate of 85 and at 70 years and older the normal rate is 75.

DISPLAY 6-2

Laboratory Tests

Lab Test	Function Assessed	Normal Range
BUN	Renal	7-20 mg/dL
Creatinine	Renal	0.6-1.2 mg/dL
Glomerular filtration rate	Renal	Higher than 60
RBCs	Blood disorders	Women: 4.1-5.1 million/mcL Men: 4.5-5.9 million/mcL
Hemoglobin	Blood disorder	Women: 12-15.5 g/dL Men: 13.5-17.5 g/dL
Platelets	Blood clotting	150,000-450,000/mL
Prothrombin time	Blood clotting	10-14 seconds
Partial thromboplastin	Blood clotting	30-40 seconds

Blood Disorder Assessment

Doctors select tests to help diagnose blood disorders based on the person's symptoms and the results of the physical examination. Sometimes a blood disorder causes no symptoms but is discovered when a laboratory test is done for another reason. For example, a complete blood count (CBC) done as part of a regular check-up may reveal a low RBC count (anemia). When a blood disorder is suspected, a CBC and other tests may need to be done to determine the specific diagnosis. The blood test most commonly done is the CBC. The CBC is an evaluation of all the cellular components (RBCs, white blood cells, and platelets) in the blood. Automated machines do this test in less than 1 minute on a small amount of blood. There are other blood tests that are performed for different types of symptoms that may be presenting. The radiographer must be aware of these tests and what the values can mean, particularly when performing computed tomography (CT) procedures.

Red Blood Cells

The main job of RBCs, or erythrocytes, is to carry oxygen from the lungs to the body tissues and carbon dioxide as a waste product, away from the tissues and back to the lungs. RBCs contain hemoglobin and should comprise 40% of the blood volume. The life span of an RBC averages 120 days with the liver processing and eliminating the worn-out and dead cells. The bone marrow is continuously making new RBCs to preplace the dead ones. Too few RBCs may indicate anemia, and too many cells create thicker blood that leads to clotting and heart attacks. Normal ranges are 4.1 to 5.1 for women and 4.5 to 5.9 for men.

Hemoglobin

Hemoglobin, abbreviated Hb or Hgb, is the iron-containing oxygen transport metalloprotein in the RBCs (erythrocytes). Hemoglobin in the blood carries oxygen from the lungs to the tissues of the body. A healthy female has 12 to 15.5 g of hemoglobin in every 100 mL of blood, whereas a male has a normal range between 13.5 and 17.5 g/dL.

Hemoglobin is involved in the transport of respiratory carbon dioxide (about 20% to 25% of the total), in which CO_2 is bound to the heme protein. The molecule also carries the important regulatory molecule nitric oxide releasing it at the same time as oxygen.

Clotting Factors

During invasive procedures, it is often times important to know if the patient has a disorder of the blood that may cause problems with excessive bleeding. During interventional radiology procedures, the femoral artery can be catheterized in order to see blood vessels in other parts of the body. Once the catheter is removed, the patient may bleed from the puncture site. With a low number of platelets, the site may not clot successfully. Other blood tests that are performed to determine clotting time and ability are prothrombin and partial thromboplastin.

Platelets

Platelets are counted as part of a CBC. These cells help in the clotting process by gathering at a bleeding site and clumping together to form a plug. A normal range of platelets is between 150,000 and 450,000 platelets per milliliter of blood. Too few platelets (<150,000) may impair blood clotting. A high number of platelets (>450,000), known as thrombocytosis, can lead to excessive clotting in the smaller vessels, especially in the heart or brain.

Prothrombin Time

A prothrombin time (PT) is a test used to help detect and diagnose a bleeding disorder or excessive clotting disorder. It measures the number of seconds it takes for a clot to form in a blood sample after certain substances are added. This is used to monitor how well the blood-thinning medication, known as an anticoagulant, is working to prevent blood clots. The PT is often performed along with a partial thromboplastin time (PTT), and the two tests assess the coagulation factors that are an important part of proper blood clot formation. These are especially important if the patient is on any blood-thinning medication such as heparin or warfarin. Normal range for PT is 10 to 14 seconds, and the normal range for PTT is 30 to 40 seconds. Anything less than these ranges may indicate that the patient has a bleeding tendency.

 Cultural Considerations

The technologist must always be mindful that certain cultures do not touch others even if it is to determine heart rate, respirations, and pulse. Provide a complete explanation about what is going to occur and ensure, through professionalism, that there is no reason to be fearful. Make sure, through proper communication, that this is only for medical purposes and lasts only for a few minutes.

CASE STUDY

As a student radiographer, you are exposed to many different situations in the health care field. On this particular day, you were asked to observe in the angiography room. The technologist has asked if you could assist with the preprocedural vital signs on Mr. Hawkins. Eager to be a part of the team, you take Mr. Hawkins to the area where vital signs are taken. As you try to carry on a light conversation and outwardly attempt to seem confident, you take his radial pulse, respirations, and blood pressure. You notice that the blood pressure seems high, but not knowing Mr. Hawkins' average values, you continue with the preprocedural workup.

ISSUES TO CONSIDER

1. Should you report your suspicion about a high blood pressure to someone? Why, or why not?
2. How will you find out what Mr. Hawkins' normal blood pressure is?
3. What should be done as a follow-up to this preprocedural assessment?

Summary

1. Vital signs consist of:
   a. Body temperature
      i. Common places to take the temperature include temporal, tympanic, and oral.
      ii. There are now contactless-type temporal thermometers that allow a quick assessment of the patient's temperature.
      iii. Normal rates for adults are 98 to 99° F.
   b. Pulse
      i. Places to take pulse include apical, radial carotid, femoral, popliteal, temporal, dorsalis pedis, posterior tibial, and brachial, with carotid and radial being the most common.
      ii. Normal rates include adults between 60 and 90 bpm, infants 120 bpm, and children between 90 and 100 bpm.
      iii. Use the first two fingers to count the patient's pulse and count for a minimum of 30 seconds, then multiply by two.
      iv. Tachycardia: more than 100 beats per minute.
      v. Bradycardia: less than 60 beats per minute.
   c. Respiration
      i. Not often used in radiography.
      ii. Normal rate is 12 to 16 breaths per minute.
   d. Blood pressure
      i. Equipment includes a stethoscope and sphygmomanometer.
      ii. Systolic is the pumping action of the heart and is the highest number recorded on the top. Normal is 120 mm Hg.
      iii. Diastolic pressure is the relaxation phase of the heart and is the bottom number. Normal is 80 mm Hg.
      iv. Pressures greater than 120/80 indicate hypertension.
      v. Pressures less than 50 mm Hg diastolic represent hypotension and may be indicative of shock.

2. Variables that affect vital signs:
   a. Time of day: Temperature, pulse, and blood pressure are usually lower in the morning than in the afternoon or evening.
   b. Gender: Men tend to have higher blood pressure than women until menopause, at which time women have higher blood pressure than the same age group of men.
   c. Age: Older patients tend to feel colder than when they were younger; this does not necessarily mean that their body temperatures change. Studies have shown that mean body temperatures are a few degrees lower than in younger patients.
   d. Weight: The more a patient weighs, the higher the temperature and blood pressure.
   e. Illness: Vital sign changes are an indication of illness or infection. Radiographers must take note of changes from the baseline taken at the beginning of a procedure.
   f. Environment: The heat of the day increases a person's temperature.
   g. Physical activity: Increased physical activity increases temperature and blood pressure.

h. Emotions: Patients who are nervous, upset, or stressed may have increased blood pressure.

3. Oxygen administration

  a. Nasal cannulas, face masks, and nasal catheters are used to provide oxygen.

  b. Delivery systems

    i. Oxygen concentration is not affected by the delivery system used. The flow rate of a desired concentration is what is regulated by the delivery system.

    ii. High-flow systems are humidified and used for patients with acute respiratory failure and require assistance with respiration to stabilize breathing. An example is a Venturi mask. High-flow delivery systems are capable of delivering oxygen concentrations as low as 0.24.

    iii. Low-flow systems provide oxygen at flow rates lower than the patient's demands. An example is a non-rebreather face mask that can deliver oxygen concentration as high as 0.8.

  c. Normal rates average at 2 LPM but can be anywhere from 1 LPM to 4 LPM.

  d. Hazards

    i. Oxygen administration cannot be started without a physician's order.

    ii. Oxygen supports fire, so care must be taken when oxygen is in use.

    iii. Oxygen use can be toxic to patients with certain diseases because of incorrect flow rates and concentrations.

  e. Pulse oximetry

    i. Probe placed on fingertip, ear lobe, or toe.

    ii. Assesses the amount of oxygen in the blood.

    iii. Normal rates

      1. SaO_2 should be between 95% and 100%.

      2. Less than 92% consistently indicates potential hypoxemia.

4. Laboratory assessments

  a. Kidney function

    i. Creatinine

      1. This is a waste by-product of muscle metabolism that is eliminated from the body by the kidneys through urine output.

      2. Levels too high indicate that the kidneys may not be able to eliminate contrast injected into a patient during a CT.

      3. Normal range is 0.6 to 1.2 mg/dL.

    ii. BUN

      1. Indicates how much urea nitrogen (waste from eating) is left in the blood after liver or kidneys work to remove it.

      2. Normal range is 7 to 20 mg/dL.

    iii. GFR

      1. Indicates kidney failure and is especially important in patients with diabetes.

      2. Adult patients have a normal rate of over 90, but that rate declines as the patient ages, reaching a normal rate of 75 at the age of 70.

  b. Blood disorder assessment

    i. RBC

      1. RBCs carry the important component, hemoglobin. RBCs live up to 120 days and make up 40% of the blood volume.

      2. Normal ranges are 4.1 to 5.1 million/mL for women and 4.5 to 5.9 million/mL for men.

    ii. Hemoglobin

      1. Hemoglobin in the blood carries oxygen from the lungs to the tissues of the body.

      2. Normal range for women is 12 to 15.5 g/dL and for men is 13.5 to 17.5 g/dL.

  c. Clotting factors

    i. Platelets

      1. Platelets come together to form a plug within a vessel to stop bleeding through an opening or cling to a vessel wall to form a thrombus.

      2. Normal range of platelets is 150,000 to 450,000 platelets per mL of blood.

      3. Lower than 150,000 platelets may indicate a problem with the patient being able to form clots to stop bleeding.

      4. Higher than 450,000 platelets may indicate the patient may have a tendency to form clots in the smaller vessels.

    ii. Prothrombin time

      1. It measures the amount of time it takes for the blood to form a clot.

      2. Normal clotting time of a healthy individual is 10 to 14 seconds.

    iii. Partial thromboplastin

      1. It measures the amount of time it takes for the blood to form a clot when a patient is on a blood-thinning medication.

      2. Normal range for an individual on heparin is between 30 and 40 seconds.

5. Cultural considerations

  a. Being professional at all times and providing excellent communication usually eliminates any culturally related concerns.

CHAPTER 6 REVIEW QUESTIONS

1. Which of the following are essential parts of the initial assessment of a patient who is in the diagnostic imaging department for an invasive procedure? (Circle all that apply.)
   a. Taking a blood pressure
   b. Taking a pulse
   c. Listening for rales in the lungs
   d. Taking a respiration rate
   e. Doing blood gas assessment
   f. Determining the oxygen saturation level
   g. Taking a temperature

2. Why is the initial assessment, defined in Question 1, so important to perform?

3. Systolic blood pressure can be defined as:
   a. The lowest point to which the blood pressure drops during relaxation of the ventricles
   b. The highest point reached during contraction of the left ventricle
   c. The difference between the systolic and the diastolic blood pressure
   d. The pressure in the pulmonary vein

4. What range of breaths per minute is the normal adult respiratory rate?
   a. 8 to 10
   b. 15 to 20
   c. 20 to 30
   d. 80 to 90

5. An adult patient is considered to be hypertensive or to have hypertension if the systolic blood pressure and diastolic blood pressure are consistently greater than:
   a. 100 systolic and 60 diastolic
   b. 120 systolic and 80 diastolic
   c. 130 systolic and 86 diastolic
   d. 140 systolic and 90 diastolic

6. Oxygen can be toxic to patients if it is incorrectly used. State two reasons why this is so.

7. A patient may be considered to have tachycardia if the pulse rate is higher than:
   a. 72 beats per minute
   b. 85 beats per minute
   c. 90 beats per minute
   d. 100 beats per minute

8. Which of the following items must be in the diagnostic imaging department and in working order? (Circle all that apply.)
   a. Suture kit
   b. Digital clock to tell the time
   c. Oxygen (usually wall-mounted)
   d. Blood pressure equipment

9. What is the normal temporal body temperature of an adult?

10. Match the following:
    a. Sphygmomanometer
    b. Temporal thermometer
    c. Stethoscope
    d. Brachial artery
    e. Radial pulse

    i. Point where the blood pressure is most often measured
    ii. Measures apical pulse
    iii. Cuff that goes around the arm to measure blood pressure
    iv. Measures body temperature at the forehead
    v. Point where the pulse is most often measured

11. Name the two types of equipment used to deliver oxygen.

12. List the hazards of oxygen administration.

13. Explain why the pulse rate goes up when the blood pressure drops.

14. What are the two laboratory values that must be considered when performing a contrast procedure of the kidneys?

15. Which of the following laboratory values are assessed for clotting of the blood? (Circle all that apply.)
    a. BUN
    b. Platelets
    c. Prothrombin time
    d. Creatinine
    e. Partial thromboplastin time
    f. Hemoglobin

Patient Populations

7

KEY TERMS

Actinic keratosis: A slow, localized thickening of the outer layers of the skin as a result of chronic, excessive exposure to the sun

Adolescent: The period of life beginning at puberty and ending with physical maturity

Alzheimer disease: An illness characterized by dementia, confusion, memory failure, disorientation, restlessness, speech disturbances, and an inability to carry out purposeful movements; onset usually occurs in persons 55 years or older

Baroreceptors: Receptors that are sensitive to the changes of pressure in the blood

Child abuse: The psychological, emotional, and sexual abuse of a child

Code Pink: A hospital code used to convey an infant or child abduction

Culture: A shared system of beliefs among a group of people

Dementia: Organic mental syndrome characterized by general loss of intellectual abilities involving impairment of memory, judgment, and abstract thinking

Depression: A morbid sadness, dejection, or melancholy

Disinfectant: A solution capable of destroying pathogenic microorganisms or inhibiting their growth

Ethnicity: A grouping of people who share backgrounds like religion

Hypothermia: Significant loss of body heat below 98.6° F

Image Gently: A campaign initiated to bring awareness and promote radiation protection in the imaging of children

Infant: A newborn up to 1 year of age

Isolette: A special enclosed unit used in newborn intensive care to keep babies warm and protected from the environment

Kyphosis: An abnormal condition of the vertebral column in which there is increased convexity in the curvature of the thoracic spine

Neonate: A newborn infant up to 1 month of age

NICU: Neonatal intensive care unit

Preschooler: A child who is not old enough to attend kindergarten

Presbyopia: Farsightedness caused by the loss of elasticity of the lens of the eye

Proprioception: The body's ability to sense movement, action, and location

Psychosis: A mental condition in which contact with reality is lost

School-age: Age at which the child who is considered to attend school

Toddler: Young child learning to walk

Urinary incontinence: Inability to control urinary functions

PEDIATRIC PATIENTS

Pediatric patients range in age from infancy to 15 years. As of the 2020 U.S. Census, people under the age of 5 years equal 6% and those under the age of 18 years equal 22.3%. This means that 72,918,842 people are considered to be in the pediatric or young adult range. To help put this in perspective, this is eight times the number of people in Los Angeles, CA, which has a population of 9.8 million (as of 2020).

Children in this broadly defined group require specific care, depending on their age and ability to comprehend the radiographic imaging procedure(s). In order to be both sensitive and effective in performing the imaging procedure, radiographers must use age-appropriate methods of communication and execution of the required procedure according to a child's age. Caring for infants and children demands special safety and effective communication techniques and approaches that are different from those of adult radiography. It also requires a sensitive approach toward the accompanying parent(s) or guardian(s) to develop a rapport. Display 7-1 outlines the developmental stages as a child ages. In addition to imaging pediatric patients in the diagnostic imaging department, mobile procedures are performed on pediatric patients in the hospital room, emergency room, operating room, and neonatal intensive care nursery.

The pediatric patient includes **neonates** in neonatal intensive care unit **(NICU)**, **infants**, **toddlers**, **preschoolers**, and **school-age** children. The immaturity of the neonatal immune system, in particular, dictates adherence of health care personnel to infection control practices. Preventative measures to reduce infections in the pediatric patient begin with basic practices such as proper handwashing and hygiene to prevent the spread of infections.

Almost 18% of all hospital stays are of children and adolescents 17 years and younger. Neonates are kept in the hospital after birth because of respiratory problems, infections, or complications from hemolytic jaundice, prematurity, or birth defects. The cause of admission to the hospital is most commonly because of infectious diseases and asthma. Those seen in the emergency department (ED) are adolescents with injuries to the extremities or head from sports. Another reason in the older adolescent is drug poisoning.

Children of all ages respond in a positive manner to honesty and friendliness. A small child may be very frightened when entering the imaging department and seeing the rooms with massive equipment. If the radiographer spends a few moments establishing a rapport with the child and acquainting the child with the new environment, the procedure would proceed more smoothly in a nonthreatening manner, and the child leaves the department with a positive attitude about the imaging process. The room should be prepared completely before the child is brought in for the procedure. This eliminates delays that can create agitation in the child.

Most children resist immediate close contact with strangers. Therefore, it is best to talk to the child from a comfortable distance and allow the child to become accustomed to one's presence before approaching them. The technologist must explain what is going to happen before and during the procedure to the child who is old enough to understand. The technologist should also give the child an estimate of how long the procedure would last and what is expected. In addition, the technologist must explain the procedure and the process to the parent or guardian. The child should be prepared for any discomfort that may be felt. If the child is to receive contrast media or medications, the method of administration needs to be explained to both the parent/guardian and the child. Explanations to children are most effective if they are brief, simple, and to the point. The child should not be given choices when it is not appropriate because it may be confusing.

DISPLAY 7-1

Developmental Stages by Age

Age	Developmental Stages
Neonate	Senses respond to the environmental conditions
1-12 months	Infants have limited language—not fearful of strangers
1-3 years	Toddlers follow simple commands—initial fear of strangers
3-6 years	Preschooler—age of initiative—socialization and verbal activity increase
6-12 years	School-age—a period of cognitive growth; can solve problems; understands cause and effect
12-19 years	Adolescence—age of identity; able to use abstract concepts

The radiographer should speak to the child at eye level even if they must sit or stoop down to do so. To avoid misunderstandings, only one person should explain and direct the child. It is important to explain the process to the parent or guardian and to ask for their assistance during the procedure when possible. Using a soft tone of voice with the child and speaking in terms that are simple and familiar enhances communication and cooperation. The radiographer must be certain that the child understands what is being said. If the child wishes to carry a toy or security item to the imaging room, this should be allowed if at all possible. If it is not practical, explain to the child that the toy will be placed so the child can see it during the procedure. Return the toy to the child immediately after the procedure.

When explaining a procedure to a child, specify what part of the body is to be examined, why, and who is performing the procedure. Also explain how the examination will proceed, what part of the child's body must be touched to properly position the patient to accomplish the procedure, and why it is important to hold still during the process. Before the procedure is started, the parent/guardian must give consent.

Some children are very modest. If a child's body must be exposed for an examination, only the necessary part should be exposed. The technologist must guard against allowing the child to become chilled while in their care. This is particularly important for infants because they lose body heat rapidly and **hypothermia** may occur.

Explicit instructions must be provided in all aspects for the adult involved in the procedure. The adult holding the child must ensure the child does not fall from the x-ray table. If the parent or guardian is holding the child during the imaging procedure, they must wear proper protective apparel, which includes a lead apron and possibly lead gloves. In addition to explaining the importance of wearing the protective apparel, the technologist should explain how to secure the apron and assist them with the garments. Make sure that the child is not left unattended while this is being done. The radiographer must never assume that the parent is watching the child on an x-ray table and must instruct the parent/guardian about the exact measures they need to take. The following is an example of how this may be done.

RADIOGRAPHER: *I would like you to stand on this side of the table with your hands on "Maggie" at all times. It is necessary for you to wear this lead apron for protection. Let me hold her while you put on the apron. The apron fastens with Velcro attachments on the sides. Now, please keep your hands on Maggie at all times.*

On occasion, if the child refuses to follow directions and is emotionally distraught, it may be necessary for the accompanying adult to leave the room. The parent/guardian must agree to leave the x-ray room. In this case, let the child know that getting the x-ray helps with getting better and that the parents want it done. Then, repeat the directions and proceed. Do not belittle or criticize the child's behavior; remain nonjudgmental and matter of fact and accomplish the task as quickly as possible. Display 7-2 summarizes the steps in caring for children during the imaging procedures.

The High-Risk Newborn Infant

Many hospitals have special care units for high-risk newborn infants. In many areas of the United States, infants are transported to such facilities for special care from the hospital in which they were born. Infants may be considered to be at high risk for life-threatening problems if they are of low birth weight or if they have other perinatal problems.

Infants whose lives are at risk require special care considerations in highly specialized NICUs. Here, they are protected from threats to their nutritional status, environmental problems such as changes in their body temperature, and infection by being placed in **isolettes** with environmental and thermal control and by the practice of meticulous infection control measures.

Infection prevention and control practices are the responsibility of all health care personnel, including the radiographer. The NICU patient, in particular, has an immature immune system and, therefore, is more susceptible to infection. The radiographer must follow and adhere to the pediatric unit's standard precautions, policies, and procedures. Hand hygiene is the basic important practice that reduces the risk of infection transmission. A surgical scrub, or a 2-minute scrub as for medical asepsis, may be required of all health care personnel entering these nurseries. Personal protective equipment such as gowns, gloves, masks, and eye protection may be required. The technologist must have proper education and training on pediatric standard precautions for the prevention of the transmission of infection. The prevention of infection includes cleaning the x-ray equipment, which includes the mobile x-ray machine, the image receptors or detectors, gonadal shielding, and right or left markers. The mobile machine must be wiped clean with a **disinfectant** solution and must be free of dust before entering the nursery. Specific procedures must be followed in regard to the imaging equipment and accessories.

The nurse in charge of the infant's care must be consulted. The nurse should be asked to assist by positioning and immobilizing the infant. Care must be taken to prevent chilling the infant or dislodging any catheters or tubing while performing the radiographic procedure, as seen in Figure 7-1. The technologist should provide a protective apparel apron to the nurse who is assisting to hold the infant; provide the infant with gonadal shielding when appropriate. However, with the low radiation doses with digital imaging, protective apparel for personnel may not be necessary.

DISPLAY 7-2

Caring for Pediatric Patients during Imaging

Always identify every patient with two methods and explain the procedure to the parents/guardians and/or the patient before beginning. Obtain a complete history from the appropriate person.

Neonate (birth to 1 month)	Keep the patient warm and never leave unattended. Make sure the parents/guardians know what to expect.
Infants (1-12 months)	Maintain trust, assess needs, maintain safe surrounding, and never leave unattended. Make sure the parents/guardians know what to expect.
Toddlers (1-3 years)	Assess needs and level of independence, have concern for privacy, maintain safe surroundings, and never leave unattended. Determine if parents/guardians are appropriate for completion of exam. If not, obtain assistance from another radiographer.
Preschoolers (3-6 years)	Assess needs, support independence, protect privacy, maintain safety, and never leave unattended. Obtain assistance if parents/guardians are not able to stay with 3- to 4-year-old patients; 5- and 6-year-old patients should be able to maintain position for 2 minutes.
School-age (6-12 years)	Assess any needs and protect privacy. At this age, there should be no need for assistance. Honest explanations and answers to questions are important to establish trust.
Adolescence (12-19 years)	Assess any needs and address the possibility of pregnancy with female patients. Protect the patient's privacy as this is critical for teens. Be respectful and discreet.

 ## Cultural Considerations

If the parents or guardians are non-English speaking, it is important to ensure both the parents and the child have an understanding of the procedure. The technologist must secure a translator before beginning the procedure to make sure that the parents understand the procedure, understand the directions, and know what will occur during the procedure. Hospitals have procedures to access a translator; therefore, one must be acquainted with the protocol in advance.

Practices should be in place to accommodate the patient's beliefs about modesty, scheduling of exams, and considerations for special prayers. In Hispanic culture, little girls have their ears pierced in infancy. It may not be possible to remove these earrings for some radiographic procedures. Older children may wear religious articles around their necks that should not be removed without permission from the parent. Be prepared if this permission is denied.

If the radiographer has any sort of respiratory infection or infected cuts on either hand, another technologist should be asked to take the NICU assignment to prevent introduction of infectious microorganisms into the protective environment of the NICU.

The Adolescent or Older Child

The older child or early **adolescent** is often expected to act as an adult would under similar circumstances. This is not a fair expectation because children of this age are not yet adults. When they are threatened by illness or injury, they return to the more familiar role of being a child.

The teenager is apt to be perceived as hostile and self-centered. Communication ceases if a health care worker conveys a feeling of disapproval. The radiographer can overcome this behavior by conveying a nonjudgmental attitude and using the therapeutic communication technique described in Chapter 3. Communication strategy approaches appropriate to the comprehension level of the

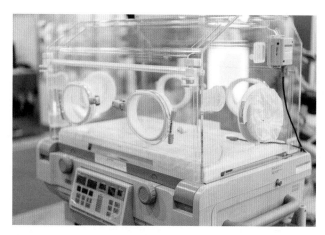

FIGURE 7-1 An isolette that is used in the neonatal intensive care unit. Notice the slot under the isolette for the placement of the image receptor. (Photo courtesy of Shutterstock/Petrychenko Anton.)

patient must be modified according to the patient's and/or the parent's needs. The interview with the teenager must include the following basic points:

- Establish a rapport
- Verify the procedure
- Identify the patient
- Explain the procedure
- Educate the patient
- Maintain the patient's concern for privacy
- Provide aftercare directions

When caring for the older child, the radiographer should be as direct and as honest as possible in explanations of what will occur during the procedure. Use simple terms and allow the patient to ask questions and express fears and apprehension. It is important to explain what the requirements are for the technologist in terms of positioning for the examination and which landmarks must be touched to achieve the images. If the child feels more secure with a parent or guardian accompanying them, this should be encouraged and allowed, if it is permitted under hospital policy. If not, the adult may stay close by and be with the child between radiographic images or as often as is appropriate and safe. The child's privacy must be respected. No part of the child's body should be exposed without an explanation of the necessity for doing so. If the patient is able to make informed decisions, allow it. This gives the older child a feeling of having some control of the situation.

TRANSPORTING INFANTS AND CHILDREN

The technologist may be responsible for transporting infants and children from one area to another in the imaging department in addition to transporting them

to the department from the hospital rooms. Additional safety measures to prevent injuring the very young patient are required. In addition, standard precautions must always be followed while the pediatric patient is being transported.

Care must be taken to ascertain the identity of the patient using at least two patient identifiers. The type of procedure that the child is to receive must be verified and confirmed, and the appropriate gowning and removal of artifacts must be considered. The identification band on the wrist or ankle must be checked with the nurse in charge of the patient before the child is taken from their room and checked again against the patient chart, electronic medical record, and/or the requisition for the procedure when the child arrives in the department.

The method of transfer depends on the child's size and the nature of the illness or injury. Under most circumstances, it is safe to carry infants and very small children for short distances (e.g., from one diagnostic imaging room to another). For longer distances, it is necessary to place the child in a crib with all sides up and locked.

Some cribs come with tops to prevent the active child from climbing over the crib rails. Crib rails must never be placed in a half-raised position because an active child can climb over them and may fall from a greater height than if the rails had not been raised at all. When an infant is transported in the hospital, if a monitoring system is in place, the proper individuals must be notified before transporting the infant, and the proper hospital procedures should be followed. Otherwise, a **Code Pink** could be initiated that would trigger a warning that a possible abduction is taking place.

CALL OUT

As an essential part of patient safety practices, compliance with the hospital protocol for transporting infants and children must be ensured.

Older children may be transported on a gurney with the side rails up and locked and a safety belt securely fastened. The parent or guardian may accompany the patient to the imaging department. Some older children may prefer to be transported in a wheelchair. If this means of transportation is appropriate, make sure that the safety belt is securely fastened for the entire time that the child is seated in the wheelchair. Children must never be left alone while in the imaging department. If they are placed on a radiographic table, their parent/guardian or an attendant must be at their side until the procedure is completed and they are taken from the imaging room. If children must wait in an outside corridor, they must be attended at all times.

Infants or very small children must have back support if they are being held or carried. This can be done in a horizontal hold with the child supported against the body and the head supported on the arm at the elbow with a hand grasping the patient's thigh (Fig. 7-2). Another method is to hold the child upright with the buttocks resting on the arm with the other arm around the infant supporting the back and neck.

When a child is returned to a hospital room, the technologist or transporter must be certain that the side rails of the crib are up and must ascertain that they are locked. The bedside stand should not be at close range to prevent the child from using it as a stepping place to climb out of the crib. No unsafe items or liquids should be within reach of the child's crib. The nurse in charge of the child must be notified that the child has been returned to the room.

IMMOBILIZATION OF INFANTS AND CHILDREN

Occasionally, a child is not able to stay quietly in one place long enough for a successful diagnostic procedure to be completed; therefore, careful immobilization methods must be initiated according to the department's policies and procedures. For certain radiographic procedures, it is easier to use an immobilization device while the image is taken. Immobilizers should be used only when no other means are safe or logical and should be of a quality that does not cause injury to the patient or compromises the outcome of radiographic images.

There are several methods of immobilizing children. An immobilizer can be made by folding a sheet in a specified manner or may be a commercial immobilizer. The child may also be held in position by one or two assistants, provided they are given the proper radiation protective apparel. Several commercial immobilizers are available that are safe and effective for specific procedures. Whatever type of immobilizer is chosen, the child who is old enough and the parent/guardian must be made to understand, before the immobilizer is applied, that this is not a method of punishment and that it will be removed as soon as the procedure is completed.

📢 CALL OUT

Explain to the parents the immobilization method that is to be used and assure them of their child's safety. Explain the importance of immobilization that reduces the possibility of motion, and, in turn, reduces additional exposure to their child.

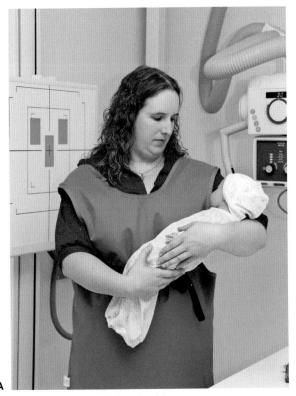 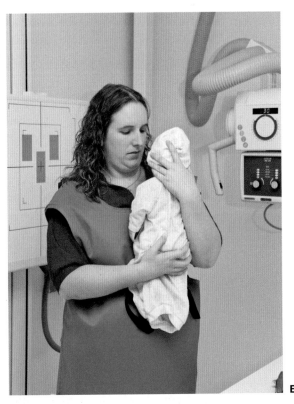

A   B

FIGURE 7-2 The mother is holding and supporting the infant's back and head in **(A)** horizontal and **(B)** upright position.

Commercial Immobilizers and Other Positioning Aids

The Pigg-O-Stat (Fig. 7-3A) is commonly used during chest radiography. It is important to prepare the parents and the child before beginning the procedure. Effectively informing the parent of the use of the immobilizer and the reasons for it reduce the anxiety associated with observing their child in the device.

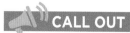
CALL OUT

When the pediatric patient cannot hold still to achieve specific positions during the exposures, it may be necessary to immobilize the patient for safety and/or to reduce radiation.

RADIOGRAPHER: *It is important to immobilize "Johnny" during the x-rays. (At this time, explain and demonstrate how the child will be immobilized without actually placing the pediatric patient in the device. Explain that the unit does not hurt the child.) By safely and carefully placing him in the unit, I can get quality images and eliminate the need for repeat exposures because of motion. If he cries, his lungs will fill with air and that is what I need. I will be as quick as possible. I would like you to stay with him and wear a lead apron to help me take the x-rays. (Explain where to stand so that the child can see the parent and know they haven't been left alone.)*

Ask if there are any questions before proceeding with the immobilization technique. Some department protocols provide the parent with protective apparel, allowing the parent to stand close to the child in the Pigg-O-Stat as seen in Figure 7-3B, because this reassures both the parent and the child and lessens anxiety and fear.

Another commercial device for immobilizing a pediatric child is the Pedia-Poser chair (Figure 7-4A). This is more user-friendly as it allows the child to sit in it like a chair instead of a saddle seat. The seat bench can be adjusted to accommodate an infant up to a toddler of age 4 years. A Pedia-Poser chair (Fig. 7-4B) has a stable base with locks on the wheels. After moving it to the desired location, it can be securely locked.

With the advent of digital imaging, the Pigg-O-Stat device is no longer used consistently. Many technologists lay the baby flat, taking a recumbent radiograph; however, this is not be the best method of allowing the lungs to expand fully.

If a child must be physically immobilized by another technologist or a parent during the examination, it is important to follow the department's pediatric

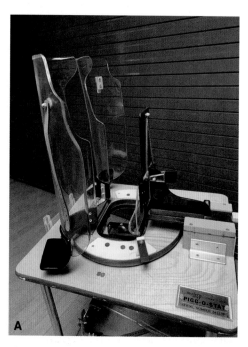
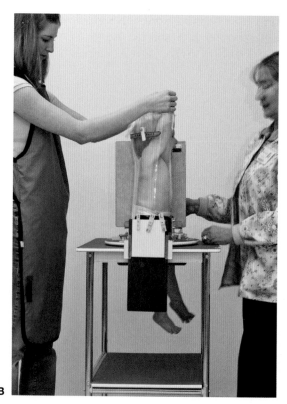

FIGURE 7-3 **(A)** A Pigg-O-Stat is used to image infants in a safe manner. **(B)** Here the mother is able to stand close to the child for reassurance.

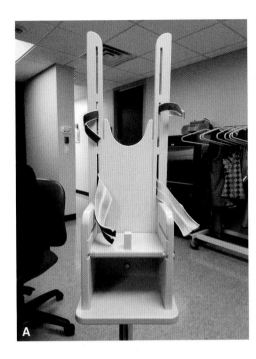

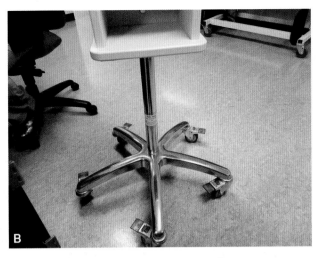

FIGURE 7-4 **(A)** The Pedia-Poser Chair is a convenient method for holding pediatric patients up to the age of 4 years. **(B)** The wheels can be locked securely to ensure that the chair does not move.

immobilization protocol. Under no circumstances should anyone use undue force when immobilizing the child; take care not to pinch or bruise the child's skin or interfere with circulation. It is better to use a sheet or commercial immobilizer than to use force.

To prevent a small child from rolling their head from side to side during skull radiography (Fig. 7-5), the person holding the child should stand at the head of the table and support the child's head with sponges between the hands, making sure to exert no pressure on the child's ears or fontanelles. When imaging the infant's and toddler's upper or lower extremities, it is important for the parent or the assistant to use lead gloves in addition to the lead apron when holding an extremity (Fig. 7-6). As with any imaging procedure, the pediatric patient must be provided with appropriate gonadal shielding.

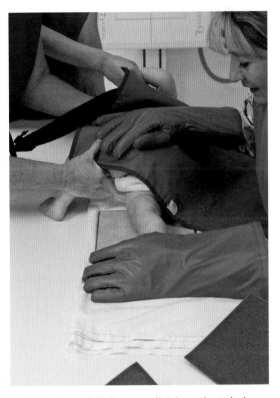

FIGURE 7-6 Immobilizing a pediatric patient during a lower extremity image.

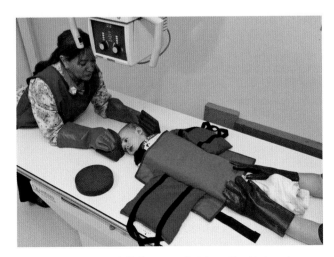

FIGURE 7-5 Immobilizing a pediatric patient's head during skull radiography.

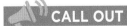
CALL OUT

Make sure to watch the pediatric patient at all times, especially during the x-ray exposure prep time to avoid repeat x-rays because of motion.

Sheet Immobilizers

Sheet immobilizers are effective and can easily be formed into any size or fashion, depending on which anatomy is imaged. To make a sheet immobilizer, fold a large sheet. Then, place the top of the sheet at the child's shoulders and the bottom at the child's feet. Leave the greater portion of the sheet at one side of the child. Bring the longer side back over the arm and under the body and other arm. Next, bring back the sheet over the exposed arm and under the body again. This method of immobilization keeps the two arms safely and completely immobile (Fig. 7-7).

Mummy-Style Sheet Wrap Immobilizer

Another method of immobilization is the mummy-style immobilizer approach. It is accomplished by folding a small sheet or a blanket into a triangle and placing it on the radiographic table, as seen in Figure 7-8. The distance from the fold to the lower corner of the sheet should be twice the length of the child. Place the child onto the sheet, with the folds slightly above the child's shoulders, making sure that the child's clothes are loosened or removed before being placed on the sheet if necessary. Bring one corner of the sheet over one arm crossing the child's body. If an upper extremity is to be imaged, tuck the corner under the baby. Bring the bottom corner up over the straightened legs, tucking the corner behind and under the infant. If both arms are to be immobilized, bring the remaining corner across the body with the arm snug against the body. Tuck the corner under the child. This immobilization method can be used for radiographic imaging procedures of the upper or lower extremities by leaving the extremity of interest unwrapped.

Other positioning aids and devices are available that aid in immobilization such as commercial devices that completely secure an infant. Creativity and patient

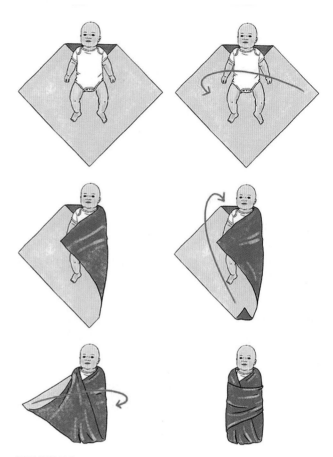

FIGURE 7-8 Mummy-wrapping an infant is an excellent way to immobilize an infant for imaging.

safety are limitations for positioning aids that include the use of sandbags, plexiglass, tape, Velcro, lead, and lead aprons.

RADIATION PROTECTION

Radiation protection is a priority for infants and children because of the radiosensitivity of their rapid and changing cell growth. The radiographer is responsible for using effective radiation protective measures during pediatric imaging procedures. The ALARA (as low as reasonably achievable) concept should be practiced in all aspects of the various procedures. Gender- and examination-appropriate shielding reduces the patient's exposure to radiation. In particular, gonadal shielding, either the contact or the shadow type, reduces patient radiation dose. The departmental protocol regarding shielding should be implemented for all pediatric procedures. In addition, the most appropriate imaging systems for pediatric procedures with the shortest exposure times and precise collimation greatly reduce the patient's radiation exposure (Fig. 7-9).

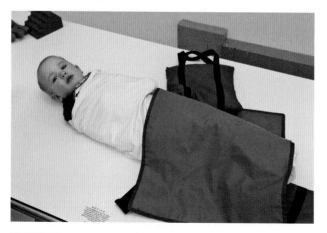

FIGURE 7-7 Use of a sheet for immobilization along with lead aprons and sandbags.

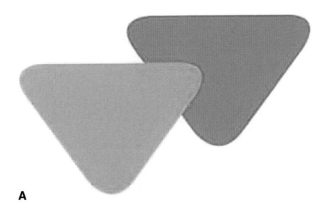

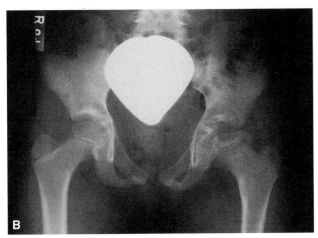

FIGURE 7-9 **(A)** The use of pediatric gonadal shielding is appropriate. This demonstrates a triangular shield that can be turned point down for a female or point up for a male. **(B)** The gonadal shield is used for a female patient in this pelvis image. (Reprinted with permission from Linn-Watson T. *Radiographic Pathology*. 2nd ed. Wolters Kluwer; 2014.)

The **Image Gently** campaign was founded in 2007 by the Alliance for Radiation Safety in Pediatric Imaging, the American College of Radiology, the American Association of Physicists in Medicine, and the American Society of Radiologic Technologists (ASRT) to raise awareness of the need to improve patient safety outcomes in pediatric imaging with an emphasis on computed tomography (CT) scanning initially. In 2014, all CT technologists underwent annual training on radiation dose reduction. The Image Gently campaign goal is to ensure that every technologist selects and uses the appropriate exposures when performing imaging and interventional procedures in children as safely as possible to reduce radiation dose.

ADMINISTERING MEDICATION TO THE PEDIATRIC PATIENT

Administering medications to children in the imaging department is a sensitive issue. The medical care of children is most frequently the role of physicians and registered nurses who have specialized education in pediatrics. Medicating children can be life-threatening and must not be undertaken by the radiographer. However, if a registered nurse is not available to administer the contrast media to patients under 18 years of age, the technologist may, with proper education and certification, administer the contrast media. Drug absorption, biotransformation, distribution, use, and elimination are different in infants, children, and early adolescents than in adults. For this reason, knowledge of pediatric medication administration is required to administer drugs accurately and safely to patients in these age groups.

The technologist must be aware of the potential for overmedication or for an adverse reaction to a drug or contrast agent in children. Before an infant or child receives medication or a contrast agent, they must be assessed for allergies and other medications that they take and that might not be compatible with the contrast. The information should be passed on to the physician who then prescribes the type and amount of contrast media.

As the technologist, make certain that the child who is receiving drugs or contrast media in the department is carefully monitored and is not released from the department until there is no risk of complications. Before being discharged, the patient must be assessed by a physician and authorized to leave with a parent or guardian. If the child is sleeping, they must remain in the department until awakening.

CHILD ABUSE

Child abuse is any act of omission or commission that endangers or impairs a child's physical or emotional health and development. There are 4 million cases of abuse and neglect reported each year. It involves over 7 million children, with the highest rate of abuse in babies less than a year old and another 25% involving children under the age of 3 years.

- Physical abuse—occurs when a child is purposely physically injured by another person
- Neglect—failure to provide adequate food, shelter, affection, supervision, education, or medical care
- Emotional abuse—injuring a child's self-esteem or emotional well-being through isolation, ignoring, or rejecting the child. Constant belittling or berating a child can also be classified as emotional abuse.
- Sexual abuse—any sexual activity with a child, such as fondling, oral-genital contact, intercourse, exploitation, or exposure to child pornography

- Medical abuse—occurs when someone gives false information about illness in a child that requires medical attention, putting the child at risk.

Child abuse usually is not a single act of physical abuse, neglect, or molestation, but is typically a repeated pattern of behavior. A child abuser is most often a parent, stepparent, or other caretaker of a child. A child abuser can be found in all cultural, ethnic, occupational, and socioeconomic groups.

The technologist may be assigned to image injuries that are the result of child abuse. It is the radiographer's ethical and perhaps legal obligation to report child abuse to the person at the institution who makes the inquiries and the required reports in such cases. In some states, all health care personnel are obligated to report suspected cases of child abuse. In other states, designated health care providers are obligated to do so. Technologists must learn the legal parameters of this obligation in the state where they practice. Each institution also has a policy and procedure with protocols that dictate the method of processing suspected cases of child abuse, which a radiographer is also obliged to know and use if the situation arises.

Any technologist assigned to image a child's injuries and who notes bruising, burns, or possible fractures that seem out of proportion to the history obtained of how the injury occurred may need to consider abuse.

Perhaps an older child tells a story about how the injuries occurred that does not correspond with what the caretaker has related. A child may report not having eaten for an inordinately long time because the parents have not provided food. Whatever form the suspected abuse takes, the radiographer must report it to the designated person in the workplace. In most states, the health care worker who reports suspected child abuse is protected from legal action if the report proves to be false; however, take care to refrain from false accusations. Often, children misjudge what is a safe action and suffer accidents because of their own mistaken judgment. Display 7-3 outlines common indications of abuse.

GERIATRIC PATIENTS

In 2020, 16.5% of the U.S. population was 65 years or older. It is expected to reach 22% by 2050. By 2060, it is expected that there will be 94.7 million people over the age of 65 years. This dramatic change is occurring because the baby boomer (born between 1946 and 1964) are entering their senior years. In 2020, the oldest of this group turned 74, with the youngest turning 54. It is expected that by 2030, all boomers will be at least 65 years old. Age 65 years is an arbitrary age designated for convenience as the age at which a person is eligible for Medicare benefits, Social Security benefits, and retirement

DISPLAY 7-3

Indicators of Physical Child Abuse

History	Child states the injury was caused by abuse
	Knowledge that the injury is not age appropriate
	Parent is unable to explain cause of injury
Behavior indicators	Child is excessively passive, compliant, and fearful
	Child is excessively aggressive or physically violent
	Child or caretaker attempts to hide injuries
	Child makes detailed/age-inappropriate comments regarding sexual behaviors

from many positions. The average life expectancy as of 2020 is 79.83 years, meaning that people who reach 65 years can expect to live another 15 years, but many people live much longer.

Persons aged over 85 years (Fig. 7-10) constitute one of the fastest-growing portions of the population (Display 7-4). By the year 2040, the population aged 85 years and over could increase by 123% from 2018. Many persons at this age are still quite youthful and productive; therefore, all persons must be assessed on an individual basis, not merely by their chronologic age (Display 7-5).

People 65 years or older are about three times more likely to be hospitalized than individuals in younger age groups. Also, the length of stay increases slightly with ages. Most older adults have at least one chronic condition.

The human body undergoes normal physiologic and anatomic changes as it ages. These changes do not occur uniformly in all people, so it is not correct to say that all persons begin to demonstrate the changes of age at the same time. Lifestyles, culture, and hereditary factors contribute to the aging process. When an elderly patient is admitted to the imaging department, the radiographer must be able to differentiate between the normal changes of aging and what may be pathology.

The elderly person is more frequently burdened with major illnesses that are chronic rather than acute in nature. Heart disease, cancer, and strokes are the cause of 80% of deaths in persons aged over 65 years. Hypertension, arthritis, diabetes mellitus, pulmonary disease, and visual

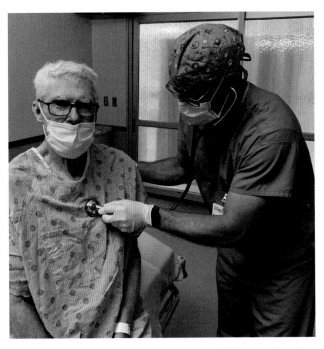

FIGURE 7-10 This young man who turns 85 years in a few days was having a hard time breathing. COVID required the use of mask wearing in all medical facilities.

DISPLAY 7-4

Aging Americans

Number of people 65 years or older	73 million or 16.5%
Number of people 85 years or older	6.5 million or 4.24%
Life expectancy for women	81.2 years
Life expectancy for men	76.2 years

Excerpted from the United States Census Bureau. *Quick Facts*. Available at www.census.gov/quickfacts /US. July 21, 2021. Accessed on March 28, 2022.; Centers for Disease Control and Prevention and the Alzheimer's Association. Alzheimer's Disease and Healthy Aging. Available at http://www.cdc.gov/aging. Accessed March 14, 2022; Federal Interagency Forum on Aging-Related Statistics. *Older American 2020: Key Indicators of Well-Being*. U.S. Government Printing Office; 2020.

and hearing impairments are also common conditions requiring long-term care. These conditions result in a great deal of physical discomfort and a multitude of social and psychological problems.

Depression is a common and debilitating emotional problem of the aged person. The threat of becoming a

DISPLAY 7-5

Categories of Young-Old to Elite-Old

Young-old	65-75 years
Old	75-85 years
Old-old	85-100 years
Elite-old	Over 100 years

burden to one's family, the fear of losing one's good health, or the necessity of giving up an independent lifestyle because of chronic disease results in feelings of helplessness and hopelessness that can give rise to a major depressive episode. Symptoms of depression in the elderly person are often confused with **dementia**. Symptoms of dementia, including disorientation, confusion, gross memory deficits, paranoid ideation, hallucinations, and depression, are not part of the normal aging process. When these symptoms are present in an elderly patient, the radiographer must remember that they are indicative of a disease process. **Alzheimer disease** is not part of the normal aging process, but growing older is the single greatest risk factor for the disease. It presents with symptoms of dementia, which may occur in persons aged over 65 years, although it may occur at an earlier time. Recent studies have indicated that of people aged over 85 years, about 50% suffer from Alzheimer disease at various stages.

📢 CALL OUT

Risk for specific diseases increases with age, but it is incorrect to make assumptions about diseases or cognitive function based solely on age.

When caring for a patient who exhibits symptoms of dementia, remember that the person may not be able to understand or retain directions. The radiographer has to explain to the patient what is to be done and then assist with following those directions. The patient who is confused or has a paranoid ideation may become frightened when confronted by the forbidding atmosphere of the radiographic imaging department. Allowing a familiar person to be present in the examination room to assist the patient may make the patient feel more secure and allow the procedure to be accomplished more effectively.

Persons who are depressed may be so preoccupied that they do not respond to outside stimuli. It may be necessary to give the same instructions a number of times to a depressed person and then to assist the patient in following directions.

The radiographer must assist the geriatric patient when the exam is over and make sure that the patient is attended to before leaving. The elderly patient must not be left alone in the radiographic imaging room, as there may be a danger of falling from the examining table.

CHANGES ASSOCIATED WITH AGING

Older adults may not have the same symptoms of a disease as a younger adult. They may have nonspecific symptoms, such as dizziness, falls for no apparent reason, infections without fever, or **urinary incontinence**. These are symptoms of disease and not a part of the normal aging process. The radiographer must be able to differentiate what is normal from what is pathologic. As aging progresses, the body systems change in a gradual manner. A brief overview of how the body systems change with normal aging, as well as the precautions the radiographer must consider because of these changes, follows.

Skin Changes

- The skin wrinkles, becomes lax, and dries out.
- Skin on the back of the hands and forearms becomes thin and fragile and veins enlarge (Fig. 7-11).
- Nails lose their luster and may yellow and thicken, especially the toenails.

Actinic keratosis occurs on different areas of the body, and if become thick enough, may show on digital images.

These changes do not occur in every ethnicity, but the implications for the radiographer remain the same for every patient, that is, to ensure that the skin of the elderly patient is not damaged.

Aging skin is susceptible to break down from shearing friction, which occurs in transfers over rough surfaces or from movement back and forth over wrinkled sheets. As collagen changes with age, the skin can't recover as quickly from injury. Older patients are more vulnerable to skin infections because of decreased vascularity, which lessens natural defenses.

Implications for the Radiographer

The radiographer must ensure that the elderly patient is protected from injury to the skin during transfers or while lying on the radiographic table for long periods of time. If this is the case, use a full-length pad on the table covered by a sheet. This helps prevent pressure on bony prominences.

Sensory Changes

- There is mild loss of visual acuity, particularly **presbyopia**.
- There may be age-related macular degeneration, which is the leading cause of vision loss in the elderly.
- Other changes to the eyes include cataracts and glaucoma.
- The lens of the eye thickens, making the pupils of the eye appear smaller.
- The light-sensing threshold is affected, and adaptation from light to dark and color perception diminishes.
- Tear production is either reduced or increased.

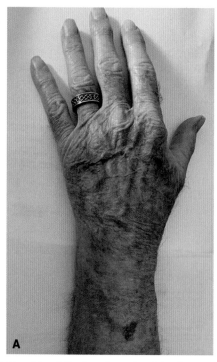 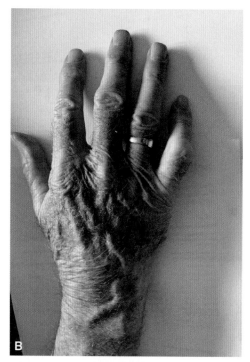

FIGURE 7-11 **(A)** The skin of the hands and wrists changes as a person ages. It loses elasticity, the veins enlarge, and age spots appear. **(B)** Joints also begin to fuse, leaving them crooked or immobile. Notice the 5th digit is not able to straighten.

- The skin of the eyelid loosens, and muscle tone decreases.
- Sensory, neural, and conductive changes occur in the ear.
- Hearing loss is common.
- The senses of taste and smell decrease.

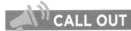

CALL OUT

Ensure and protect the patient from injury during radiographic examinations. Assist and observe as they are getting on and off the x-ray table at all times.

Implications for the Radiographer

Rapid changes in lighting, such as moving from a brightly lighted waiting room into a darkened examining room, may cause the elderly patient momentary blindness. Offer patients assistance so that they do not fall.

The radiographer must assess that the patient is able to hear directions. Do not assume that all older persons have a hearing deficit and need to be spoken to in an abnormally loud voice. If it is determined that the patient has diminished hearing, step closer to the patient (if culturally acceptable) or speak just loud enough for the patient to hear. Do not shout as that actually makes it harder to understand what is being said.

Pulmonary Changes

- Pulmonary function changes with age; lung capacity diminishes because of stiffening of the chest wall, among other changes.
- Cough reflex becomes less effective.
- The normal respiratory defense mechanisms lose effectiveness.
- Chronic obstructive pulmonary disease (COPD) or emphysema is seen more often in the elderly patient because of the years of abuse to the lungs from smoking or environmental conditions.
- Lung cancer is more common in people aged over 65 years and in former smokers. In fact, lung cancer causes more deaths than any other cancer in this age group.

Implications for the Radiographer

The patient becomes short of breath and fatigues more easily. Because of the decreasing effectiveness of the cough reflex, the patient is more apt to aspirate fluids when drinking. A patient with COPD cannot be expected to lie flat for more than brief periods because this position increases dyspnea.

During chest radiographic examination, when possible, ask the geriatric patient to take in a deep breath, exhale, and take in another deep breath and hold their

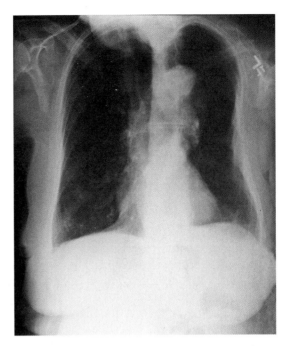

FIGURE 7-12 Posteroanterior (PA) chest image of a geriatric patient showing full lung expansion.

breath on the second full inhalation to ensure full lung expansion (Fig. 7-12).

Cardiovascular Changes

- Structural changes occur in the heart as aging progresses.
- The coronary arteries calcify and lose elasticity (Fig. 7-13).

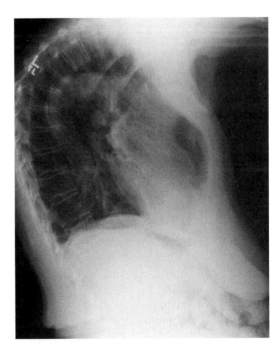

FIGURE 7-13 Lateral chest shows a female patient with severe kyphosis and atherosclerosis of the aorta. It also demonstrates where *not* to put the letter marker!

- The heart continues to pump the same amount of blood, but there is a decline in coronary blood flow.
- The aorta and its branches dilate and elongate; the heart valve thickens.
- The **baroreceptors** in the aorta and internal carotid arteries become less sensitive to blood volume and pressure changes.
- About 85% of patients over the age of 80 years have cardiovascular disease (CVD).
- Hypertension is common and can lead to other processes such as chronic heart failure (CHF) or stroke.

Implications for the Radiographer

Because of normal cardiovascular changes of aging, the elderly patient tires more easily; imaging examinations and procedures should be conducted in as efficient a manner as possible to avoid fatigue.

Hypothermia and complaints of feeling cold are common problems for the elderly patient because of decreased circulation; therefore, it is important to avoid chilling.

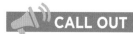

CALL OUT

Additional or warm blankets are helpful to prevent discomfort during radiographic examinations.

One-fourth of people aged over 65 years have postural hypotension (a drop in systolic blood pressure of 20 to 30 mm Hg) for 1 to 2 minutes after changing from a prone to a standing position. Rapid position changes result in a feeling of dizziness, and the patient may fall. The radiographer must always assist the elderly patient to a sitting position for a short time before they stand and step off the radiographic table. This allows the patient to adjust to the new position before walking.

Gastrointestinal Changes

- Gastric secretion, absorption, and motility decrease.
- There is a predisposition to dryness of the mouth, and the swallowing reflex becomes less effective.
- The abdominal muscles weaken.
- Many elderly patients do not have teeth, or the teeth present are decayed or gums diseased. Many have full dentures or partial plates.
- Esophageal motility declines.
- The tone of the internal anal sphincter decreases.
- Common conditions for the geriatric patient include diverticulitis and pancreatitis.
- Gastrointestinal (GI) malignancies are the second highest cause of cancer mortality and include cancers of the pancreas, stomach, and colon.

Implications for the Radiographer

If the patient is required to fast before a diagnostic examination, schedule the examination for the early morning so that the patient can have breakfast close to the usual time.

The elderly patient's ability to drink liquid contrast media may be affected because of a decline in esophageal motility. Instruct the patient to drink slowly to avoid choking. The patient who must drink liquid in the imaging department may need to be positioned in an upright position to prevent aspiration.

If a patient's dentures must be removed for some reason, place them in a plastic denture cup and in a secure location where they will not be broken or lost. Return them to the patient as soon as it is possible to do so safely.

The elderly patient may have a difficult time retaining the contrast media (Fig. 7-14) during a lower GI examination because of loss of sphincter control. This potential problem must be considered when planning for the procedure.

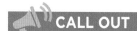

CALL OUT

The use of an enema tip with an inflatable cuff (Fig. 7-15) facilitates lower GI examination in patients with loss of sphincter control.

Genitourinary Changes

- Muscle tone and bladder capacity decrease.
- Pubic hair becomes sparse.
- Vaginal atrophy occurs.

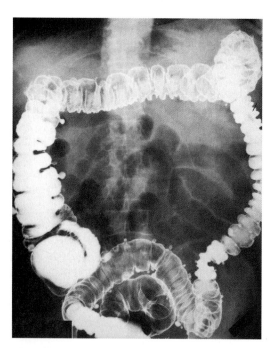

FIGURE 7-14 Double-contrast lower gastrointestinal image of an elderly patient demonstrating diverticula.

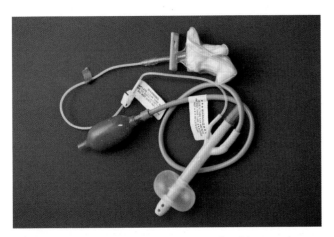

FIGURE 7-15 Double-contrast enema tip with an inflatable cuff is used to help patients retain the contrast during a lower gastrointestinal exam.

- Involuntary bladder contractions increase.
- The prostate gland enlarges, and the tone of the bladder neck increases.
- The size of the penis and testes is decreased because of sclerosis of blood vessels.
- Urinary incontinence is a common problem.

Implications for the Radiographer

Loss of muscle tone in the female genitourinary system may make the patient more susceptible to urinary incontinence in stressful situations. Both the elderly male and the female patient may have a limited bladder capacity and may need to urinate more frequently. Have a bedpan and urinal available for elderly patients who cannot use the lavatory easily.

Musculoskeletal Changes

- Bone mineralization is reduced, and bones become weaker. This is known as osteoporosis.
- Muscle mass decreases. Muscle cells decrease in number and are replaced by fibrous connective tissue.
- Muscle strength decreases.
- Tendons lose some of their water content, making structures more susceptible to pain or injury from stress.
- Ligaments become less elastic, reducing flexibility.
- Articular cartilage erodes and joint spaces collapse. Figure 7-11B demonstrates how joints can become immobile, such as the fifth digit.
- Intervertebral discs shrink, and vertebrae collapse, resulting in shortening of the spinal column (Fig. 7-16).
- There is an accentuated forward upper thoracic curve, which may result in **kyphosis**, as seen in Figure 7-13.
- The normal lordotic curve of the lower back flattens.
- Flexion and extension of the lower back are diminished.
- Placement of the neck and shaft of the femur changes.

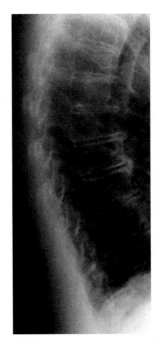

FIGURE 7-16 Lateral T spine shows loss of intervertebral space in an elderly female patient.

- Posture and gait change. In men, the gait narrows and becomes wider. In women, the legs bow, and the gait is somewhat waddling.

Implications for the Radiographer

Increased muscular weakness increases patients' discomfort when they are expected to assume positions necessary for imaging procedures. Painful joints and deformities accompanied by decreased tolerance for movement also increase discomfort. The radiographer must assist the patient to the required position and then use positioning sponges to facilitate maintaining that position. The risk of falling is greater when caring for elderly patients because of musculoskeletal changes. It is the radiographer's obligation to assist patients in positioning and getting on and off the radiographic table to prevent falls.

Neurologic Changes

- Brain weight changes, which may be because of reduced size of neurons (Fig. 7-17).
- The ability to store information changes very little in the absence of disease; however, some short-term memory loss occurs.
- Sensorimotor function decreases.
- Reaction time to both simple and complex stimuli decreases.
- The time needed to perform activities increases.
- There is a decrease in postural stability that is greater in women than in men.
- A decrease in **proprioception** creates problems with spatial relations.
- There is loss of sensitivity to deep pain.

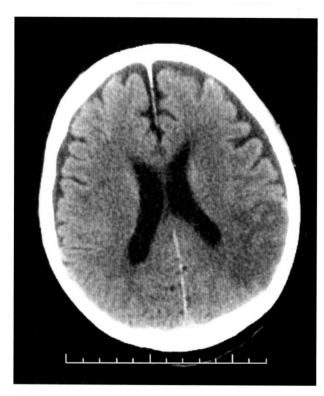

FIGURE 7-17 Computed tomography (CT) of the brain shows atrophy of the brain tissue away from the inner skull margin.

Implications for the Radiographer

Remember that the elderly patient is less responsive to painful stimuli and is not aware of a painful stimulus until an injury has occurred. The radiographer must increase awareness of potential for patient injury.

The elderly person processes information and direction in a slower manner. The radiographer must be certain that the patient understands directions and allow more time to execute moves.

FALL RISK

Physical changes can increase the risk of falling. Hearing deficits increase the risk of a fall because the brain is focused on trying to hear and not on walking. The patient with osteoporosis has an increased risk of a serious injury from a fall. Many elderly patients that have fallen are afraid of falling again.

The environment within the imaging department should be assessed for potential dangers that may cause a patient to fall. Is the floor free of obstacles that the elderly patient must navigate? One of the most common cause of falls in the radiography room is using a stool that has wheels. These should not be used but should be replaced with chairs if it is necessary to have wheels in order to move the patient while imaging an upper extremity or

 WARNING!

Never allow a patient to sit on a stool on wheels as it is too easy to fall off of. If wheels are required, use a chair with a back to provide stabilization for the patient.

doing upright head and neck images. To prevent injury, the locks on the chair wheels should be used, or the technologist should stand behind the chair to prevent it from moving backward as the patient sits down.

RADIATION SAFETY

The biologic changes that occur in an old or very old patient make them vulnerable to the harmful effects of radiation. Because organ mass decreases, less dose of radiation is necessary. The radiographer must assess the patient's body habitus and any related pathologic conditions that require adjustments to the technical factors of radiation. Just as in the pediatric patient with the campaign of "Image Gently," the ASRT advocates that the radiographer uses critical thinking skills and "Image Wisely." Avoid forming the habit of dose creep that was discussed in Chapter 4. Use the knowledge learned from the radiologic sciences and pathology classes to be ethical when it comes to setting the kVp, mAs, or choosing the processing algorithm.

ELDER ABUSE

It is estimated that 1 of every 20 seniors experiences elder abuse; the abusers are family members, caregivers, strangers, men, and women. Elder abuse is the neglect, mistreatment, or exploitation of anyone 65 years or older (or any disabled dependent adult). Unfortunately, the prevalence and reporting of elder abuse have increased in recent years. Elder abuse can involve:

- Physical abuse or violence: the use of physical force that may result in bodily injury, physical pain, or impairment.
- Sexual abuse: nonconsensual sexual contact of any kind with an elderly person.
- Emotional or psychological abuse: the inflicting of anguish, pain, or distress through verbal or nonverbal acts.
- Isolation or caregiver's neglect or self-neglect: the refusal or failure to fulfill any part of a person's obligations or duties to an elder or self.
- Financial abuse: occurs when anyone takes or keeps an elder's property with the intent to defraud.

CHAPTER 7: Patient Populations | 161

DISPLAY 7-6

Recognizing the Signs of Abuse

- **Physical abuse:** Injuries are incompatible with the explanations; bruises, scratches, or other injuries; inappropriate use of physical restraint or medication.
- **Sexual abuse:** The elder patient communicates acts of sexual abuse; bruising on the breast or genital areas with or without bleeding.
- **Emotional or psychological abuse:** Elderly person or dependent adult is withdrawn or secretive or is hesitant to talk freely around caregiver; family members or caregivers isolate the elder; restricting contact with other family members or friends; the elder verbally reports mistreatment.
- **Neglect:** Poor hygiene; dirty or torn clothes or lack of appropriate shelter; medical conditions that go untreated; malnutrition or dehydration
- **Financial abuse:** Unusual bank account activity; unpaid bills, eviction notices, or discontinued utilities; changes in spending patterns often accompanied by the appearance of a new "best friend"; the elder reporting financial abuse in various forms

Recognizing the warning signs of elder abuse is laid out in Display 7-6.

There are three subcategories of elder abuse:

1. Domestic elder abuse: This is a pattern of violence by someone who has a special relationship with the elder, such as a spouse, child, sibling, or caregiver.
2. Institutional elder abuse: This occurs in residential care facilities, such as assisted living or board and care; the perpetrators are usually the paid caregivers, staff, and professionals. Display 7-7 provides indicators to look for when institutional abuse is suspected.
3. Self-neglect or self-abuse: This does not involve a perpetrator, but rather the neglect is because of the elder refusing to accept care. Self-neglect can lead to illness, injury, or death.

Victims of elder abuse often remain silent and do not report incidences of abuse. They may fear retaliation or do not wish to report an abusive family member to protect the abuser from legal consequences.

Implications for the Radiographer

While it is not the duty of the radiographer to determine if there is elder abuse present, the radiographer should alert the radiologist who might be reading the images to any suspicions that may occur. With a history from the radiographer, the radiologist may be able to correlate a physical history with pathology seen on the images. While radiologists pay close attention to the clinical history in pediatric cases, they may need to rely on the critical thinking skills of the radiographer to make a differential diagnosis.

Display 7-8 provides information on how a radiographer can avoid being accused of abuse or neglect while imaging a patient.

DISPLAY 7-8

Care of the Elderly during Imaging Procedures

- Avoid pinching patient's skin, rough handling, or shoving while transferring the geriatric patient from a gurney or wheelchair onto the radiographic table.
- When immobilizing elderly patients, utilize the standards of care for immobilizing the geriatric patient as prescribed by the institution during imaging procedures.
- Assist geriatric patients when they ask for help.

DISPLAY 7-7

Indicators of Caregiver Elder Abuse

- Caregiver responds for the elder, preventing the patient from responding.
- Caregiver is flirtatious in an inappropriate sexual approach to the patient.
- Caregiver lacks affection toward patient.

PATIENTS WITH DISABILITIES

More than 40 million Americans have some form of disability. Increasing number of children are being diagnosed with asthma, which limits their physical activities; and more adults are suffering from some form of work-related activity. As noted in the previous section, seniors are living longer and many suffer from various health conditions that limit their abilities.

Disability should not be confused with the older term "handicapped," which suggested a negative connotation. Rather, disability is an umbrella term for impairments, limitations, and restrictions. Disabilities can be caused by trauma, disease, or a condition that interferes with a person's normal body processes. It also addresses how a person participates and interacts within the environment. As an example, a child may not be able to participate in sports such as baseball, football, and the like because of asthma.

There are different classifications of disability that might be seen in the imaging department. Mobility limitations can be caused by injury to the brain or spinal cord, or illness such as COPD. Sensory limitations affect a person's ability to speak, hear, or see. These can affect communication and safety in a medical facility or social environment. Patients with neurologic disorders such as Huntington disease, Parkinson disease, cerebral palsy (CP), or multiple sclerosis (MS) may present challenges for the radiographer unless there is a clear understanding of how these conditions affect a person.

Huntington disease begins when the brain's neurons start to deteriorate. Seen more often in patients 35 to 50 years of age, the symptoms can include involuntary movement of the feet, fingers, face, or trunk. Other complications are problems with coordination and balance. Radiographers need to be attentive to the needs of these patients and stand by to provide assistance as needed. Some type of immobilization may be necessary when imaging the extremities.

Parkinson disease, like Huntington disease, is a degenerative illness affecting the central nervous system that eventually leads to trembling of the upper and lower extremities. People may also experience muscle rigidity in their limbs. In the end stage of Parkinson, people need help standing and walking. This means that the radiographer needs to provide complete assistance for the patient when getting them on the radiographic table. Use of the critical thinking skills of how imaging can be done using various positioning methods needs to be employed.

MS usually occurs in people over the age of 20 years but rarely over the age of 40 years. People with MS start to have vision changes, muscle weakness, and difficulty walking because of weakness in the legs. It becomes difficult for people with MS to coordinate voluntary muscle activity and begin walking with jerky movements. Because of the movements and lack of coordination, the radiographer must always be at the ready to assist the patient. Always ask if a patient needs help before assuming that it is needed. It may be necessary to acquire help so that the patient is not left alone on the radiographic table.

CP involves injury to the brain, which affects movement, balance, and posture. CP is the most common motor limiting disability affecting children. Eighty percent of the people with CP have what is known as spastic CP where the muscles contract and cause tightness and stiffness. This interferes with walking and movement of the limbs. As with all the other forms of motor limiting disabilities, the radiographer must always be diligent to the patient's needs and constantly monitor the patient for any possibility of falling. If assistance is required, ask the caregiver or family member who may have come with the patient for help. If one is not available, get another radiographer for help. The patient's safety is the most important part of the radiographic exam in these cases.

Rearrange the room if the patient is in a wheelchair in order to provide the space necessary for the wheelchair to move. When speaking to a patient in a wheelchair, sit down so that eye contact can be made, which improves communication. The wheelchair should be considered part of the patient's personal space. It is not appropriate to use the patient's personal wheelchair as a resting spot for radiographic equipment needed during the examination. The radiographic table should be positioned to accommodate the patient's wheelchair if the patient can remain seated for the imaging.

Sensory disabilities such as hearing and visual impairment are common in adults and children. In the health care setting, meeting the needs of these patients ensures communication that improves patient-centered care. Many children do not receive vision screening soon enough to prevent visual impairment. Of course, visual impairment prevents these children from doing well in school, leaving many with poor educational outcomes. Additionally, people with low vision report that health care staff seldom ask how communication can be better accommodated while involved with exams and tests within a health care facility. Another consideration is the presence of a caregiver accompanying the patient. The radiographer must remember to speak to the patient and not the caregiver. It is important to also be mindful of the Health Insurance Portability and Accountability Act (HIPAA) and not violate the patient's privacy rights.

Hearing loss in children is usually a congenital condition or from chronic otitis media. One in five adults may have some hearing loss. Patients who are deaf or hard of hearing experience poor communication in the health care facility usually because of a lack of sign language interpreters. Although the law has improved the ability to have access to hearing impaired devices for communication while in the hospital, communicating with patients is still a problem as the patient may understand parts of the message while speaking with the health care worker, and, therefore, the radiographer may not realize that not all of the communication was understood or even heard.

Intellectual and developmental disabilities that are seen in children can range from minor to severe. Nearly 1 of 68 children is diagnosed with autism, which causes social, behavioral, and communication problems. Attention-deficit hyperactivity disorder (ADHD) is the most common neurobehavioral disorder in children. Children with this disorder have learning, language, coordination, mood, and anxiety problems. Different cultures perceive ADHD differently, creating additional knowledge needed on providing quality patient care.

Although any disability that the patient may have is a main consideration during imaging, it is important to remember that the patient is a person despite the disability. These patients are unique as any other individual that enters the imaging department for any type of examination. Involve the patient in all transfers after careful assessment of mobility and fall risk. Communication is critical in this assessment.

📢 CALL OUT

Do not assume that all patients with physical and sensory disabilities need assistance when walking, standing, or moving from a wheelchair to the table. It is wiser to ask the patient if assistance is needed.

THE AGITATED OR CONFUSED PATIENT

Patients with emotional problems may come to the ED for treatment that requires diagnostic radiographs, or patients who are hospitalized in mental health units may require diagnostic imaging procedures. These patients are frequently agitated or confused and may become combative.

Patients who react in a combative or aggressive manner usually do so because they are frightened or feel that they have no control over what is happening to them. They resort to violent behavior as a means of self-protection. This behavior may be brought on by chemical abuse or by **psychosis** of varying causes. The confused elderly patient may not understand what is happening and become violent because of a sense of fear. Precautions to ensure safety must be taken when threatened with this type of behavior.

Patients who are more likely to demonstrate combative behavior are those who have a history of such outbursts or a history of growing confusion and disorientation. Other warning signals are increasing agitation demonstrated by rapid pacing back and forth across the room; a patient in animated and increasingly noisy conversation with a person who is not present; a demonstration of illogical thought processes; refusal to be cooperative; or distrust of the medical personnel and explanations of the procedure or fear of the examining room and equipment. Patients who are combative occasionally display no emotion at all.

Before approaching a patient who is not reacting in a rational manner, discuss the case with nursing personnel if applicable. Request assistance if the patient is behaving in a combative manner or has a history of combativeness. It is wise to trust first instincts about a patient's behavior. Do not become isolated with a potentially assaultive patient. Always leave a door open and clear a direct path so that leaving a room quickly is an option if necessary. Do not begin the procedure without assistance from security or some other protective personnel.

At times, patients who are agitated or confused react more favorably to persons of a specific gender. If this seems to be the case, having a radiographer of the preferred gender conduct the procedure is helpful.

It is best to approach a patient who is agitated or confused from the side, not face-to-face. Never touch a patient who is behaving in this manner without first asking for permission to do so and explaining what is going to happen. Use simple, concise statements to explain the purpose of the procedure. Call the person by name. Give the angry patient an opportunity to express the anger, but make no attempt to defend or try to reason with the patient.

If a patient is speaking in a delusional or irrational manner, it is important not to become involved in the conversation, as doing so might increase the patient's agitation. If the patient refuses to proceed, simply stop and return the patient to the area from which they originated. Explain that the procedure will be continued at a later time. To continue to work with an agitated and confused person who is belligerent may cause injury to all persons involved. If the diagnostic images are essential to the patient's treatment, the patient has to be immobilized and supervised by persons in the hospital who are educated to care for such patients.

📢 CALL OUT

Do not become involved in a conversation with a delusional patient because this only validates the patient's concept of reality, which may not be correct.

CASE STUDY

While working the 3:30 PM to midnight shift at an acute care hospital, you are getting ready to perform skull radiographs on a 34-year-old male patient named Tony. Tony is an outpatient who had been waiting in the waiting room for almost 30 minutes by the time you came on shift and called him back for his exam. He seems to follow directions well and complies with requests to lie on the table on his back. However, when you ask that he turn over onto his stomach for the last two images, Tony suddenly starts shouting that you are trying to kill him by excess radiation to his brain.

ISSUES TO CONSIDER

1. What is the first response that should be made?
2. As you are soon to be the only technologist in the department, what should you do?
3. How should you end this examination?

THE INTOXICATED PATIENT

Patients who are intoxicated are often involved in accidents that result in injuries to themselves and to others. Intoxicated patients brought to the ED for care may be quarrelsome and reluctant to cooperate, may be unable to follow all rules of safety while being treated, and may inadvertently fall from a gurney or radiographic table.

The technologist caring for an intoxicated patient must keep the communication simple, direct, and non-judgmental. Do not become involved in the patient's attempt to argue. If the patient refuses treatment or becomes increasingly difficult to manage, call for help immediately. Do not attempt to complete the assignment until adequate assistance has arrived. It may be best to simply stop the procedure. Before doing so, get direction from the referring physician. Do not leave the patient alone, and observe the patient at all times to prevent falls. More than one strong assistant may be required to complete the diagnostic images of an intoxicated person.

Often, an intoxicated patient is accompanied by someone who is also intoxicated and belligerent. The companion may become aggressive and combative. In this instance, do not allow the companion to come into the examining room with the patient. Simply inform the companion that it is against the rules of radiation safety to be present and direct them to wait outside. If the companion chooses to argue, stop the procedure and call for assistance. Although this may not be a concern for the radiographer, under no circumstances should an intoxicated patient be allowed to leave the health care facility accompanied by an intoxicated companion. If necessary, notify security to prevent this.

CULTURAL CONSIDERATIONS

Race and **ethnicity** are often considered to be the same, but this is not the case. Race is considered to refer to all persons who have the same physical characteristics, such as skin coloration, body structure, hair color and texture, and facial appearance. It is the biologic or distinctive genetic traits of a group of people. Ethnicity is the grouping of people by shared backgrounds such as religion, culture, tribal, and other social factors. To put it another way, race is related to biology; ethnicity is how people identify with others.

Culture is defined as a shared system of beliefs, values, and behavioral expectations that provide social structure for daily living. This includes beliefs, habits, likes and dislikes, and customs and rituals of a particular group of people. Do not assume the cultural context of a patient based on race or ethnicity as it could offend the patient.

Culture affects how patients understand health, illness, and illness prevention. Culture backgrounds affect how people express pain or even if and when they seek help. When the health care worker doesn't consider this or is unaware of this while caring for the patient, the quality of care can be affected.

A group within a particular culture usually shares the same ethnicity or characteristics of social and cultural heritage. For example, the 2020 U.S. Census identified racial categories, as well as ethnic and cultural areas. Display 7-9 shows the different cultures and categories.

There are more than 100 ethnic groups and 562 federally recognized Native American tribes in North America. Each tribe is ethnically, culturally, and linguistically diverse. The population of ethnically diverse people is increasing rapidly. The U.S. Census Bureau believes that the population of the United States remains

DISPLAY 7-9

Race and Ethnicity for Federal Statistics

Population, Census April 1, 2020

Race and Hispanic Origin	Definition	% of Population
American Indian or Alaska Native	Persons having origins in any of the original peoples of North and South Americas who maintain tribal affiliation or community attachment	1.3
Asian	Persons having origins in any of the original peoples of the Far East, Southeast Asia, or the Indian subcontinent	5.9
Black or African American	Persons having origins in any of the Black racial groups of Africa	13.4
Hispanic or Latino	A person of Cuban, Mexican, Puerto Rican, South or Central American, or other Spanish culture or origin, regardless of race	18.5
Native Hawaiian/other Pacific Islanders	A person having origins in any of the original peoples of Hawaii, Guam, Samoa, or other Pacific Islands	0.2
White	A person having origins in any of the original peoples of Europe, the Middle East, or North Africa	60.1
Two or more races	A person who identifies with two or more of the above-listed categories	2.8

predominately White; however, based on the 2020 Census results, other groups are increasing disproportionately. Hispanics are now the largest minority group, replacing African Americans.

The implications of this influx of varying peoples into the health care system are significant. Culture and ethnicity play a major role in the assessment of the patient. The radiographer must not stereotype any person based on cultural or ethnic background. The patient who has been reared and educated in the United States has an understanding of the Western health care delivery system, whereas those from other countries may have little or no understanding of this system and may wish to return to their own traditions in health care. Critical thinking is demanded of the radiographer in assessing the patient and planning care. The patient's reactions to treatments offered, reaction to pain, and other aspects of health care may not be those to which the radiographer is accustomed. Aspects of this assessment include the following:

Culture: What are the customs and values of this patient that may affect treatment?

Sociologic: What is the patient's economic status, educational background, and family structure?

Psychological: How will the patient's self-concept and sexual identity affect a plan of care?

Physiologic and biologic: Are there anatomic or racial aspects of this patient that may affect a plan of care?

The radiographer must realize that there can be no standard model of assessment, plan, and intervention for care for all patients. North America is multicultural, meaning not all cultures have assimilated to the thinking of the area in which they live. Canada embraced this concept in the early 1970s and has accepted the differences among peoples. The United States, however, continues to live under the concept of the "Melting Pot." There are many different races, ethnicities, and cultures, but there is a belief of national culture, a homogeneous American society. Rather than embracing multiculturalism as in Canada and other countries, the United States encourages different cultures to assimilate into the American culture. Although people from all over the world are welcome, they are encouraged to integrate themselves into American society. The question is, with the U.S. population made up of peoples from all over the world with their own beliefs and cultures, what is the American culture?

This belief in health care has significant implications. Using only the Western-derived model for all patients may lead to a poor assessment and poor outcome of treatment.

All aspects of cultural and ethnic diversity must be a part of the radiographer's assessment and plan of care.

Cultural Considerations and Aging

Radiographers are aware of the challenges that may be experienced when imaging the elderly because of physical limitations, such as impaired vision, hearing, and/or limited mobility. Equally important is the need for the radiographer to develop cultural knowledge, awareness, and sensitivity when imaging the elderly in order to provide the best care. The word "culture" defines human behavior and beliefs, which include thoughts, communicated words, actions, and customs of various social, ethnic, religious, and economic groups. The importance of respecting the patient's beliefs and values improves patient care and provides a positive outcome for the imaging procedure. Otherwise, cultural insensitivity and intolerance may have an adverse effect on patient care.

The culture of the patient is reflected in an attitude toward aging, illness and its treatment, pain, death, and dying. Some elderly patients are accepting of whatever treatment the physician and other health care workers offer. Others require a detailed explanation and reassurance at every step. The relationship between the patient and the caregiver also varies with the cultural beliefs of the patient and family. It is important for the technologist to seek consent from the elderly patient to discuss the procedure or treatment with the caregiver to ensure that HIPAA is not violated. Some caregivers are highly solicitous and anxious concerning the treatment that their relative is to receive. Others leave the patient in the health care worker's hands and attend to other affairs.

Radiographers must perform the procedure by following an approach with sensitivity to the patient's cultural differences. In some societies, it is understood that the adult child who is the caregiver attends to every detail of a parent's medical treatment, whereas in other cultures, patients are expected to know and understand how to conduct their own care. If a caregiver is to oversee the patient's care, the radiographer should include them in the procedure based on their appropriate expectations to engage in the imaging procedure according to the departmental protocol. If this is not the case, the patient needs careful and complete direction that is appropriately and effectively communicated. Whatever the culture of the patient, one must be sensitive and take differences into consideration to provide the best possible patient care. The examination or procedure will be more comfortable for the patient, which facilitates the procedure for the elderly patient as well as the health care provider.

Cultural Competence

Culture competence in health care refers to the ability of the health care worker to demonstrate competence toward patients with diverse values, beliefs, and behaviors. To accomplish this, consideration of the individual social, cultural, and linguistic needs of patients must be met. It involves more than having sensitivity to the different cultures. It requires active learning and a development of skills that are reevaluated over time. A step toward being competent is to have an understanding of the different cultures that make up the patient populations. The Joint Commission (TJC) requires hospitals to provide orientation to all staff on cultural diversity.

Respecting a patient's cultural and personal values and preferences is an important part of each patient's rights. Understanding what these are goes a long way in providing quality patient care in a competent and friendly manner.

In Asian and Pacific Islanders, the extended family has significant influence. The eldest male is often the decision maker and spokesperson. Elders are respected, and their authority is often unquestioned.

Hispanics share a strong heritage that includes family and religion. Older family members are respected and consulted on important matters involving health and illness.

Native Americans are oriented in the present and value cooperation. They also place value on family and spiritual beliefs.

African Americans place importance on family and church. There are extended bonds with grandparents, aunts, uncles, and cousins. Usually, a key family member is consulted for important health-related decisions.

Any issues that arise can be minimized if the radiographer is aware of the differences between cultures. Although there are many different cultural issues that play a major role in patient compliance, only a few are presented here to help identify some of the major differences:

Language: Asian cultures are hierarchical, and it is not appropriate for a younger person to tell an older person what to do. The eldest male is at the top of the social hierarchy, so instructions to the patient may have to be conveyed through that family member.

Eye contact: Middle Eastern cultures avoid eye contact between men and women out of propriety. Direct eye contact may be interpreted as sexually suggestive. In Native American cultures, the eyes are the window of the soul. To look directly into the eyes could be seen as an attempt to steal the patient's soul. In Asian cultures, looking someone in the eyes directly implies equality. Also, Hispanics avoid direct eye contact as a way of demonstrating respect, although this is not as rigid as in most Asian cultures.

Gender: In Middle Eastern cultures, it is the role of the husband to protect his wife. The technologist must be aware of this when performing certain radiographic procedures.

Legal Concerns: A Case Study

Radiographers must be aware of the cultural beliefs of the patient population of the facility where they work. The highest diversity can be found in the larger metropolitan areas. Radiographers that do not consider the beliefs of their patient may find themselves in a legal situation. Just such a situation occurred in a large city where there is a high population of Asians. The patient arrived for a CT examination of the head. The history documented on the request was "dizziness." The radiographer called the patient back from the waiting room and observed that the patient did not walk with any difficulty and was able to get on the CT examination table without aid. After explaining the procedure to the patient, the technologist began the study. When it ended, the technologist went to the patient's side opposite that from the beginning of the examination. As he began to return the gantry to the upright position and lower the table, the patient tried to dismount the table. Unfortunately, the technologist did not stop this patient, who fell from a height, fracturing her hip. Through the discovery phase of the lawsuit, it came to light that Asians have a high degree of independence; they rarely ask for help unless it is absolutely necessary. Although there were other factors that were involved in the suit, the court ruled that the patient did not receive the expected standard of care from the technologist and ruled in favor of the patient. This case demonstrates the importance of an understanding of the cultural diversity of patients by the radiographer.

Summary

1. Pediatric patients range in age from newborn to 15 years. Older adolescents are aged 15 to 19 years.

   a. The technologist must relate to all patients in an appropriate and specific manner, regardless of age.

   b. The infant is usually accompanied by parents. The technologist should attempt to ease the parents' anxiety by giving them an explanation of the procedure to be performed and the approximate amount of time it takes.

   c. If it is necessary to immobilize the child, explain the reasons to the child (if appropriate), as well as to the parents. A soft material such as a sheet may be used. If the child is to be held, it should be done in a firm, safe, and nonthreatening manner to prevent injury. A commercially manufactured immobilizer is more effective. Protective apparel and shields should be worn.

   d. Child abuse usually is not a single act of physical abuse, neglect, or molestation, but is typically a repeated pattern of behavior. The abuser is most often a parent, stepparent, or other caretaker. Abusers are found in all cultural, ethnic, occupational, and socioeconomic groups. Pay close attention to the child and parent or caregiver for behavioral clues if child abuse is suspected.

   e. Medicating children can be life-threatening. If a registered nurse is not available to administer contrast media to pediatric patients, the radiographer may do so after receiving proper education and certification.

2. Each elderly patient should be assessed to determine any special needs and not generalize the disabilities of aging as they vary in each individual.

   a. Realizing the limitations that an elderly patient may have and adjusting the procedure to accommodate any needs of the limitation greatly facilitates the completion of the exam.

   b. The elderly are more likely to suffer chronic illnesses than acute ones, with heart disease, cancer, and strokes being the cause of 80% of the deaths in people over the age of 65 years.

   c. Depression is often confused with dementia in the elderly patient. However, do not confuse depression for dementia just because of the patient's age.

      i. Patients with either process may not fully understand directions. The radiographer must make sure that the patient is safe during an exam by assessing the patient's abilities.

      ii. These patients are at a higher risk for falling.

   d. Changes that occur with the aging process include changes with the skin, the sensory organs, respiratory and vascular system, the GI and urinary systems, and musculoskeletal and neurologic systems.

      i. Changes in the skin occur at varying ages but are usually noticeable by the age of 65 years. The skin becomes thin and is easily torn. The skin is susceptible to break down from pressure or laying in wet material. Use a pad on the table for the patient to lay on.

      ii. Sensory changes include vision and hearing, and the radiographer should be alert to the patient's movements to prevent falls. Do not assume that just because the patient is past the age of 65 years that there is a loss of hearing. If there is, stand closer and speak louder, but do not shout as that actually makes it harder for the patient to understand.

   iii. Lung capacity diminishes and the cough reflex is less effective. COPD and emphysema are common ailments seen in the elderly patient.

   iv. There are changes in the heart and the greater blood vessels as the patient ages. The heart valves thicken. Eighty-five percent of patients over 80 years have CVD. Hypertension is common and can lead to CHF or strokes.

   v. The abdominal muscles weaken and the swallowing reflex is less effective. GI cancers are the second highest and include pancreas, stomach, and colon. Rectal sphincters are less effective, so this must be taken into consideration with lower GI exams. Urinary incontinence is also a common problem.

   vi. The bones and muscles become weaker and many people have osteoporosis, which affects the technical aspects of the exam. Intervertebral disc spaces shrink and vertebrae collapse onto each other. This is a common cause of kyphosis. Patients experience more aches and pain in their joint spaces than in their younger years.

   vii. Neurologic changes cause increased reaction time to such things as driving a car. There may be short-term memory loss. Spatial relations may be affected because of depth perception changes.

  e. Elder abuse includes physical, emotional, sexual, financial, or neglect. These can occur as institutional, domestic, or self-abuse. The radiographer must be mindful of injuring an elderly patient so as not to be accused of abuse during imaging.

3. There are over 40 million Americans with a disability. Patients with mobility disabilities such as Parkinson disease, MS, and CP are often seen in the imaging department. The radiographer must make the imaging room accommodating for these patients to reduce any fall risks.

  a. Other disabilities include sensory, intellectual, and developmental disabilities, any of which might bring a patient into the imaging department. Remember that the patient with a disability is a patient despite the disability.

4. Agitated, confused, or intoxicated patient:

  a. Causes of the agitation or confusion may include chemical abuse, psychosis, or stress. Elderly patients may also be confused or agitated in the unfamiliar environment of the imaging department.

  b. If patients refuse the exam, do not argue and comply with their wish.

  c. Get a supervisor involved in order to determine if the images are critical to the care of the patient.

  d. If the patient is intoxicated, remain nonjudgmental and make sure that you and the patient can continue in a safe manner. If not, security assistance may be required.

5. Ethnicity is how people identify with others, whereas race is the color of the skin, facial appearance, and body structures—all things related to biology. Culture is a shared system of beliefs and values that provide social structure.

  a. Do not stereotype any person based on cultural or ethnic background. It is too easy to inadvertently insult or embarrass the patient, which has an adverse effect on patient care.

  b. Cultural competence requires an understanding of the different cultures that make up patient populations. TJC requires orientation to all staff on diversity.

  c. Language, eye contact, and gender are all issues that one should have some knowledge about when working in a multicultural environment.

CHAPTER 7 REVIEW QUESTIONS

1. Confusion and other symptoms of dementia are to be expected in an elderly patient because they are part of the normal aging process.
  a. True
  b. False

2. Which of the following statements is *not* considered part of the definition of cultural competence?
  a. It is an evolving process.
  b. Self-assessments are required.
  c. It requires a set of measurable skill and goals.

  d. It requires that organizations and their workers value diversity.

3. The World Health Organization's disease classification that encompasses an individual's limited ability to learn and function is known as:
  a. Mental retardation
  b. Cognitive disorder
  c. Intellectual disability
  d. Mental disability

4. Eighty percent of deaths in persons aged over 65 years are due to:
   a. Trauma, peritonitis, and emphysema
   b. Fractures, chemical abuse, and schizophrenia
   c. Cancer, heart disease, and strokes
   d. Diabetes mellitus, arthritis, and hypertension

5. Social determinants of health might include (1) education level, (2) income level, or (3) physical environment.
   a. 1 and 2
   b. 1 and 3
   c. 2 and 3
   d. 1, 2, and 3

6. Which of the following is true regarding individuals who have a learning disability?
   a. They have difficulty with at least two aspects of learning.
   b. As many as one in five American has a learning disability.
   c. People with learning disability usually have IQs in the normal range.
   d. Prevalence of learning disability remains constant in all age groups.

7. On average, people who reach age 65 years can expect to live nearly ____ more years.
   a. 5
   b. 10
   c. 15
   d. 20

8. Reports from the Agency for Healthcare Research and Quality have shown which of the following?
   a. Worsened access to care for minorities
   b. Worsened quality of health care for minorities
   c. Improvement in health disparities for minorities
   d. No change in quality of or access to care for minorities

9. Children who have ADHD are typically treated with which type of medication?
   a. Psychotropics
   b. Antidepressants
   c. Stimulants
   d. Anticonvulsants

10. The leading cause of vision loss in the elderly is:
    a. Presbyopia
    b. Cataracts
    c. Macular degeneration
    d. Glaucoma

11. Which of the following is NOT a culturally appropriate service in the health care field?
    a. Arrangement of language services in the patient's preferred language
    b. Knowledge of concerns the patient might have about touch and modesty
    c. Knowledge of potential discomfort with opposite gender workers helping the patient
    d. Obtaining appropriate religious paraphernalia for the patient during a procedure

12. Which of the following statements is true regarding aging and CVD?
    a. Veins become more elastic with age.
    b. The heart continues to pump the same amount of blood as it ages.
    c. The elderly always develops coronary disease.
    d. About half of people 80 years and older have CVD.

13. When communicating with children who have a mental health disorder, health care workers should: (1) address the parents instead of children, (2) address children directly, or (3) involve parents only as appropriate to assist with assessing a child's communication needs.
    a. 1 and 2
    b. 1 and 3
    c. 2 and 3
    d. 1, 2, and 3

14. To confirm understanding of information such as informed consent discussions, health care workers should:
    a. Ask patients if they understand and agree to the consent
    b. Have the family members respond for the patients and sign the consent
    c. Ask the patient to "teach back" what was discussed regarding the consent
    d. Give the patient various materials to read before asking them to sign the consent

15. Fall risk in the elderly is increased by all of the following *except*
    a. Physical changes
    b. Poor nutrition
    c. Decreased ability to regain balance
    d. Hearing deficits

16. About one-half of infants are hospitalized if they get which of the following?
    a. Asthma
    b. Respiratory virus infections
    c. Chickenpox
    d. Pertussis

17. Seniors living with family or in long-term care facilities are less at risk for elder abuse and neglect.
    a. True
    b. False

18. Which of the following are signs of autism? (1) Avoiding eye contact. (2) Disinterest in pretend games. (3) Problems with language
    a. 1 and 2
    b. 1 and 3
    c. 2 and 3
    d. 1, 2, and 3

Imaging Beyond the Outpatient

OBJECTIVES

After studying this chapter, the student will be able to:

1. Demonstrate the steps in performing various mobile procedures.

2. Explain how to manage various types of trauma situations.

3. List the precautions a radiographer should take when the patient has a head or spinal cord injury.

4. List the precautions a radiographer should take with a patient with a fracture.

5. Describe the special care needed to image a patient with wounds or burns.

6. Explain the radiographer's responsibilities while in the surgical suite.

KEY TERMS

Abrasion: A scraping or rubbing away of the surface skin by friction

Cervical: Of or pertaining to the neck

Concussion: Brain injury caused by a blow to the head that may or may not cause unconsciousness

Debride: Debridement is the removal of damaged tissue or foreign objects from a wound. It may include removal of dead tissue that prevents the wound from healing

Fracture: A disturbance in the continuity of a bone

Hemothorax: Collection of blood in the pleural cavity

Pneumothorax: Accumulation of air or gas in the pleural cavity, resulting in collapse of the lung on the affected side

INTRODUCTION

Mobile (portable) imaging procedures are performed on patients who cannot be transported to the imaging department because of a serious injury, illness, or other condition. Therefore, many patients are imaged with the use of mobile radiography equipment in the emergency department (ED); in intensive care, coronary care, neonatal intensive care units (ICUs); in special care rooms; in the patient's room; or in the operating rooms (ORs).

The trauma patient may be strapped to a backboard with a cervical collar and splints in place. These patients commonly have oxygen, intravenous (IV) tubing, or life support equipment when the radiographer is to perform trauma mobile radiographic procedures. Because these patients cannot be transported to radiology, the radiographer must adapt all skills to achieve diagnostic images according to the patient's condition and needs. Specifically, a radiographer must adapt positioning and technical considerations (the central ray [CR], image receptor [IR], and exposure factors) during the course of performing trauma mobile radiography. In addition, the radiographer must analyze each patient situation in relation to the procedures requested by the physician, while at the same time keeping in mind general radiation protection measures. Preplanning is essential for achieving diagnostic outcome images under trauma or mobile circumstances.

MOBILE RADIOGRAPHY

Student radiographers, no doubt, hear the term "portable" x-ray. This term has been in use since wheels were put on a unit so that x-ray could be performed outside of the imaging department. However, this is not an accurate term and mobile radiography is the correct description of exams using this type of equipment. Mobile radiographic units allow images to be taken under conditions that keep a patient from coming to the imaging department. Almost any radiographic exam can be performed with a mobile unit. Surgical radiography cannot be performed without a mobile unit (with the exception of cystography tables); chest radiography in the ICU or critical care unit (CCU) is completed every morning with a mobile unit; and trauma radiography in the ED is performed with mobile units until the patient is stabilized and able to come to the imaging department for further evaluation in computed tomography (CT) or magnetic resonance imaging (MRI). Many times, rather than bringing the patient to the imaging department from the ED, patients are imaged with the mobile unit while on the stretcher (Fig. 8-1). This allows the patient to remain connected to the various equipment used to monitor heart rate, pulse, and oxygen levels.

Radiographic mobile units (Fig. 8-2) operate on batteries that must be recharged by plugging the unit into a

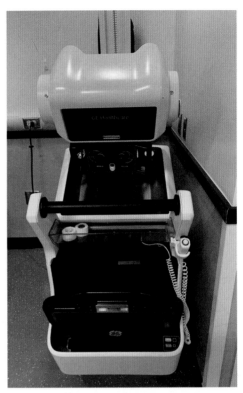

FIGURE 8-2 A mobile unit "parked" in the emergency department ready for use. Notice that it is plugged in and is charging to be ready for its next use.

wall outlet. Fluoroscopic mobile units (most often used in the OR or in the ICU for pacemaker insertions) are known as C-arms because of the configuration of the unit, as can be seen in Figure 8-3. These allow images to be viewed on a monitor in real time (dynamic) or as a stationary (last image hold) image for comparison. It is a large portion of the radiographer's workload and is therefore critical that students are well versed in manipulating the equipment so as not to hit a patient's bed (or the patient!) with the mobile unit, as well as learning how to place the C-arm over a surgical patient without destroying the sterile field.

Mobile radiography can be challenging in terms of positioning. Patients in a hospital bed or on a stretcher in the ED must have the IR placed behind or underneath them (Fig. 8-4). There is no "Bucky" tray in which the IR can be placed and aligned to the CR. Radiographers must be able to determine the amount of angle to place the x-ray tube in order to match it with the IR. Sometimes, it is necessary to reposition the IR because of patient body habitus (Fig. 8-5A and B). Cross-table lateral images are not as easily performed while in the ED as many times, there is limited space and only a curtain between patients. The radiographer must be creative and use the critical thinking skills that come with experience. Determining how the image can be taken without moving the body part and only angling the tube and IR requires "thinking outside the box" and comes with practice.

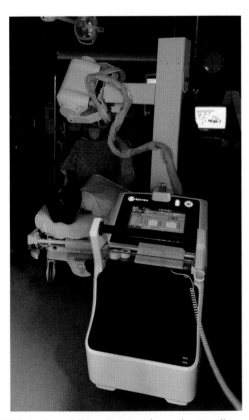

FIGURE 8-1 A mobile unit setup for a chest radiograph in the emergency department.

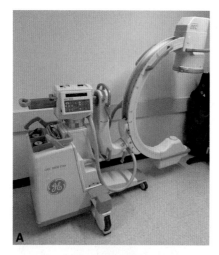

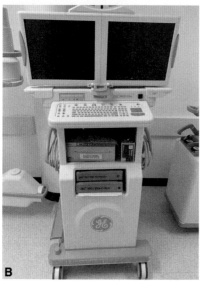

FIGURE 8-3 **(A)** A C-arm is used most often in the surgical suite. It gets the name from the configuration of the tube over the image receptor that is always aligned. **(B)** These double monitors allow images to be saved on one side while dynamic images occur on the other.

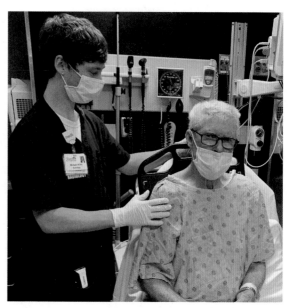

FIGURE 8-4 The image receptor goes behind a patient's chest for a mobile chest x-ray in the Emergency Department.

Guidelines for Radiographers

The following guidelines can be used when performing mobile radiographic procedures:

1. Review the radiographic request for a mobile procedure and gather any special equipment that may be needed prior to starting the exam (Fig. 8-6).
2. Confirm the patient's identity with two identifiers and confirm the procedure to be completed with the patient and/or nursing staff or physician if there is any discrepancy.
3. Assess the patient for ability to follow directions and assist with positioning. Obtain assistance, if needed.

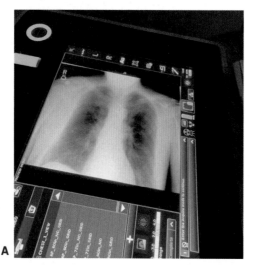

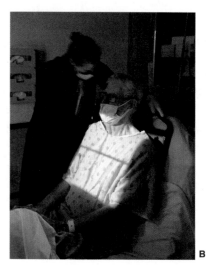

FIGURE 8-5 **(A)** A patient with long lungs requires adjustment of the IR to get the angles on one image. **(B)** Repositioning the image receptor (IR) and keeping the alignment with the central ray (CR) does take practice.

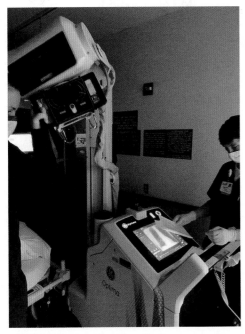

FIGURE 8-6 Before performing the image, make sure to check the request once more to ensure that the correct patient and exam are being performed. (Illustration courtesy of Shutterstock/Madmeow.)

4. Have visitors leave the area while the images are being performed. Attend to radiation protection as necessary.

5. After the images have been taken, clean the IR and the mobile unit with a disinfectant wipe approved for this type of use (Fig. 8-7A and B).

6. Be sure to leave the patient in a safe environment with the bed rails up as applicable.

TRAUMATIC INJURIES

Traumatic injuries are caused by external force or violence (Fig. 8-8). Injury (trauma) is the leading cause of death among all persons under the age of 44 years. The injuries may be the result of:

Motor vehicle accidents (MVAs)	Choking
Pedestrian accidents	Industrial accidents
Motorcycle accidents	Suicide
Falls from heights	Drowning
Assaults (stabbings and gunshot wounds [GSWs])	Smoke inhalation
Blunt trauma	Sports injuries

The trauma patient presents a wide variety of challenges for the radiographer. The nature of the injury and the patient's condition require the radiographer to use critical thinking and judgment of a knowledgeable radiographer. Technical knowledge combined with the ability to adapt creatively is required to provide the physician(s) with the necessary diagnostic information to treat the patient. In some cases, trauma radiographs are obtained rapidly to screen for life-threatening injuries.

The radiographer is one of the first members of the health care team to see the patient once the patient is admitted to the ED after traumatic injury or acute

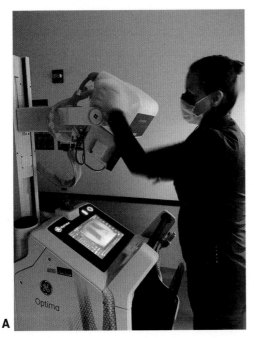

A

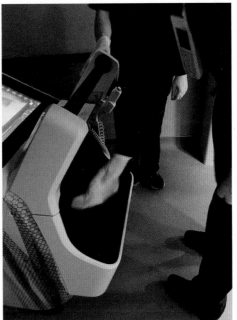

B

FIGURE 8-7 After each use, the **(A)** mobile unit and the **(B)** image receptor must be cleaned with a disinfectant.

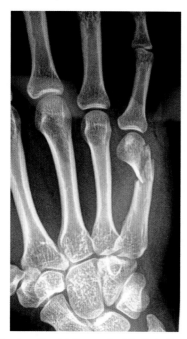

FIGURE 8-8 A patient hit a wall with their fist, fracturing the fifth metacarpal. A Boxer's fracture is a traumatic injury.

illness (Display 8-1). Trauma patients can have a single injury or multiple injuries. When the radiographer is called to the ED to perform diagnostic radiographic images, it must be assumed that exposure to the patient's blood or body fluids is likely. To avoid infecting oneself or the patient, always maintain standard precautions by having clean disposable gloves available before beginning the procedure. The appropriate personal protective equipment must be worn if applicable.

DISPLAY 8-1

Emergency Team Members

Emergency physician, attending physician, and resident/medical student	Respiratory therapist
General and/or specialty surgeon available (if indicated)	Phlebotomist
Two emergency registered nurses	Anesthesiologist
Pediatric nurse (if required)	Admitting clerk
Radiology technologist	House supervisor

This may include gloves, mask, goggles, a protective gown, and a lead or lead equivalent apron when caring for a patient who is hemorrhaging or vomiting. If it is necessary to touch an open wound, wear sterile gloves. In addition, the IR must be protected with an impermeable covering or bag.

Many patients admitted to the ED are in severe pain. Depending on a patient's injuries, the radiographer is required to assist in diagnosing the extent of injuries or illness by taking a series of images. This requires patience and skill. The radiographer needs to accomplish the procedure without extending present injuries or increasing the patient's discomfort. Usually, time for achieving the goal is brief because the patient's life may be at risk. In trauma radiography, general radiation safety measures must be combined with speed and accuracy.

If the injured or acutely ill patient is transferred from the ED to the diagnostic imaging department for images, the radiographer must observe the patient for symptoms of shock. The radiographer assesses the patient's neurologic status and level of consciousness before beginning any procedure, and then reassesses every 5 to 10 minutes while the patient is in the department. If any changes in the patient's condition are observed, the physician and the emergency team are quickly alerted, and the radiographer prepares to assist with emergency measures, as outlined in Chapter 9.

Guidelines for Radiographers

The following are the general guidelines when caring for a patient who has traumatic injuries:

1. Do not remove dressings or splints.
2. Do not move patients who are on a stretcher or backboard until ordered to do so by the physician in charge of the patient.
3. When performing an initial cross-table lateral **cervical** spine radiograph, never move the patient's head or neck or remove the cervical collar. The physician must interpret the radiograph and "clear" the cervical spine for injury before removing the collar or moving the patient. Many patients now go directly to CT for imaging without radiographs.
4. Request direction from the ED team when planning moves and assemble adequate assistance to move the patient safely and as painlessly as possible.
5. Do not disturb impaled objects. Support them so that they do not move as the patient is imaged.
6. Do not remove pneumatic antishock garments.
7. Have oxygen, suction equipment, and an emesis basin ready for use (Fig. 8-9A and B).
8. Work quickly, efficiently, and accurately to minimize repeat images.

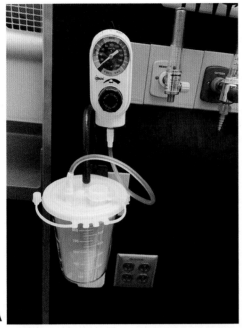
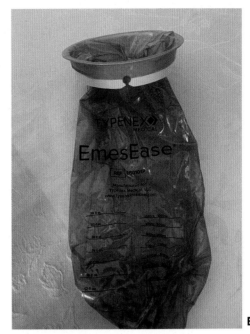

FIGURE 8-9 **(A)** Suction equipment is usually located on the wall of the emergency department alongside an oxygen flow meter. **(B)** Emesis containers allow a larger volume without the mess of the old basins.

Basic Rules for Trauma Radiography

The following are the basic rules for trauma radiography:

- Assess the situation and develop an action plan for the imaging procedure.
- Verify the patient's identification with two patient identifiers.
- Verify the x-ray examination with the physician's order.
- Make introductions to the patient.
- Determine patient mobility and explain the procedure to the patient.
- Predetermine equipment and accessories needed for the procedure (Display 8-2).
- Announce "x-ray" before making an exposure to allow personnel to leave the area for mobile procedures.
- Take at least two radiographs at 90° to one another for each body part (Fig. 8-10A and B).
- Make sure that the CR and IR alignment approaches routine positioning applications, adapting to the patient's condition.
- Include all anatomy of interest.
- For long-bone radiography, include both the joints; two exposures may be required with overlap (1.5 to 2 inches) to ensure that the entire bone is included.
- Provide radiation safety protective apparel for anyone who asks for it. Digital imaging has reduced the need for this measure; however, it must still be offered and provided if desired.

DISPLAY 8-2

Equipment and Accessories Needed in a Trauma Situation

- Lead aprons and other protective apparel for those involved in the procedure
- Universal precaution supplies (gloves, gown, and mask as needed)
- Impermeable IR covers
- IRs and grids (if required)
- Letter markers
- Positioning sponges with impermeable covers
- Mobile (portable) or C-arm unit

A cooperative environment with all personnel involved in the emergency procedure facilitates proper care of the patient.

Head Injuries

The term "head injury" may refer to any injury of the skull, brain, or both that requires medical attention. Radiographers are not called to perform radiographic images as often as in the past because of the effectiveness of CT, which allows the physicians to diagnose head, brain, and facial injuries (Fig. 8-11). All head injuries are potentially serious because they may involve the brain, which is the seat of consciousness and controls every human action.

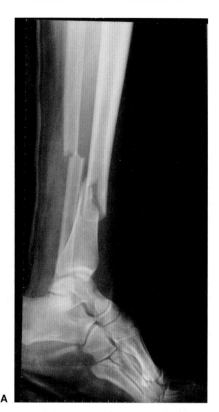 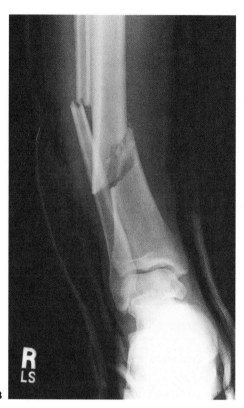

A   B

FIGURE 8-10   **(A)** Lateral and **(B)** anteroposterior right ankle. These trauma radiographs are taken at right angles to each other to demonstrate the deviation of the bone fragments that are not seen in the lateral projection.

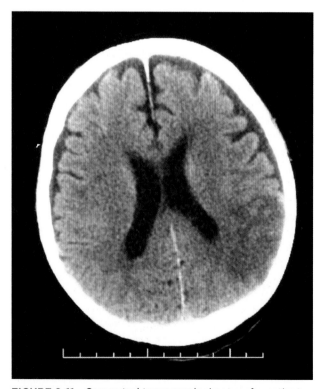

FIGURE 8-11   Computed tomography image of a patient suffering a head trauma.

The two basic types of head injury are open and closed. With an open injury to the skull or meninges, the brain is vulnerable to damage and infection as its protective casing has been broken. If the injury is closed (also called a *blunt injury*), the brain tissue may swell. The swelling is limited by the confines of the skull, and the resulting pressure may cause extensive brain damage. The brain has little healing power, so any injury to it must be considered potentially permanent and serious.

Fractures at the base of the skull (*basal skull fractures*) often have accompanying fractures of the facial bones. This type of injury may result in a tear in the *dura mater*, the outer membrane surrounding the brain and spinal cord, and a leakage of the cerebrospinal fluid (CSF) may result.

Consider all patients with head injuries to have accompanying cervical spinal injuries until it is medically disproved. Take precautions to alleviate potential extension of these injuries. It is vital for the radiographer to be knowledgeable in understanding the signs and symptoms of patients with a variety of injuries. It is important to report any observable changes in the patient's status to the emergency physician and/or team.

With a head injury of any magnitude, the patient is assessed by the Glasgow Coma Scale (discussed in detail in Chapter 9). This provides a score that places a patient at one of four levels of consciousness: (1) alert and conscious; (2) drowsy; (3) unconscious but reactive to stimuli; or (4) comatose. Patients scoring high have a minor brain injury, and a low score (3 to 8) indicates a severe brain injury.

Radiographer's Response

1. Keep the patient's head and neck immobilized until the physician rules out injury to the spinal cord.
2. Do not remove sandbags, collars, or dressings. Take all radiographic images with these in place.
3. Do not flex the patient's neck or turn it to either side. Rotation of the head may increase intracranial pressure.
4. Keep the patient's body temperature as normal as possible. Do not allow the patient to become chilled or overheated.
5. Check the patient's pulse and respirations frequently while performing the procedure.
6. Observe for airway obstruction.
7. Apply a sterile pressure dressing if bleeding becomes profuse, and call for emergency assistance.
8. Observe the patient for signs and symptoms of hypoxia and changes in level of consciousness. If a patient who is initially alert and cooperative suddenly appears to be drowsy or slow to respond, immediately notify the physician in charge of the patient.
9. Be prepared to assist with oxygen administration and other emergency treatments. Patients with head injuries must not be suctioned through nasal passages.

Traumatic Brain Injuries

There were 64,000 traumatic brain–related deaths in the United States in 2020. These injuries affect how the brain works and are caused by head injuries substantial enough to cause swelling or bleeding to the brain itself. Falls, firearms, MVAs, and assaults account for the majority of traumatic brain injuries. Brain injuries that do not cause death may need ongoing care as disabilities are often permanent when the injury is moderate or severe.

A **concussion** occurs when the brain is jolted, hitting the inside of the skull. Individuals suffering from repeated concussions can suffer from personality changes, depression, and anxiety. Radiographers must be watchful of the patient who has suffered some type of head injury as it very well may have caused a brain injury. Although a Glasgow Coma Scale test does not have to be performed, the radiographer must be able to determine any changes in the patient's ability to respond to directions.

WARNING!

Never leave a head trauma patient alone in the radiographic room.

Medical Interventions

Although most head injuries are mild and require only rest and minimal observation to allow time for the brain to heal, some may have lingering effects such as persistent emesis, loss of consciousness, or some form of amnesia. These patients should be evaluated with a CT scan of the head. If the CT scan reveals no pathology, the patient can be discharged but must be observed for up to 8 hours. Those patients with a moderate-to-severe head injury must be watched for hypotension, as they have a mortality rate twice that of patients without hypotension. Patients with these types of head injuries are usually intubated and require a chest image to make sure the tube is located in the correct place. Certainly, these patients receive a CT scan of the head and neck, and possibly chest, if the injuries stem from an MVA. As mentioned earlier, the radiographer may not be called upon to take mobile radiographic images in the ED as often as in the past. Once patients are stabilized to be transported to the CT department, this type of imaging is faster and more effective than radiography.

Spinal Injuries

The spinal cord carries messages from the brain to the peripheral nervous system. It is housed in the vertebral canal, which extends down the length of the vertebral column. The spinal column is protected by the fluid in the canal and by the vertebrae—the bony structures encircling the canal. Motor function depends on the transmission of messages from the brain to the spinal nerves on either side of the spinal cord. Injury to or severing of the spinal cord causes message transmission to cease. The result is a cessation of motor function and partial or complete cessation of physical function from the level of damage to the cord to all parts below that level.

The severity of the injury to the cord is dependent on the location of the injury and if there is complete or incomplete severing. Most spinal cord injuries occur in the cervical or lumbar areas because these are the most mobile parts of the spinal column. The cause of spinal injuries is often the result of MVAs, falls, or GSWs. The spinal cord loses its protection when there is injury to the protective vertebrae. Spinal cord tissue, like brain tissue, has little healing power; injuries to it usually cause permanent damage.

Assessment

The radiographer is among the health care workers to attend to the patient with a possible spinal cord injury, to assist in making the diagnostic assessment of the injury. If signs or symptoms of cervical spine injury are present, the patient may need a cervical spine series. Take great care in obtaining these radiographs to prevent extending the existing damage to the spinal cord. A mobile cross-table lateral cervical spine radiographic image with a horizontal beam may be taken in the ED without moving the patient or removing the backboard, collar, or sandbags used to immobilize the spine (Fig. 8-12). Remember that any movement can result in bone fragments or unstable vertebrae compressing the spinal cord and extending the injury. If this is cleared, the patient most likely is taken to the CT or MRI department for further examinations. However, if all seven cervical vertebrae cannot be seen on the cross-table lateral image (Fig. 8-13), it may be necessary to perform a "swimmers" projection (Fig. 8-14) to see the lower portion of the cervical spine. It is extremely important that the patient not move the neck but only the arm. Figure 8-15A and B, although not the best quality image, demonstrates the importance of seeing all seven vertebrae. This image is "dark" as the technologist was trying to demonstrate C-7 through the shoulders. It can be seen faintly but enough to show the subluxation of C-6 over C-7. If this patient had been moved without determining the seriousness of the spine injury, they could have been paralyzed.

Symptoms

Patients with spinal cord injuries typically have some level of paralysis and decreased motor sensation, depending on the severity of the injury and its location. Those with complete transection of the spinal cord experience paralysis of the skeletal muscles with a loss of sensation (touch, pain, and pressure) below the level of the injury. There may also be respiratory distress, bradycardia, unstable blood pressure, and bladder and bowel incontinence.

If only a partial transection of the spinal cord has occurred, there is some sensory retention such as feeling pain, pressure, and touch. Loss of reflexes and paralysis are asymmetric below the level of the injury. The blood pressure is more stable.

Radiographer's Response

If the patient is a trauma patient and is unconscious, assume that there is a spinal cord injury until disproven. Most often, the radiographer is required to take the images in the ED with the mobile unit; however, if the patient must come to the imaging department, the radiographer must:

1. Monitor vital signs.
2. Maintain an open airway. If respirations change, notify the physician at once and call for assistance. If in respiratory failure, use jaw downward movements. Do not tilt the head.
3. Do not allow or request the patient to move when performing radiographs. Do not move the patient's head or neck.

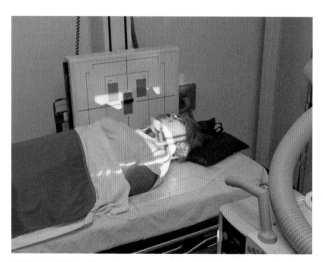

FIGURE 8-12 Do not move a patient with a suspected spinal cord injury until a lateral, cross-table image has been taken and cleared.

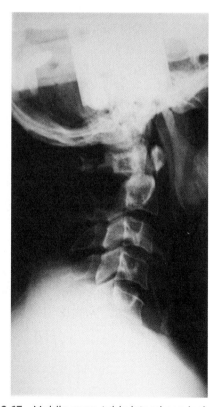

FIGURE 8-13 Mobile cross-table lateral cervical spine image. Only five vertebrae are shown so another type of image must be obtained.

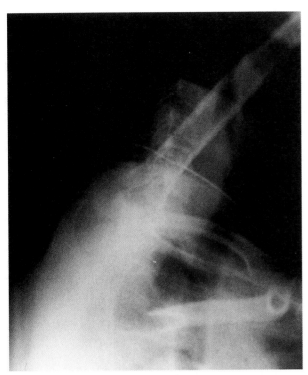

FIGURE 8-14 If C-7 and the top of T-1 cannot be demonstrated, a Swimmer's projection can be performed.

4. Do not remove sandbags, collars, antishock garments, backboard, or other supports until diagnosis is confirmed and a physician supervises the removal.

5. Observe for signs and symptoms of shock.

6. Keep the patient warm.

Transporting the Patient with a Spinal Injury

The best means of moving a patient is with a log roll, discussed in Chapter 5. However, if it is necessary to move a patient from gurney to the radiographic table, it is best to use a lateral transfer board. If the patient is not on a backboard, it is necessary for the radiographer to obtain three assistants to assist with the log roll. The lead person stands at the head and directs the other three members of the team. The lead person places hands on both sides of the patient's head alongside the neck with the hands under the shoulders. One person places hands across the patient's body under the shoulder and hip, the next person places hands under hip and knee (from the inside), while the last person places hands under the lower leg and ankle from the inside (Fig. 8-16A). On direction from the lead radiographer, the first two movers roll the patient's body in unison, whereas the last two movers lift the leg to keep the spine in a straight line, as seen in Figure 8-16B. At this time, a scoop board or transfer board can be placed under the patient along with a sheet if there isn't one already under the patient. Be sure to roll the patient back in unison and check alignment of the spine from neck to sternum to symphysis pubis to ensure it is in a straight line. Once the patient is on the board with a sheet, it is quite easy to move the patient from side to side or up and down as the sheet slides on the surface of the radiographic table.

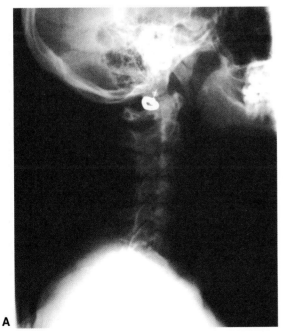
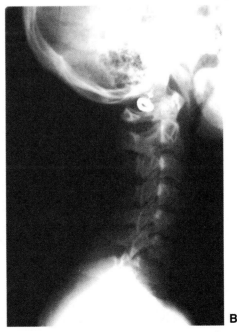

FIGURE 8-15 **(A)** Cross-table lateral C-spine image only shows six cervical vertebrae. **(B)** After pulling the shoulders down, this image shows the subluxation of C-6 over C-7. (Reprinted with permission from Linn-Watson T. *Radiographic Pathology.* 2nd ed. Wolters Kluwer; 2014.)

Logroll method

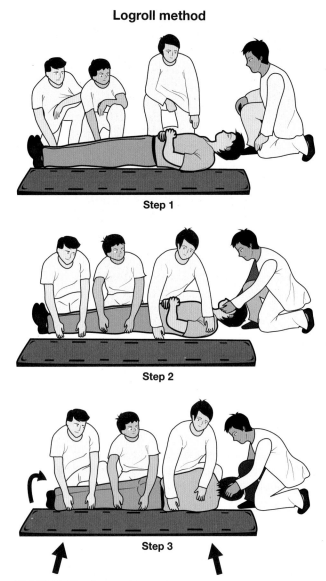

FIGURE 8-16 Step 1: Obtain four individuals to perform a log roll. Step 2: Proper hand placement of each of the three assistants and the radiographer at the head is shown. Step 3: On cue from the lead person, everyone turns the patient toward themselves. (Illustration courtesy of Shutterstock/Madmeow).

Fractures

A fracture may be defined as a disturbance in the continuity of a bone. Fractures can be classified simply as open or closed. An open fracture indicates a visible wound that extends past the skin surface. The broken bone itself often breaks through the soft tissue, making the fracture clearly visible.

A closed fracture may not be obvious to the untrained eye. Often, there is swelling around the injured areas, pain, and deformity of the limb. All or some of these symptoms may be absent, and a closed fracture still may be present. Figure 8-17 shows a slight deformity

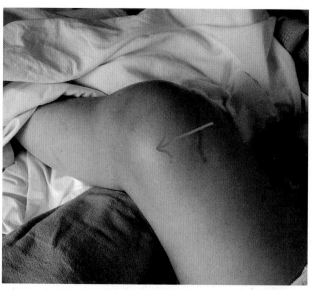

FIGURE 8-17 Deformity of the distal femur indicating a femur fracture.

on the lateral aspect above the knee of this patient who fell down the stairs fracturing her femur above the prosthesis of total knee replacement. Figure 8-18 A and B shows the actual fracture, which is more severe than would be anticipated from looking at the patient. This again illustrates why it is so important to do two images at 90° to each other. After going to surgery, an intramedullary rod was placed into the femur and screwed into place (Fig. 8-19).

Internal injuries caused by fractures of the pelvic bones are a leading cause of death after MVAs. Always consider the possibility of a fractured pelvis when caring for patients with multiple traumatic injuries. Use extreme caution when making initial diagnostic radiographs because the slightest movement may initiate hemorrhage or irreparable damage to a vital organ. Patients with suspected pelvic fractures may be on a backboard or in pneumatic antishock garments. These are radiolucent and must remain in place during initial assessment radiographs. At times, it may be feasible to move the patient to the radiographic table on the backboard that has been placed by the emergency team because this device allows the patient to remain immobilized.

A large number of trauma deaths result from blunt or penetrating trauma to the thorax. Multiple rib fractures can cause a flail chest, which in turn may result in **pneumothorax** (air or gas in the pleural space that collapses the lung) (Fig. 8-20) or **hemothorax** (blood in the pleural space). Fractured ribs are extremely painful and can be life-threatening. Stab wounds and GSWs can also cause fractures to the ribs and hemorrhage into the pleural cavity. When working with patients who have suffered this type of trauma, work quickly while observing the patient for symptoms of shock because

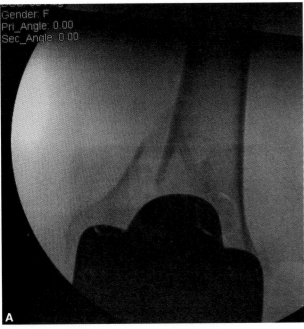
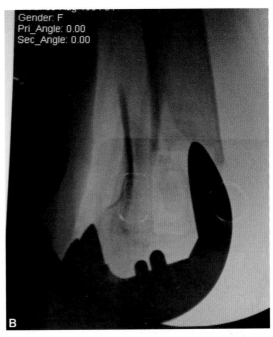

FIGURE 8-18 **(A)** Anteroposterior image taken in surgery shows how the femur has been fractured with the distal portion moving laterally. **(B)** Lateral image shows just how far displaced the femur became. These images are the radiographs of the patient from Figure 8-17.

of hemorrhage. Also, avoid causing further pain or extending injuries.

Hip fractures and fractures of the femur are common among elderly patients as a result of bony changes related to age and disease (Fig. 8-21). These fractures are a common result of home accidents in elderly patients,

and these patients must be treated with utmost care to prevent extension of the injury. With a practiced eye, the radiographer is able to assess patients that come from the ED on a stretcher with a knee slightly bent and rotated externally. If the patient is an elderly female with a history of a fall, it is likely the hip is fractured.

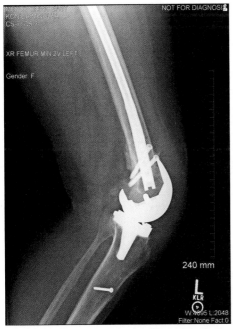

FIGURE 8-19 The patient had to have the fracture repaired in surgery with the use of an intramedullary rod.

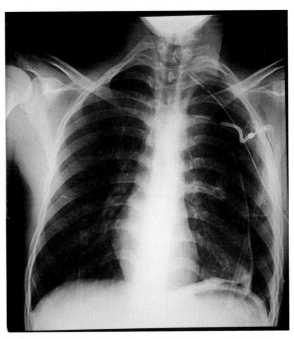

FIGURE 8-20 Chest radiograph showing a chest tube inserted to alleviate a left pneumothorax.

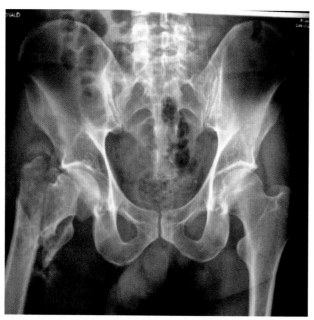

FIGURE 8-21 Pelvis showing a hip fracture. This patient was homeless and walked with a fractured hip for over a month causing it to become severely displaced.

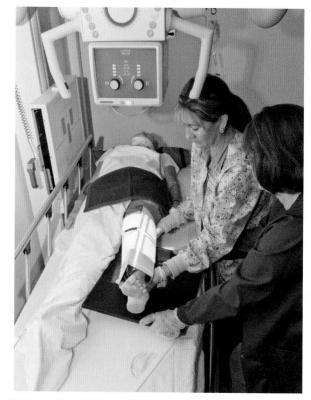

FIGURE 8-22 Support the limb at both joints to raise it enough to place the image receptor.

Symptoms

- Pain and swelling
- Functional loss
- Deformity of the limb
- Grating sound or feel (crepitus) if moved
- Discoloration of surrounding tissue because of hemorrhage within tissue (closed fracture)
- Overt bleeding (open fracture)
- Possible signs and symptoms of shock

Radiographer's Response

1. Keep affected limb or body part immobilized.
2. Inform the patient of any intended moves to enlist support.
3. Do not remove splints or other supportive devices.
4. When moving a splinted limb, support the limb at both joints above and below the fracture (Fig. 8-22).
5. If the patient has an open fracture, wear sterile gloves if in contact with the wound, and use standard precaution measures.
6. Observe the patient for signs and symptoms of shock, and be prepared to act if such an emergency occurs.

Follow-up studies ordered on patients following the initial examination are usually performed in the radiology department, but may also be performed as a mobile procedure. In some cases, the patient may require surgery after initial examination.

Wounds

There are multiple types of wounds that may be seen in the ED and/or the imaging department. Wounds that pierce the skin and go into the body are known as penetrating wounds. This would include such things as puncture wounds (stepping on a nail) or surgical wounds made by the physician during an operation. Wounds that injure the layers of the skin (such as burns, chemical, or thermal) may need special care as will bites and stings from animals that break the skin surface. Patients involved in bicycle or motorcycle accidents may have **abrasions**, lacerations, and skin tears that are blunt force trauma type of wounds. Wounds caused by pressure sores such as a decubitus ulcer are often chronic and require special treatment and care, especially if moving the patient onto the hard surface of a radiographic table.

Wounds on patients coming through the ED have almost always been treated, even if only temporarily, before the radiographer is required to take images. If the wound has dirt and debris in it, the area must be cleaned before closing it. If not, infection can set in, causing complications. Antibiotics may be required or even anesthesia to **debride** the wound. Hospital glue may be used to repair a small opening and comes off after a few weeks, which is usually enough time for the wound to heal. Steri-Strips are a special type of bandage that can be used to pull the skin edges tightly together. These are left on until they fall off. Stitches must be removed by the physician (or assistant) after approximately 7 days. These are a more stable method of closing the wound until it heals. Regardless of the wound treatment used, the radiographer must be aware of it and be careful not to remove any bandages that have been placed over the area. If it appears on the radiographic image, make a note of it on the requisition for the radiologist.

Burns

Burns are a common injury seen in adults and children. Many combat victims have acute burns that can be fatal if the severity of the burn is significant. As of 2020, almost 400,000 burn victims were treated in the United States. Recent research is defining how ultrasound imaging modality is able to assess burn depth. Developing this technique of classifying burns would greatly improve care and decrease associated complications.

Burns are classified in degrees, depending on the depth of penetration of the skin's surface. First-degree burns affect the outer layer. A sunburn without blisters is a first-degree burn. Second-degree burns penetrate a bit further down than the first-degree burn. It causes the skin to turn red and blister and may be painful and swollen. Third-degree burns go into the innermost layer of skin known as the subcutaneous tissue. The skin looks either white or turn black and look charred. Fourth-degree burns are the most severe as they may involve muscle and bone. The nerve endings are destroyed, leaving the patient with no feeling in the area.

Patients who have been burned or exposed to smoke from a fire manifest pulmonary complications because of the inhalation of smoke. Mobile chest radiographs are an important diagnostic tool to determine adult respiratory distress syndrome (ARDS). Patients do not show signs of ARDS immediately after the incident, but rather, several days after exposure. It is usually the pulmonary complications, along with other organ crisis, that cause patient mortality. If the radiographer is required to perform a mobile chest radiograph on a burn patient, it is critical that precautions be taken to prevent infection. The protocol for infection control for burn victims must be followed very carefully and patients with burns are susceptible to septicemia.

SURGICAL RADIOGRAPHY

In addition to conventional mobile x-ray equipment, a radiographer must be prepared to use the C-arm fluoroscopic mobile unit for a variety of procedures as part of the health care team in the OR. The radiographer's role during OR procedures is to provide the physician with images of the site of interest for determining the exact location, position, and alignment for appropriate fixation or approach for patient treatment and care.

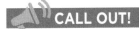 **CALL OUT!**

The technologist may be asked to image patients prior to the operation (pre-op), during the operation (intraoperative), or in the recovery room (postoperative).

The Surgical Team

The surgical team consists of a variety of staff members who serve the patient before and during surgery. They are:

Surgeon: The physician who plans and performs the surgical procedure and makes surgical decisions.

Surgical assistant: Usually, another surgeon or surgical resident. There may be several assistants if the patient's surgical needs require this.

Anesthesiologist: A physician with special education in anesthesia who makes the decisions concerning the type of anesthesia required.

Nurse anesthetist: A registered nurse who has had special education in anesthesia who administers anesthesia and monitors the anesthetized patient under the supervision of the anesthesiologist.

Circulating nurse: Oversees the safety of the patient and maintains the surgical environment; is attired in scrub suit, cap, mask, and shoe covers, but is not clothed in sterile attire.

Scrub nurse or scrub technician: Dons sterile attire and sets up the sterile fields for the operation. Assists the surgeon by presenting sterile instruments and sterile equipment needed during the procedure.

Radiologic technologist: Present at the request of the surgeon to perform imaging procedures; is clothed in a scrub suit, cap, mask, and shoe covers.

The Surgical Environment

Every possible effort is made in the surgical suite and in special procedures areas to protect the patient from infection. Barriers that limit the source of contamination are used for this purpose. All persons who enter the surgical suite or special procedures areas are expected to follow the rules established to maintain these barriers. There are theoretically three zones designated in the surgical suite to help decrease the incidents of infection. They are:

Zone 1: An unrestricted zone—persons may enter in street clothing.

Zone 2: A semi-restricted zone—only persons dressed in scrub dress with hair covered and shoes covered may enter.

Zone 3: A restricted zone—only persons wearing scrub dress, shoe covers, and masks are allowed to be present. If a surgical procedure is in progress, the doors to this area are kept closed, and only persons directly involved in the procedure may be present. Those directly involved in the operation are dressed in sterile gowns and sterile gloves. They are often referred to as *"being scrubbed."*

Surgical departments have dress and behavior protocols that are strictly enforced. The radiographer who is assigned to work in this area is expected to follow these protocols as designated by the Occupational Safety and Health Administration. They are:

1. Shoes must be comfortable with closed heel and toe and not cloth covered. Cloth-covered shoes may allow blood, body fluids, and other liquids to permeate. Cloth-covered shoes will not protect the feet should a heavy object fall on them, such as an IR or detector.

2. Personal hygiene must be meticulous. A shower should be taken shortly before beginning a workday in the OR or special procedures area.

3. Jewelry, long or artificial fingernails, and nail polish are prohibited. Jewelry harbors microorganisms as do long, polished, or artificial nails.

4. Any body-piercing jewelry must be removed because it may become loose and fall onto the sterile field.

5. All persons who expect to proceed from the unrestricted zone into the semi-restricted zone must obtain and put on a scrub suit. Tuck the top of the scrubs into the pants or wear a scrub top that fits close to the body. Many facilities now have a unit (Fig. 8-23) that dispenses the pants and tops. Individuals must have a code to retrieve the garments, and when they are returned to the dispenser, it is credited back to the person's code. This deters the theft of surgical pants and tops that was fairly common because of the comfort of these items!

6. All hair, beards, or mustaches must be covered with a surgical cap and mask. Hair must be confined because it sheds microorganisms with movement (Fig. 8-24). Shoe covers must be placed over shoes to reduce contamination and to protect shoes from coming in contact with blood and body fluids.

7. Before proceeding into Zone 3, all persons must scrub hands and arms for medical asepsis. It is believed that bare skin may shed microorganisms. In many institutions, all who are not scrubbed for the surgical procedure must wear a scrub jacket to cover bare arms.

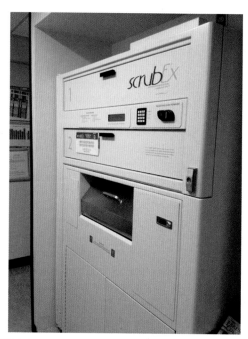

FIGURE 8-23 Unit dispenses surgical tops and pants after an individual enters a code.

8. Before entering a room where a surgical procedure is in progress, a mask must be securely worn. The masks worn in the OR must be single, high-filtration masks. These masks protect the patient from droplets expelled by personnel and protect the health care

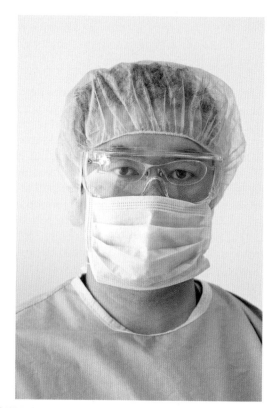

FIGURE 8-24 Make sure that the mask covers all facial hair.

worker from pathogenic organisms in the surgical environment. The mask must cover the nose and mouth and must not gap. The ties should not cross because it may create venting (Fig. 8-25). Because they are regarded as highly contaminated, masks must be worn for only one procedure and then discarded by touching only the ties of the mask and dropping into the receptacle for this purpose. A mask must not be placed around the neck to be worn again (Fig. 8-26).

Sterile drapes and other equipment and supplies used for sterile procedures must be packaged in a particular manner to be considered safe for use. They are also stored in a particular manner that protects them from contamination. Any break in sterile technique increases the patient's susceptibility to infection. Those involved in carrying out a sterile procedure must constantly be aware of which areas and articles are sterile. If a sterile article is touched by a nonsterile one, it must be replaced by an article that is sterile. The radiographer must learn correct methods of opening sterile packs and donning sterile gown and gloves.

The use of contaminated instruments or gloves, a wet or damp sterile field, or microorganisms blown onto a surgical site are the most common causes of contamination. Ventilating ducts in the OR must have special filters to prevent dust particles from entering the room.

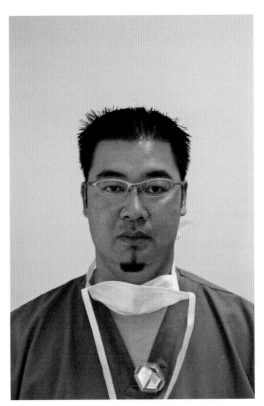

FIGURE 8-26 A mask that has been untied and allowed to touch an unsterile top must not be reused. Do not allow the mask to hang around the neck.

Airflow and humidity must be controlled to prevent static electricity. Doors must remain closed, and traffic into and out of the room must be carefully controlled. When radiographers need to use mobile radiographic equipment that is not stationed in the OR, they must carefully clean it with a disinfectant solution before bringing it into the suite.

Conversation in the OR or special procedures room is kept to a minimum. The radiographer must always be aware that the surgeon is in charge while performing a surgical or invasive procedure. The environment is often tense as the patient's life is at risk, and needless conversation is not welcome.

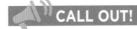 **CALL OUT!**

The technologist must be ready to follow the physicians' instructions during imaging in the OR at all times to ensure that the mobile x-ray or the C-arm is positioned correctly to facilitate the procedure.

The radiographer whose work involves sterile procedures must develop a sense of responsibility and maintain the highest standards possible when practicing surgical asepsis. The patient's welfare depends on this.

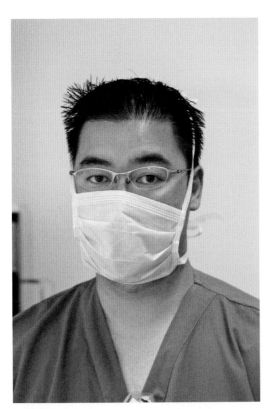

FIGURE 8-25 The mask must be securely tied behind the neck and on top of the head so there is no gap at the sides.

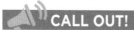
CALL OUT!

When mobile imaging is required, all individuals present during x-ray exposures should wear radiation-protective apparel or stand behind mobile shielding.

The radiographer is responsible for making certain that any radiographic equipment used during a sterile procedure is clean and dust-free before use. The following are some guidelines for working in the OR and special procedures areas:

1. Mobile machines or C-arms must be cleaned with a disinfectant solution, and if IRs are to be used, they must also be cleaned with a disinfectant solution.
2. Sterile technique must be maintained for all items and persons involved in the invasive procedure.
3. If possible, when using imaging receptors, place them before draping the patient for the procedure.
4. If the IRs must be placed after the procedure is begun, the radiographer may pass the IR to the scrub nurse who receives the IR in a sterile plastic bag and places it in the radiographer's direction.
5. If the radiographer places the IR, the surgical team must make room. The radiographer may place the IR by raising the sterile drapes, touching only the inside of the drape, or the circulating nurse may lift the drapes and assist in placing the IR into the holder. However, most imaging in the OR is now performed with the mobile C-arm. If the mobile C-arm is used, a sterile cover is placed over the components when it is placed over the patient during fluoroscopy (Fig. 8-27).

   If multiple images or fluoroscopic imaging is used, all personnel who are not scrubbed must stand behind the mobile shield. The scrubbed members of the team must wear radiation-protective apparel. They may also step behind protective lead-lined shields (Fig. 8-28).
6. When hands are directly exposed to radiation, leaded sterile gloves as well as all other protective equipment must be worn.
7. Pregnant female personnel should not be present in the OR when radiographic or fluoroscopic imaging is in progress.
8. The radiographer must wear the radiation detection monitor on the outside of the lead apron and under the sterile gown during imaging procedures.

Imaging in the OR can be rewarding or it can be stressful. If the radiographer is experienced in the use of the equipment, is knowledgeable of the sterile fields, and is confident in positioning, the experience can be one of acceptance and fulfillment. Don't be afraid as it takes time to become competent in this arena. Take time to

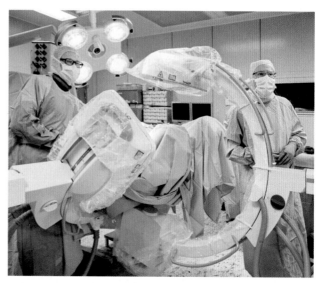

FIGURE 8-27 Because the image receptor and the tube of the C-arm may very well be placed over the open wound in surgery, a sterile plastic cover is placed over both to keep the area sterile. In this case, the patient is having hip surgery and there are two C-arms in use for the anteroposterior and lateral images.

learn the physician's routine and mannerisms, and speak with the surgical team for ideas on how to be useful when needed. This goes a long way to provide an atmosphere that is enjoyable, even though the situation is serious.

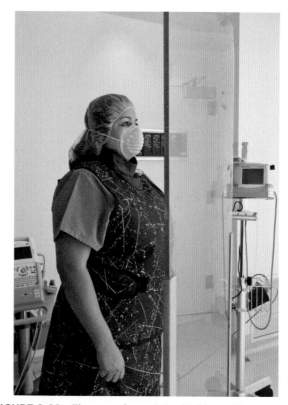

FIGURE 8-28 The use of a mobile shield provides protection for those individuals in the operating room.

Summary

1. Trauma injuries are caused by a variety of accidents, assaults, choking, or suicide.
   a. It is the leading cause of death of those under 44 years.
   b. Critical thinking is necessary to work quickly to get quality images and think creatively to alter routine positioning to obtain the required images.
   c. The patient may be in pain, and if transferred to the imaging department, the patient must be observed for shock.
   d. Follow the guideline of C-spine precautions and long-bone radiography.
2. Head injuries can be open or closed and are serious if they involve the brain.
   a. Consider spine injuries with head injuries.
   b. Patients are assessed with the Glasgow Coma Scale.
   c. CT and MRI are now used almost exclusively to determine the extent of injuries.
3. The severity of spinal injuries is dependent on locations of the injury and if there is complete or partial severing of the cord.
   a. Clear the C-spine before moving the patient.
   b. C-7 and the top of T-1 must be seen to clear the spine.
   c. There may be some form of paralysis and motor sensory loss along with respiratory distress.
   d. When moving the patient with a spinal injury, do so on a board. If there is no board, log roll the patient to place a board under the patient.
4. Fractures are either open (break the skin) or closed.
   a. Be aware there may be internal injuries because of fractured bones, such as lung injures as a result of fractured ribs.
   b. Hip fractures are common in elderly women. Assess the patient for positioning before moving.
   c. Support the limb at both joints.
5. Wounds are usually treated before coming to the imaging department. Note any dressing artifacts seen on an image.
6. Burns are classified in degrees from 1 to 4 depending on depth of the burn.
   a. Patients suffer smoke inhalation and need a chest radiograph.
   b. Follow burn infection control protocol carefully.
7. Surgery can be a rewarding part of radiography or it can be stressful.
   a. Know what is sterile and how to work around it.
   b. Know the zones within the OR area.
   c. Know how to dress according to policy.
   d. Know how to place the IR without breaking the sterile field.
   e. Provide protection for all individuals in the OR.

CHAPTER 8 REVIEW QUESTIONS

1. When called to the emergency room, supplies needed may include: (Circle all that apply)
   a. Gloves
   b. A mask
   c. A protective gown
   d. Goggles
2. List the guidelines that should be followed when caring for a patient with a traumatic injury.
3. List possible members of the emergency room health care team.
4. A radiographer must consider that all patients with head injuries may also have:
   a. Facial fractures
   b. Seizures
   c. Shock
   d. Cervical spine injuries
   e. Changes in vital signs
5. What precaution(s) must be followed when taking radiographic exposures of a patient who has a head injury? (Circle all that apply)
   a. Keep the head and neck immobilized until the physician in charge rules out cervical spine injury.
   b. Wear sterile gloves if the patient has open wounds.
   c. Check the patient's vital signs frequently.
6. What precaution(s) must a radiographer take when caring for a patient with a fractured extremity? (Circle all that apply)
   a. Support the joint above and below the fracture and at the joints if moving a splinted limb.
   b. Do not remove splints without the direction of the physician in charge.
   c. Inform the patient before moving the fractured limb.
   d. None of the above

(continued)

7. Special care is necessary when caring for a patient whose brain or spinal cord might be injured because:

    a. Extreme pain may result from the movement.

    b. This type of injury heals slowly.

    c. The incidence of infection is high.

    d. These tissues have very little ability to heal.

8. What is the leading cause of death for all persons under 44 years?

    a. Cancer

    b. Stroke

    c. Trauma

    d. Drowning

9. Explain when the cervical collar may be removed on a trauma patient.

10. When entering a surgical suite and preparing to enter Zone 2, the radiographer must: (Circle all that apply)

    a. Change into a scrub suit

    b. Change shoes

    c. Wear a mask

    d. Put on a hair cover

11. What are the responsibilities of a radiographer in the OR? (Circle all that apply)

    a. Know what is sterile and what is not.

    b. Provide radiation protection for all persons involved.

    c. Take diagnostic images as directed by the surgeon.

    d. Act in the role of the circulating nurse when that person is not present.

12. Patients with severe burns (Circle all that apply):

    a. Require protective isolation

    b. May experience no sensation

    c. May be in extreme pain

    d. None of these are true

Medical Emergencies

9

INTRODUCTION

Many patients come to the diagnostic imaging department in poor physical condition. This may be because of illness, injury, or a lengthy preparation for a diagnostic examination. When a person is in a weakened physical condition, physiologic reactions may not be as expected. Many abnormal physiologic reactions occur quickly and without warning and may be **life-threatening** if not recognized and treated immediately. Nontraumatic-related medical emergencies that are most likely to occur while the patient is undergoing diagnostic imaging are shock, anaphylaxis (a type of shock), pulmonary embolus (PE), reactions related to diabetes mellitus, cerebrovascular accident (CVA), cardiac and respiratory failure, syncope, and seizures. As the first member of the health care team to observe these reactions in the imaging department, the radiographer must be able to recognize the symptoms and initiate the correct treatment.

The technologist must be able to assess the behaviors that determine a patient's level of neurologic and cognitive functioning on admission for a diagnostic procedure. If this initial assessment is performed, the technologist is able to recognize changes in the patient's mental status if they occur.

The first action that should be taken in a life-threatening emergency is to call the hospital emergency team, the physician conducting the procedure, and a coworker for assistance. Every technologist must learn the correct procedure for calling the hospital emergency team in the institution of employment. In many health care institutions, this procedure is dubbed "calling a code" or CODE BLUE. Memorize the emergency team number, and be prepared to explain the exact location of the emergency and the problem that has occurred.

All imaging departments have an emergency cart that contains the medications and equipment that are needed when a patient's condition suddenly becomes critical. This is often called the "crash cart." Know where to obtain this cart quickly, and know who is responsible for maintaining the cart and having all its equipment and supplies in working order. Be familiar with the oxygen administration equipment so that assistance can be provided quickly. If an automatic defibrillator is not attached to the crash cart, its location must be known and quickly retrieved for any life-threatening emergency.

Although imaging technologists are not the health care workers who are responsible for a patient's pain management during the majority of medical care, the technologist must be sensitive to complaints of pain and discomfort while the patient is in the imaging department.

ASSESSMENT OF NEUROLOGIC AND COGNITIVE FUNCTIONING

The technologist must be able to quickly assess the patient's neurologic functioning. If a patient's condition deteriorates, it must be quickly recognized on the basis of changes in the initial assessment data. Neurologic assessment can be highly technical and complex and is not within the scope of a technologist's practice. However, a rapid neurologic assessment tool that is used frequently in health care institutions is the Glasgow Coma Scale. This scale addresses the three areas of neurologic functioning and quickly gives an overview of the patient's level of responsiveness. It is simple, reliable, and convenient to use.

Three areas can be readily observed—eyes opening, motor response, and verbal response. A patient can be rated a maximum of 15 points for neurologic functioning. If the patient's score begins to drop after the initial assessment, notify the physician in charge of the patient immediately (Display 9-1).

DISPLAY 9-1

Glasgow Coma Scale

Eyes open	
Spontaneously	14
To voice	3
To painful stimuli	2
No response	1
Motor response	
Obeys commands	6
Localized pain	5
Withdraws from painful stimuli	4
Abnormal flexion	3
Extension	2
No response	1
Verbal response	
Oriented	5
Confused speech	4
Inappropriate words	3
Incomprehensible sounds	2
None	1
Total points possible	15

Another indicator that a patient's condition is deteriorating is a change in the level of consciousness (LOC). These changes can be subtle but must not be ignored. The LOC can be assessed quickly with the following three parameters:

1. Ask the patient to state certain items, such as name, date, address, and the reason for coming to the imaging department. *If the patient gives these responses readily and correctly, then it can be assumed that the patient is responding to verbal stimuli and is oriented to person, place, time, and situation. Note any undue need to repeat questions and any slow response, difficulty with choice of words, or unusual irritability.*

2. Note the patient's ability to follow directions during instruction regarding positioning for the examination. Also note any movement that causes pain or other difficulty in movement, as well as any alterations in behavior or a lack of response. Report these to the physician in charge of caring for the patient. *These measures provide a baseline against which changes in the patient's mental and neurologic status can be assessed.*

3. Assess the patient's vital signs at this time if current readings are not on the chart. Chapter 6 describes how to perform baseline vital signs and the normal ranges. Baseline readings are critical to have in order to note any changes that may occur. An increasing systolic blood pressure or widening of the pulse pressure may indicate increasing intracranial pressure. Slowing of the pulse may also indicate increasing intracranial pressure. As compression of the brain increases, the vital signs change. Respirations increase, blood pressure decreases, and the pulse rate decreases further. A rapid rise in body temperature or a decrease in body temperature is also an ominous sign.

If the patient has no complaints on initial assessment, note this. If the patient begins to complain of a headache, becomes restless or unusually quiet, or develops slurred speech or a change in the level of orientation as a procedure progresses, report this to the physician immediately, stop the procedure, stay with the patient, and summon assistance. This includes requesting the emergency cart to be brought to the patient. Then, prepare the patient for oxygen and intravenous fluid administration if warranted.

 WARNING!

Changes in a patient's neurologic status or LOC must never be ignored! Stop work and notify the physician of these changes.

SHOCK

Shock is the body's pathologic reaction to illness, trauma, or severe physiologic or emotional stress. It may be caused by body fluid loss, cardiac failure, decreased tone of the blood vessels, or obstruction of blood flow to vital body organs. Shock causes the body to suffer from insufficient blood flow to the body. It is a life-threatening condition that may occur rapidly and without warning. It may be reversible if it is not allowed to progress. The technologist may be the first health care worker to observe the initial symptoms of shock; therefore, it is important to recognize them and begin the interventions that halt its progress, which eventually leads to organ failure and death.

The Shock Continuum

The vital organs of the body depend on oxygen and other nutrients supplied by the blood for their survival. When this supply is diminished, adverse effects on normal physiologic functions occur. The shock syndrome may progress as a continuum in the patient's struggle to survive and return to a normal physiologic state.

At the onset of the shock continuum, the changes in physiologic function are in the cells of the body and are not clinically detectable except for a possible increase in heart rate. As the condition progresses, blood is shunted away from the lungs, skin, kidneys, and gastrointestinal tract to accommodate the critical need for oxygen of the brain and heart. At this stage, called the *compensatory* stage, a host of symptoms are noticeable:

1. Cold and clammy skin
2. Nausea and dizziness
3. Increased respirations (shortness of breath [**SOB**])
4. Anxiety level increases; patient may begin to be uncooperative.
5. Blood pressure is decreased, and pulse rate is increased.

If shock is allowed to progress beyond the compensatory stage, the mean arterial pressure (the average pressure at which the blood moves through the vasculature of the body) falls. All body systems are inadequately perfused, including the heart, which begins to pump inadequately. Vasoconstriction reduces arterial blood flow into organs and their tissues, causing ischemia and necrosis.

The peripheral circulation reacts to the chemical mediators released by the body in this state, and fluid leaks from the capillaries, further decreasing the amount of fluid in circulation. The patient goes into acute renal failure, and the liver, gastrointestinal, and hematologic systems begin to fail. This stage in the shock continuum is called the *progressive* stage. Progressive symptoms include:

1. Significantly decreased blood pressure with an increase in pulse rate
2. Respirations are rapid and shallow.
3. Pulmonary capillaries leak fluid into the lungs, causing severe pulmonary edema, known as acute respiratory distress or shock lung.
4. **Tachycardia** results and may be as rapid as 150 beats per minute.
5. Chest pain may occur.
6. Mental status begins to change with subtle behavior alterations such as confusion, with progression to lethargy and loss of consciousness.
7. Renal, hepatic, gastrointestinal, and hematologic problems occur.

If shock progresses beyond this point, it is called the *irreversible* stage. The organ systems of the body suffer irreparable damage, and recovery is unlikely.

Irreversible stage involves the following:

1. Low blood pressure
2. Renal and liver failure
3. Release of necrotic tissue toxins and overwhelming lactic acidosis

Display 9-2 shows the progression of shock with the corresponding symptoms. There are different classifications of shock. These include hypovolemic, cardiogenic, and distributive or obstructive shock. The following sections provide descriptions, clinical manifestations, and the technologist's response to each of these.

DISPLAY 9-2

Progression of Shock with Associated Symptoms

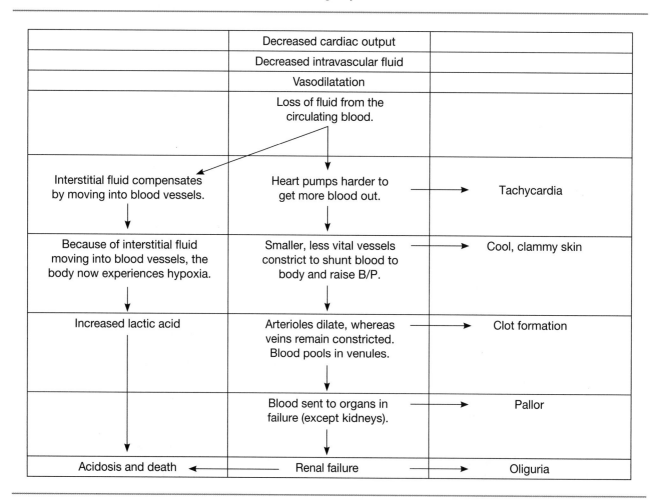

Hypovolemic Shock

Body fluids are contained within the cells of the body and are in the extracellular compartments. The extracellular fluid is further distributed to the blood vessels (intravascular) and into the surrounding body tissues (interstitial). Approximately three or four times more body fluid is within the interstitial spaces than within the vasculature of the body. When the amount of intravascular fluid decreases by 15% to 25% or by a loss of 750 to 1,300 mL, hypovolemic shock occurs. This decrease in volume may be because of internal or external hemorrhage; loss of plasma from burns; or fluid loss from prolonged vomiting, diarrhea, or medications.

Clinical Manifestations

Although the radiographer is not required to know and record what class level the patient is experiencing, it is important to know the signs and symptoms of hypovolemic shock.

Class I: A blood loss of 15%

- Blood pressure is within normal limits.
- Heart rate is less than 100 beats per minute.
- Respiration ranges from 14 to 20 per minute.

Class II: A blood loss of 15% to 30%

- Blood pressure is within normal limits.
- Heart rate is greater than 100 beats per minute.
- Respiration ranges from 20 to 30 per minute.

Class III: A blood loss of 30% to 40%

- Blood pressure begins to decrease to below normal limits.
- Heart rate is greater than 120 beats per minute.
- Respiration increases to 30 to 40 per minute.

Class IV: A blood loss of 40% or more

- Systolic blood pressure decreases from 90 to 60 mm Hg.
- Heart rate is now in tachycardia with a weak and thready pulse.
- Respiration is greater than 40 per minute.

The patient may become excessively thirsty as a result of the fluid loss from hypovolemic shock. The extremities are cold; the skin is cold and clammy with cyanosis starting at the lips and nails. If the patient is dark-skinned, cyanosis may be observed by pressing lightly on the fingernails or earlobes. If the patient is cyanotic, the color does not return to the compressed area in the usual 1-second interval. A bluish discoloration of the tongue and soft palate of the mouth is also indicative of cyanosis. If this condition is allowed to continue, cardiac and respiratory failure follows.

Response

1. Stop the ongoing procedure; place the patient supine with legs elevated 30° (if there is no head or spinal cord injury). Do *not* place the patient in the Trendelenburg position.
2. Notify the physician in charge and call for emergency assistance from the department nurse, if available.
3. Make certain that the patient is able to breathe without obstruction caused by position or blood or mucus in the airway.
4. If there is an open wound with blood loss, put on clean gloves and apply pressure directly to the wound with several thicknesses of dry, sterile dressing.
5. Bring the emergency cart to the room.
6. Prepare to assist with oxygen, intravenous fluids, and medications.
7. Keep the patient warm and dry, but do not overheat the patient because this increases the need for oxygen.
8. Assess vital signs every 5 minutes until the emergency team assumes this role.
9. Do not leave the patient unattended. If there is anxiety, explain what is happening.
10. Do not offer fluids to the patient, even if requested. Explain that any subsequent examination or treatment may require an empty stomach.

Cardiogenic Shock

Cardiogenic shock is caused by failure of the heart to pump an adequate amount of blood to the vital organs. The onset of cardiogenic shock may occur over a period, or it may be sudden. The patient who has been hospitalized for myocardial infarction, dysrhythmias, or other cardiac pathology is most vulnerable. A subcategory, obstructive shock, can be caused by a **cardiac tamponade**, a PE, pulmonary hypertension, arterial stenosis, constrictive pericarditis, or tumors that block blood flow through the heart.

Clinical Manifestations

- Complaint of chest pain that may radiate to jaws and arms
- Dizziness and respiratory distress
- Cyanosis
- Restlessness and anxiety
- Rapid change in the LOC
- Pulse may be irregular and slow; may have tachycardia and tachypnea.
- Difficult-to-find carotid pulse indicates decreased stroke volume of the heart.
- Decreasing blood pressure
- Decreasing urinary output
- Cool, clammy skin

Response

1. Summon the emergency team and have the emergency cart placed at the patient's side.
2. Notify the physician in charge of the patient.
3. Place the patient in the semi-Fowler position or in another position that facilitates respiration.
4. Prepare to assist with oxygen, intravenous fluid, and medication administration. Chest pain must be controlled.
5. Do not leave the patient alone; offer an explanation of treatment as appropriate; alleviate the patient's anxiety.
6. Assess pulse, respiration, and blood pressure every 5 minutes until the emergency team arrives.
7. Do not offer fluids.
8. Be prepared to administer cardiopulmonary resuscitation (CPR), if indicated.

Distributive Shock

Distributive shock occurs when pooling of blood in the peripheral blood vessels results in decreased venous return of blood to the heart, decreased blood pressure, and decreased tissue perfusion. This may be the result of loss of sympathetic tone. Distributive shock is characterized by the blood vessels' inability to constrict and their resultant inability to assist in the return of blood to the heart. It may also occur when chemicals released by the cells cause vasodilatation and capillary permeability, which in turn prompts a large portion of the blood volume to pool peripherally. There are three types of distributive shock: neurogenic, septic, and anaphylactic.

Neurogenic Shock

Neurogenic shock results from loss of vasodilatation of peripheral vessels. Spinal cord injury, severe pain, neurologic damage, the depressant action of medication, a lack of glucose (as in insulin reaction or shock), or the adverse effects of anesthesia can all cause neurogenic shock.

Clinical Manifestations

- Hypotension
- **Bradycardia**
- Warm, dry skin
- Initial alertness if not unconscious because of head injury
- Cool extremities and diminishing peripheral pulses

Response

1. Summon emergency assistance.
2. Notify the physician in charge of the patient.
3. Keep the patient in a supine position; legs may be elevated with physician's orders.
4. Have the emergency cart brought to the patient's side.
5. If spinal cord injury is possible, do not move the patient.
6. Stay with the patient and offer support.
7. Monitor pulse, respirations, and blood pressure every 5 minutes.
8. Prepare to assist with oxygen, intravenous fluids, and medications.

Septic Shock

Septic shock is the least likely to be observed by the radiographer in the imaging department. However, radiographers must be able to recognize septic shock. Patients in the intensive care unit or emergency room who are in septic shock may need to have a mobile radiograph performed instead of being moved to the imaging department. Radiographic studies used to evaluate patients with suspected sepsis or septic shock include chest, abdomen, and extremity radiography. Chest radiography is most common as most patients with sepsis have pneumonia (Fig. 9-1).

When invaded by gram-negative bacteria, the body begins its immune response by releasing chemicals that increase capillary permeability and vasodilatation, leading to shock syndrome.

Clinical Manifestations

The clinical manifestations of septic shock are divided into two phases:

First Phase:
- Hot, dry, and flushed skin
- Increase in heart rate and respiratory rate
- Fever, but possibly not in the elderly patient
- Nausea, vomiting, and diarrhea
- Normal to excessive urine output
- Possible confusion, most commonly in the elderly patient

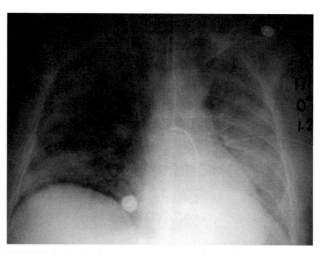

FIGURE 9-1 A 45-year-old woman admitted to the intensive care unit with septic shock secondary to spontaneous biliary peritonitis.

Second Phase:

- Cool, pale skin
- Normal or subnormal temperature
- Drop in blood pressure
- Rapid heart rate and respiratory rate
- Oliguria or anuria
- Seizures and organ failure if syndrome is not reversed

Response

The technologist is rarely the person who initiates action if septic shock is present. However, if a patient in septic shock is in the imaging department, care must be taken to ensure that the patient does not become chilled, because shivering increases the body's oxygen consumption.

Anaphylactic Shock

Because some imaging procedures use contrast media that contain iodine, to which some people are allergic, this is the most frequently seen type of shock in radiographic imaging. The radiographer must be able to recognize it at its onset to prevent life-threatening consequences.

Anaphylactic shock (**anaphylaxis**) is the result of an exaggerated hypersensitivity reaction (allergic reaction) to reexposure to an antigen that was previously encountered by the body's immune system. When this occurs, histamine and bradykinin are released, causing widespread vasodilatation, which results in peripheral pooling of blood. This response is accompanied by contraction of nonvascular smooth muscles, particularly the smooth muscles of the respiratory tract. This combined reaction produces shock, respiratory failure, and death within minutes after exposure to the allergen. Usually, the more abrupt the onset of anaphylaxis, the more severe the reaction will be.

The most common causes of anaphylaxis are medications, iodinated contrast media, and insect venoms. The path of entry may be through the skin, respiratory tract, or gastrointestinal tract, or through injection.

The technologist performing the procedure in which contrast media are injected is responsible for the patient. A meticulous history of previous allergic responses that the patient may have had to any medication or food, including previous incidents when receiving contrast agents in imaging, must be obtained. If any of these responses are reported, the radiologist must be informed before injection of any contrast media.

When iodinated contrast media are being used for diagnostic procedures, observe the patient continuously for signs of allergic reaction. If early symptoms of anaphylactic shock are observed, quick action must be taken to halt the progression of symptoms.

Clinical Manifestations

The signs of anaphylactic shock may be classified as mild, moderate, or severe.

Mild Systemic Reaction:

- Nasal congestion, **periorbital** swelling, itching, sneezing, and tearing of eyes
- Peripheral tingling or itching at the site of injection
- Feeling of fullness or tightness of the chest, mouth, or throat
- Feeling of anxiety or nervousness

Moderate Systemic Reaction:

- All the foregoing symptoms, plus:
- Flushing, feeling of warmth, itching, and urticaria
- **Bronchospasm** and edema of the airways or larynx
- Dyspnea, cough, and wheezing

Severe Systemic Reaction:

- All the foregoing symptoms with an abrupt onset
- Decreasing blood pressure; weak, thready pulse either rapid or shallow
- Rapid progression to bronchospasm, laryngeal edema, severe dyspnea, and cyanosis
- Dysphasia, abdominal cramping, vomiting, and diarrhea
- Seizures and respiratory and cardiac arrest

Response

1. Do not leave the patient. Stop any infusion or injection of contrast immediately and notify the radiologist or department physician if any of the symptoms occur.
2. If the patient complains of respiratory distress or has any of the symptoms listed in the severe reaction section, call the emergency team as well as the radiologist.
3. Place the patient in the semi-Fowler position or in a sitting position to facilitate respiration, if appropriate and safe to do so.
4. Monitor pulse, respiration, and blood pressure every 5 minutes or until the emergency team arrives to assume responsibility.
5. Prepare to assist with oxygen, intravenous fluid, and medication administration. Have large-gauge venous catheters available.
6. Prepare to perform CPR as required.

The medications usually given for anaphylactic shock are epinephrine, diphenhydramine, hydrocortisone, and aminophylline.

Many imaging departments have a standardized procedure form that must be completed before the administration of contrast media. This form may request some or all of the information shown in Display 9-3. Other facilities may have much more on the form used in the imaging department. Regardless of the form used, the radiographer is the responsible person for obtaining the history and should not rely solely on the patient filling out the form. Review the form and question the patient. There are many legal situations that could have been prevented if an adequate history had been performed.

DISPLAY 9-3

Information Requested Before Administration of Contrast Agents

Name _____

Age _____

Date _____

Have you had the study you are having today at any other time? _____

If so, did you have ANY reaction? _____ Yes _____ No

SOB? _____ Yes _____ No

Nausea? _____ Yes _____ No

Hives? _____ Yes _____ No

Chest pain? _____ Yes _____ No

Are you allergic to any food, medications, or any other substances? Please specify.

_____

Recent laboratory tests performed and results: Blood urea nitrogen and creatinine

_____

Have you had any blood in your urine? _____ Yes _____ No

Have you had or now have any of the following?

Hypertension? _____ Yes _____ No

Diabetes mellitus? _____ Yes _____ No

Asthma? _____ Yes _____ No

Sickle cell anemia? _____ Yes _____ No

Kidney disease? (explain) _____ Yes _____ No

Heart disease? _____ Yes _____ No

Have you had COVID-19 or a variant? _____ Yes _____ No

Have you had any procedures that involved use of contrast media? If so, please explain.

_____

After the examination, the physician completes a report indicating the type of contrast agent used and any unusual responses. If the patient has an anaphylactic reaction, the nature of the reaction should be written on the patient's imaging history. The person performing the injection and examination must also document the reaction in the patient's chart.

A copy of this report is kept in the patient's diagnostic imaging department file, and the department supervisor also keeps a copy. If these precautions in documentation are taken, the history of the patient's previous problem will be on record, and the correct decisions can be made if subsequent procedures using contrast media become necessary.

Patients who have received contrast media as part of the diagnostic imaging procedure should remain in the department for 30 minutes for observation if they are not patients in the hospital. If they are having no problems after 30 minutes, they may be allowed to return home, accompanied by another person. They should be clearly instructed in the signs and symptoms of an anaphylactic reaction and told to return to the hospital emergency department (ED) immediately if any of these symptoms appear. A patient who has had even a mild allergic reaction during a diagnostic procedure that involves the use of a contrast medium should be instructed to report this if there is a possibility of receiving iodinated contrast media in the future. If the reaction was severe, the patient may need to wear an alert bracelet to prevent further exposure to antigens of this sort. The pharmacology of contrast media is discussed in Chapter 12 in Section III, and special attention should be paid to this as contrast reactions are unpredictable.

 WARNING!

Radiographers must be meticulous in obtaining a history from the patient who is about to receive a contrast medium as they are responsible for the outcome and consequences of the injection.

PULMONARY EMBOLUS

A PE is an occlusion of one or more pulmonary arteries by a thrombus or thrombi. The thrombus originates in the venous circulation or in the right side of the heart and is carried through the vessels to the lungs, where it blocks the pulmonary arteries. It is the most common pulmonary complication of hospitalized surgical patients. The onset is sudden and requires immediate action to prevent severe consequences. They are fatal in more than 50% of the cases that present. PEs are associated with significant morbidity and mortality, causing approximately 120,000 deaths per year in the United States. People who have severe symptoms of COVID-19 have an increased risk of pulmonary embolism. After years showing a decline in the number of deaths attributed to PE, death rates have begun to climb once again. The biggest increase is for people under the age of 65. Deep vein thrombosis (DVT) and PE are more common as people age; therefore, the trend in younger people is worrisome.

PE is associated with trauma, orthopedic and abdominal surgical procedures, pregnancy, congestive heart failure, prolonged immobility, and hypercoagulable states. Ninety-five percent of all cases of pulmonary embolism are caused by DVT. Emboli may also be the result of air, fat, amniotic fluid, or sepsis. The severity of symptoms depends on the size or number of emboli that disturb the pulmonary circulation. Risk factors include immobilization for longer than 72 hours, recent hip surgery, cardiac disease, malignancy, estrogen use, and prior DVT. The end result is arterial hypoxemia, which may be a life-threatening emergency.

When working with postoperative patients and patients who have suffered traumatic events affecting the long bones of the body, the technologist must be aware of the complication of PE and be prepared to initiate emergency action if it occurs.

Clinical Manifestations

- Rapid, weak pulse
- Hyperventilation
- Dyspnea and tachypnea
- Tachycardia
- Apprehension
- Cough and hemoptysis
- **Diaphoresis**
- **Syncope**
- Hypotension
- Cyanosis
- Rapidly changing LOCs
- Coma; sudden death may result.

Response

1. Stop the procedure immediately and call for emergency assistance.
2. Notify the physician and bring the emergency cart to the patient's side.
3. Monitor vital signs.
4. Do not leave the patient alone; reassure the patient.
5. Prepare to assist with oxygen administration and administration of intravenous medication and fluid.

DIABETIC EMERGENCIES

Diabetes mellitus is a group of metabolic diseases resulting from a chronic disorder of carbohydrate metabolism. It is caused by either insufficient production of insulin or inadequate utilization of insulin by the cells of the body. Insulin is a hormone normally secreted by the islets of Langerhans located in the pancreas. In diabetes mellitus, either the cells stop responding to insulin or the pancreas ceases to produce insulin. In either case, the result is hyperglycemia, which leads to a series of metabolic complications. These disease processes adversely affect the structure and function of blood vessels and other organs of the body. The result is an abnormal amount of glucose in the blood (hyperglycemia). This high blood sugar produces classic symptoms of **polyuria**, **polydipsia**, and **polyphagia**.

As of 2018, 34.2 million people have diabetes in the United States. This is up from 29.1 million in 2014. Approximately one in three American adults (88 million) have prediabetes. The Centers for Disease Control and Prevention has determined that the rapid increase in diabetes is an epidemic. The American Diabetes Association estimates that diabetes costs $327 billion in the United States each year as of 2018. This represents a 26% increase in a 5-year period. Diabetes is listed as the seventh leading cause of death and rising. Only $1 out of every $7 is spent on fighting diabetes and preventing it.

There are three major types of diabetes mellitus. The causes are not identical, and the course of the disease process and the treatment vary according to the type presenting. They are:

1. *Type 1 diabetes mellitus (insulin dependent).* Type 1 usually occurs in persons younger than 30 years and has an abrupt onset.
2. *Type 2 diabetes mellitus.* This is the most common type of diabetes. It usually occurs in persons older than 40 years and has a gradual onset.
3. *Gestational diabetes.* This is a diabetic condition that occurs in the later months of pregnancy in women who have never had diabetes before. Hormones secreted by the placenta that prevent the action of insulin are the cause.

Persons with diabetes mellitus are extremely susceptible to infections and therefore require extra skin care and infection control precautions. All forms of diabetes are treatable with insulin and other medications (type 2); however, both type 1 and type 2 are chronic conditions that usually cannot be cured. Gestational diabetes is usually resolved with delivery of the infant.

Acute Complications of Diabetes Mellitus

Diabetes without proper treatment can cause complications. Acute complications include hypoglycemia, diabetic ketoacidosis, and hyperosmolar nonketotic syndrome (also called hyperosmolar nonketotic coma). The descriptions, manifestations, and technologist's responses are as follows:

- *Hypoglycemia* occurs when persons who have diabetes mellitus have an excess amount of insulin or oral hypoglycemic drug in their bloodstream, or an inadequate food intake with which to utilize the insulin. This may occur when the patient has not had anything to eat or drink before coming to the imaging department. The onset of symptoms is rapid, and immediate action is necessary to prevent coma. The technologist must use high-sugar food (like candy or even orange juice) to counteract the symptoms.
- *Diabetic ketoacidosis* occurs when insufficient insulin (type 1) causes the liver to produce more glucose, resulting in hyperglycemia. There is altered LOCs (ALOCs). The patient should be sent to the ED to be rehydrated with fluids, electrolyte replacement, and insulin therapy.
- Hyperglycemic hyperosmolar nonketotic syndrome (HHNS) (coma) is not as common a complication but is no less severe. It is more common in patients with type 2 diabetes mellitus and is the result of dehydration, or it may occur in the elderly person with no known history of diabetes mellitus. This patient must also be sent to the ED for fluid and potassium replacement.

Clinical Manifestations

The following occur in all cases:

- Tachycardia
- Headache
- Blurred or double vision
- Extreme thirst
- Sweet odor to the breath may occur in diabetic ketoacidosis.

Response

1. Stop the procedure and notify the physician in charge of the procedure.
2. Do not leave the patient unattended.
3. Monitor the vital signs and prepare to administer intravenous fluids, medication, and oxygen as needed and requested by an emergency team.

CVA (STROKE)

CVAs, also known as strokes and brain attacks, are caused by occlusion of the blood supply to the brain, rupture of the blood supply to the brain, or rupture of a cerebral artery, resulting in hemorrhage directly into the brain tissue or the spaces surrounding the brain (Fig. 9-2).

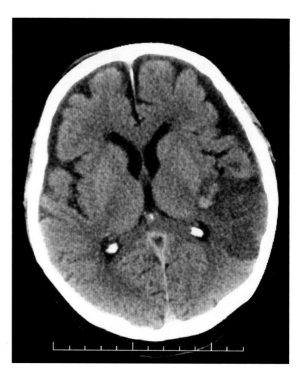

FIGURE 9-2 Computed tomography (CT) of the brain showing bleeding on the right side, which resulted in a stroke. Notice the slight atrophy of the brain away from the skull on the anterior right and left sides.

Regardless of the cause, there is a lack of blood to the brain tissue. Brain tissue suffers irreversible damage within 5 minutes or less.

Strokes vary in severity from mild transient ischemic attacks (TIAs) to severe, life-threatening situations, depending on the cause. A TIA occurs when the blood to the brain is interrupted only briefly. It is known as a "ministroke" and is a warning sign that the patient may be at risk for having a more serious stroke. There are two different types of strokes with different causes: ischemic and hemorrhagic. Ischemic strokes are the most common and is usually caused by a blood clot that blocks or plugs a blood vessel in the brain that keeps the blood from flowing to the tissues of the brain. This causes the brain cells to begin to die within a few minutes. A hemorrhagic stroke is less common and occurs when a blood vessel breaks and bleeds into the brain. CVAs occur most frequently with little or no warning and may possibly occur in the imaging department during a stressful procedure.

A stroke is an event that is as great a medical crisis as a heart attack, and it is extremely important that the stroke victim receive immediate emergency evaluation. Being started on fibrinolytic therapy reduces the neurologic damage from an ischemic stroke. The warning signs and symptoms of this medical crisis must be recognized in order to be prepared to initiate emergency care. Although the signs and symptoms depend on the location of the obstruction, the size of the artery involved, and the functional area affected, the general signs may be noted as those listed here.

Clinical Manifestations

- Sudden severe headache
- Numbness and muscle weakness or flaccidity of face or extremities, usually one-sided
- Sudden trouble seeing
- Confusion
- Dizziness or stupor
- Difficult speech (dysphasia) or no speech (aphasia)
- Ataxia
- May complain of stiff neck
- Nausea or vomiting may occur
- Loss of consciousness

Response

1. Stop the procedure immediately and notify the department physician and nurse.
2. Do not leave the patient alone.
3. Monitor the vital signs and prepare to administer intravenous fluids and oxygen because they may be needed and requested by the emergency team.

CARDIAC AND RESPIRATORY EMERGENCIES

Respiratory failure, cardiac failure (also called cardiac arrest), or an airway obstruction may occur in the diagnostic imaging department without warning and when least expected. The technologist may be the first health care worker to witness this event and thus will be the person to call the code and initiate emergency action. The human brain can survive without oxygen for only 4 to 5 minutes before there is damage. This means that there is little time to ponder over the situation before acting.

All health care staff must be prepared to perform basic CPR and the abdominal thrust maneuver. Basic life support guidelines have made early cardiac defibrillation a high-priority goal and the ability to use an automated external defibrillator (AED) a basic life support skill.

There are frequent changes in basic life support methods, and it is the technologist's responsibility to keep abreast of the changes and rules in the place of employment concerning responsibilities as a responder to a cardiac or respiratory type of emergency. The brief descriptions of CPR, the use of the AED, and the abdominal thrust maneuver do not prepare the technologist to administer these techniques. A complete basic life support course for health care professionals is mandatory and should be renewed on a yearly basis to stay abreast of new techniques, even though the CPR card is good for 2 years. Anytime the technologist is working with a patient to open the airway, clean gloves must be worn. A disposable mask with a one-way valve is recommended when performing CPR (Fig. 9-3). This type of mask should

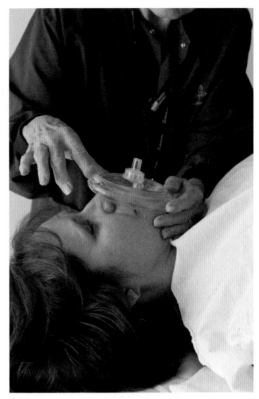

FIGURE 9-3 Disposable mask with a one-way valve. Remember that if actually performing CPR with a mask over the mouth, clean gloves must be worn. CPR, cardiopulmonary resuscitation.

be available in every diagnostic imaging department. A manual resuscitation bag may be used if available. AEDs must also be made available and ready for use for a health care worker who is competent to use them.

Cardiac Arrest

When the heart ceases to beat effectively, the blood can no longer circulate throughout the body, and the person no longer has an effective pulse. There are a number of possible causes for this type of event. The electrical activity of the heart may be disrupted, causing the heart to beat too rapidly, as in ventricular fibrillation or ventricular tachycardia. The heart may beat too slowly, as in bradycardia or atrioventricular block. Pulseless electrical activity may also result from hypovolemic shock, cardiac tamponade, hypothermia, or a PE. In addition, drug overdoses, severe acidosis, or a severe myocardial infarction may cause this to occur. Irreversible brain damage and death result within minutes of a cardiac event, depending on the person's age and health status before the arrest.

Clinical Manifestations of Cardiac Arrest

- Loss of consciousness, pulse, and blood pressure
- Dilatation of the pupils within seconds
- Possibility of seizures

Respiratory Arrest

Respiratory arrest is the cessation of breathing. This differs from cardiac arrest where the flow of blood stops. In respiratory arrest (which may also be called pulmonary arrest) there can be complete absence of breathing (apnea) or the patient may have agonal breathing where the gasps for air are completely ineffectual. Whether apnea or agonal breathing, if no air is moving through the airway, the patient is in respiratory arrest.

Clinical Manifestations

- The patient stops responding.
- The pulse continues to beat briefly and then quickly becomes weak and stops.
- Chest movement stops, and no air is detectable moving through the patient's mouth.

Response to Both Cardiac and Respiratory Arrest

1. If the patient is an adult and is unresponsive, shake the patient and ask, "Are you all right?" If there is no response, call immediately for emergency medical services (call a CODE). If no one is near, shout for help, stating the location as well. "I need help STAT in Room 102." Do not leave the patient alone.
2. Assess the carotid pulse of an adult patient. Do not waste time taking the blood pressure or listening for a heartbeat.
3. If the patient is an adult with no pulse and the CODE has been called, place the patient in a supine position on a hard surface. If the patient is already on the radiographic table, leave the patient there as the hard table is a perfect place to perform CPR.

Begin CPR

1. Chest compressions are the first step in CPR. The technologist should give 30 compressions with a depth of at least 2 inches into the patient's chest.
2. Immediately after the chest compressions, the technologist should open up the airway through the head tilt, chin lift method (Fig. 9-4). This method should be used only when it is known with certainty that the patient has no C-spine injury. This is not likely in the imaging department unless the patient originated in the ED with possible trauma. Put on gloves; remove any obvious material in the mouth or throat. If the patient has dentures that are loose, remove them. Avoid pushing a foreign object further back into the mouth or throat. Do not perform blind finger sweeps! Never sweep the mouth of an infant or small child unless the object is visible and reachable.
3. Look, listen, and feel for airway movement. If there is nothing, tightly place the bag mask or mouth mask over the patient's mouth and nose. Take a deep breath

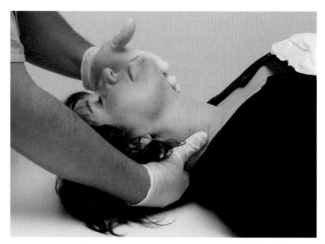

FIGURE 9-4 Direct the chin up and back.

and slowly, over 2 full seconds, with the least amount of air needed to make the chest rise, exhale into the mouth mask. Allow the patient to exhale. Repeat the maneuver. This sequence reduces the amount of air that enters the stomach of the patient to prevent the complication of regurgitation, aspiration, and pneumonia.

4. If the patient is not breathing and initial ventilation attempts are not successful, assess for foreign body in airway. If rescue ventilations have failed and an obstructed airway is suspected, use abdominal thrusts to remove obstruction (as explained later in this chapter). Recheck for breathing.
5. If the patient is breathing, place in a recovery position (Fig. 9-5).
6. Assess for signs of circulation by checking carotid pulse, and evaluate for coughing, movement, and breathing.
7. If no signs of circulation or breathing are present, the AED is not readily available, and the emergency team has not arrived, repeat the chest compressions.

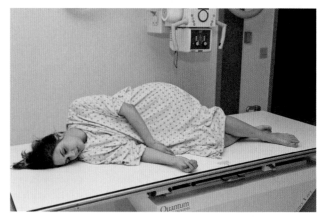

FIGURE 9-5 Patient in a recovery position. The head should be directed down so that any vomit can drain out.

Chest Compressions

Take adequate time to determine the lack of a pulse (no more than 7 seconds). Performing cardiac compressions on a person whose heart is functioning is extremely dangerous to the patient. Once cardiac compressions have been started, interruptions should be avoided. In one-person rescue, this is not possible; therefore, the interruption in compressions should not last more than 7 seconds.

The rescuer's hands must be positioned correctly to prevent internal injury while the cardiac compressions are being performed.

1. Find the lower margin of the patient's rib cage at the area where the ribs and sternum meet. Place the index finger above this junction and the heel of the other hand next to the finger. Place the second hand on top and interlace the fingers.
2. This should place the hands about 1.5 inches from the xiphoid tip toward the patient's head. The fingers should not touch the chest wall of the patient (Fig. 9-6).
3. Keep the elbows straight and use the body weight to help compress the sternum 2 inches directly downward; then release the compression completely.
4. Because it is more important to supply blood to the body, 30 compressions are given in a smooth, even rhythm before any ventilation. Do not rock during

compressions. Make sure that it is an up and down motion.

5. Inflate the patient's lungs two times.
6. Reassess the patient's carotid pulse and respiratory status. If the patient has no pulse or respiration, continue with 30 compressions followed by two inflations until the emergency team arrives.

> ⚠️ **WARNING!**
>
> **Never attempt chest compressions on a patient whose heart is beating.**

Defibrillation

Cardiac arrest may precede or follow respiratory arrest. It may also occur when the electrical activity of the heart is present but not effective in delivering oxygenated blood to vital organs. When cardiac arrest occurs and the patient is being monitored or is immediately placed on a monitor, use the quick-look paddles found on most defibrillators to determine the presence of ventricular tachycardia or ventricular fibrillation. If these are not available, apply the AED as quickly as possible to analyze the patient's heart rhythm. For every minute that defibrillation is delayed, the patient's chances of survival decline by 10%. The AED procedure is briefly described next; however, all health care professionals must be properly instructed in this procedure in a certified class with clinical practice.

1. Place the AED pack near the patient's left shoulder and open it. This should turn the power on automatically and initiate voice instruction from the pack. CPR may be continued until it is time to attach the electrodes.
2. Attach the electrodes onto the patient's anterior chest: one at the right upper sternal border below the clavicle and the other on the left chest lateral to the left nipple. Make sure that there is a tight contact with the skin by removing any excessive hair or moisture that may be present (Fig. 9-7).
3. Press the analyze button to assess the need for defibrillation. The machine states whether defibrillation shock is required.
4. If a shock is required, all persons must be totally clear of the bed or table and any contact with the patient. The machine dictates a "clear" order.
5. Press the shock button when the AED dictates the order. Do not press the shock button before the order.
6. If the AED states that no shock is indicated and the patient remains without a pulse, resume CPR.

When the patient is a child, the cause of the arrest is frequently respiratory in nature. As a result, the emergency medical team should be called after CPR is administered

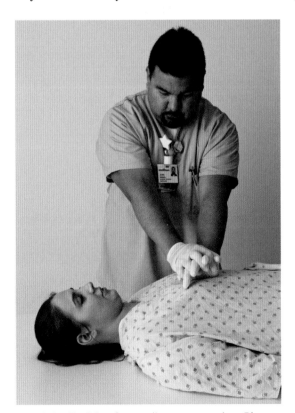

FIGURE 9-6 Position for cardiac compression. Place one hand on top of the other, keeping elbows straight.

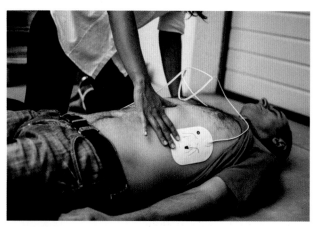

FIGURE 9-7 Attach one electrode at the right upper sternal border below the clavicle and the other on the left chest lateral to the left nipple.

for 1 minute unless another person is present who can call the CODE while the other person is administering CPR. The procedure is much the same for infants and children; however, there are some variations, which are listed in Display 9-4.

The use of a one-way mask on the infant or child for protection is desirable. If the technologist has been trained in the use of a breather bag, it may be used. The equipment must be of a size to adequately fit the patient.

Radiographers and all health care personnel must guard against becoming infected by a communicable disease while performing lifesaving procedures by wearing disposable gloves and by learning to use a manual resuscitation bag or a one-way face mask. Education in the use of this equipment must be obtained before it can be used effectively; such education should be a part of CPR training.

DISPLAY 9-4

Variations in CPR Techniques for Infants and Children

Neonate
- Head tilt, chin lift (or jaw thrust if trauma is present)
- Two effective breaths, then 30 to 60 breaths per minute
- Back blows or chest thrusts; no abdominal thrusts
- Compression landmark is the lower half of the sternum, one finger width below the inter-mammary line.
- Use two fingers for compression at approximately 1/2 inch at about 120 compressions per minute or 90 compressions to 30 breaths.

Infant Under 1 Year
- Head tilt, chin lift (or jaw thrust if trauma is present)
- Two effective breaths, then 20 breaths per minute
- Back blows or chest thrusts; no abdominal thrusts
- Brachial pulse checked
- Compression landmark is the lower half of the sternum, one finger width below the inter-mammary line.
- Use two thumbs or two fingers for compression at approximately 1/2 to 1 inch at about 100 compressions per minute.

Child Aged 1 to 8 Years
- Head tilt, chin lift (or jaw thrust if trauma is present)
- Two effective breaths in less than 10 seconds
- Check breathing by "look, listen, feel"
- Abdominal thrusts or chest thrusts
- The carotid pulse is checked.
- Compression landmark is the lower half of the sternum with the heel of the hand; the compression depth of the chest is 1 to 1.5 inches at a rate of 100 per minute or 30 compressions to two ventilations.

AIRWAY OBSTRUCTION

An airway obstruction happens when the patient is unable to move air in or out of the lungs. The obstruction may block part of the airway or the entire pathway. When only a portion of the airway is obstructed, it is known as respiratory dysfunction.

Respiratory Dysfunction

Respiratory dysfunction may precede respiratory arrest. It can be the result of airway obstruction caused by positioning, the tongue falling backward obstructing the throat of an unresponsive person, a foreign object lodged in the throat, disease, drug overdose, injury, or coma. Whatever the cause, gas exchange is no longer adequate to meet the needs of the body.

Clinical Manifestations of a Partially Obstructed Airway

- Labored, noisy breathing
- Wheezing
- Use of accessory muscles of the neck, abdomen, or chest on inspiration
- Neck vein distention
- Diaphoresis
- Anxiety
- Cyanosis of the lips and nail beds
- Possibly a productive cough with pink-tinged frothy sputum

Response to a Patient with a Partially Obstructed Airway

1. Call for assistance; do not leave the patient alone.
2. Assist the patient to a sitting or semi-Fowler position.
3. Attempt to relieve the patient's anxiety.
4. Prepare to administer oxygen.
5. Prepare to use the emergency cart.

A foreign body such as a piece of chewing gum or food may lodge in a patient's throat and produce respiratory arrest. This type of accident occurs most often in the elderly, the very young, or the intoxicated while eating. However, the radiographer must consider this possibility in any case of respiratory arrest.

When airway obstruction caused by a foreign object occurs, the patient usually appears to be quite normal and then suddenly begins to choke. The patient grabs the throat and is unable to speak. If no one is present to observe this, the patient eventually loses consciousness. Unless the early signs are observed, it is impossible to know the cause of the unconscious state. Airway obstruction may occur with the patient sitting, standing, or lying down and must be dealt with initially in that position.

Response

1. If the patient does not respond and breathlessness is established as described in the preceding paragraphs, seal the patient's nose and mouth, and ventilate as in the initial steps of CPR.
2. If the patient's chest rises and falls, proceed as for basic CPR.
3. If the patient's chest does not rise and fall, reposition the head using the head tilt, chin lift, or jaw thrust as indicated. Then attempt to ventilate again.
4. If this is unsuccessful, assume that the airway is obstructed and use the abdominal thrust to attempt to remove the obstruction.

Abdominal Thrust: Patient Standing or Sitting

Stand behind the patient and grasp with both hands above the patient's umbilicus and below the xiphoid process of the sternum. Position the lower hand with the thumb inward; the other hand firmly grips the lower hand. Make a rapid upward movement that forces the abdomen inward and thrusts upward against the diaphragm (Fig. 9-8). This maneuver forces air up through the trachea and dislodges the foreign object. Never attempt to practice this maneuver on a person who is not in distress because of the possibility of serious injury. Be sure the hands

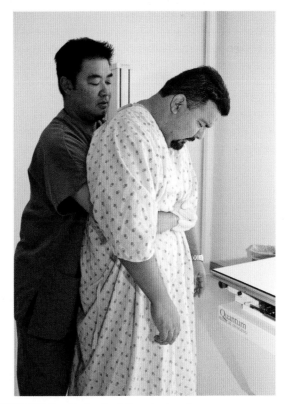

FIGURE 9-8 Abdominal thrust, standing.

are placed away from the xiphoid process to prevent internal injury.

Abdominal Thrust: Patient in Supine Position

Place the patient in a supine position. Kneel astride the patient's thighs and place the heel of one hand against the patient's abdomen above the navel and below the tip of the xiphoid process. Place the other hand over the first and quickly press the abdomen upward. Be certain to direct the thrust directly up and not deviate to the left or right. This maneuver acts in the same way for the patient who is sitting or standing.

Chest Thrust: Patient Sitting or Standing

The chest thrust is used to dislodge a foreign object only if the patient is in the advanced stages of pregnancy or is excessively obese and the abdominal thrust cannot be used effectively.

Stand behind the patient with arms under the patient's armpits and around the chest. Place the thumb side of a fist in the middle of the sternum, avoiding the xiphoid process and the margins of the rib cage. Place the other hand on top and thrust backward. Repeat this maneuver until the object is dislodged.

Never attempt abdominal or chest thrust on a patient whose airway is not obstructed. To do so may cause serious injury to the patient's diaphragm and lungs.

If the patient is an infant and an obstructed airway is suspected, place the patient face down over the forearm with the infant's legs straddling the elbow. Support the infant's head and neck between the thumb and the forefinger with the patient's head lower than the chest but not straight down. Deliver five sharp blows to the patient's back between the shoulder blades (Fig. 9-9).

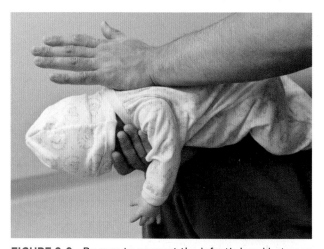

FIGURE 9-9   Be sure to support the infant's head between the thumb and the fingers when delivering back blows.

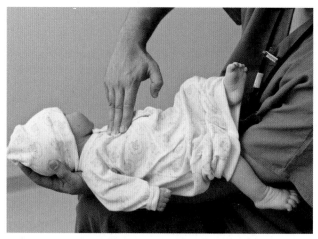

FIGURE 9-10   Chest compression on an infant to relieve complete foreign body airway obstruction.

If this is not successful, perform chest thrusts with two or three fingers on the midsternal area about one per second (Fig. 9-10).

The method of dealing with foreign body airway obstruction for infants and children also varies with their weight, age, and size.

Chest Thrust: Patient Pregnant or Excessively Obese or Unconscious

After determining breathlessness in the prescribed manner, attempt ventilation. If this is not successful and the patient is in the advanced stages of pregnancy or is excessively obese, use the chest thrust to attempt to dislodge the foreign object.

Kneel beside the patient and place hands in the same position as with thrust for external cardiac compression. Make sure that thrusts are slow and firm, and performed as many times as is necessary to relieve the obstruction.

SEIZURES

A seizure is an unsystematic discharge of neurons of the cerebrum that results in an abrupt alteration in brain function. It usually begins with little or no warning and may last only for seconds or for several minutes. A seizure is accompanied by a change in the LOC. Convulsions and seizures are interchangeable terms for the same thing. However, not all seizures result in uncontrollable shaking of the patient. Seizures can go unnoticed by both the observer and the patient in some cases.

Seizures themselves are not a disease but a syndrome or symptom of a disease. They may be caused by infections, especially those that are accompanied by high fever. They may also be caused by extreme stress, head trauma, brain tumors, structural abnormalities of the cerebral cortex, genetic defects (epilepsy), birth trauma, vascular disease, congenital malformations, or postnatal trauma. Odors and flashing lights can cause a seizure in a person who is seizure prone.

There are basically two types of seizure: generalized and partial.

Generalized Seizures

These types of seizures occur when abnormal electrical activity that causes a seizure begins in both hemispheres of the brain at the same time.

Clinical Manifestations

- May utter a sharp cry as air is rapidly exhaled
- Muscles become rigid and eyes open wide.
- May exhibit jerky body movements and rapid, irregular respirations
- May vomit
- May froth and have blood-streaked saliva caused by biting the lips or tongue
- May exhibit urinary or fecal incontinence
- Usually falls into a deep sleep after the seizure

Partial Seizures: Complex and Simple

A partial seizure occurs when abnormal electrical activity affects only a small area of the brain. Seizures that occur only in one hemisphere of the brain and impair the consciousness of the patient are known as complex partial seizures. If the seizure does not affect awareness of the seizure by the patient, it is known as a simple partial seizure.

Clinical Manifestations of a Complex Partial Seizure

- Patient may remain motionless or may experience an excessive emotional outburst of fear, crying, or anger.
- Patient may manifest facial grimacing, lip smacking, swallowing movements, or panting.
- Patient is confused for several minutes after the episode with no memory of the incident.

Clinical Manifestations of a Simple Partial Seizure

- Only a finger or a hand may shake.
- Patient may speak unintelligibly.
- Patient may be dizzy.
- Patient may sense strange odors, tastes, or sounds.
- Patient does not lose consciousness.

Response to a Patient Having a Seizure

1. Stay with the patient to prevent injury.
2. Call for assistance.
3. Do not attempt to insert anything into the patient's mouth.
4. Remove dentures and foreign objects from the patient's mouth, if possible, but do not put fingers into the mouth.
5. Place a blanket or pillow under the patient's head to protect it from injury.
6. Do not restrain the arms or legs, but protect them from injury.
7. Do not attempt to move the patient to the floor; if on a radiographic table, do not allow the patient to fall to the floor.
8. Observe the patient carefully and keep track of the time of the seizure to record later.
9. Provide the patient privacy.
10. After the seizure has ceased, position the patient to prevent aspiration of secretions and vomitus. Turn the patient to a Sims position and put the face downward, so that secretions may drain from their mouth, as seen in Figure 9-5.

SYNCOPE

Syncope, or fainting, is a transient loss of consciousness, which usually results from an insufficient blood supply to the brain. Heart disease, hunger, poor ventilation, extreme fatigue, and emotional trauma are all possible causes. The elderly patient who is asked to change positions from lying to standing too quickly may also have a syncopal reaction because of orthostatic hypotension. Orthostatic hypotension is an abnormally low blood pressure occurring when a person stands up before the blood pooled in the extremities has time to circulate to the upper body.

Patients are frequently instructed not to eat breakfast before coming to the diagnostic imaging department from their homes or hospital rooms. Often, they are ill, and a lack of nourishment may increase the likelihood of fainting. The patient cannot choose the "proper" place in which to faint, and injury can easily occur. When fainting and falling from a standing position, it is easy to hit the head quite hard on the floor or a corner of the radiography table and fracture the skull. The technologist must be able to recognize and watch for the symptoms that indicate a patient is about to faint.

If it is suspected that the patient is in a weakened condition because of a recent traumatic injury or illness, do not allow the patient to stand for an upright image and then leave the patient while the exposure is obtained. Consider other methods of obtaining the exposure, or have an assistant stand beside the patient for support, if necessary. Patients who have recently been given medication that they are not used to may also become dizzy and unable to stand for even a short while.

If caring for an elderly patient, allow the patient time to sit for several minutes before standing or walking. Always be at the patient's side for protection from falling.

Patients complaining of chest pain and dizziness must never be taken to the imaging department by wheelchair and expected to stand for even a few minutes. To do so may cause the patient to faint.

Clinical Manifestations

- Pallor, complaints of dizziness, and nausea
- Hyperpnea and tachycardia
- Cold, clammy skin

Response

1. If the patient complains of feeling dizzy or appears to be confused, have the patient lie down.
2. Place a patient who has already fainted in a supine position with legs elevated.
3. Do not try to keep a patient standing if they are about to fall. Support and assist the patient to the floor in a manner that prevents injury. Place a knee behind the patient's knee and an arm around the waist and assist the patient to the floor (Fig. 9-11).

Legalities of Failing to Identify Manifestations of Patients Presenting with Syncope

Patients that come to the imaging department may not be forthcoming with how ill they are actually feeling. In addition, patients that come in may be made to stand up, then lie down on their side, then on their stomach,

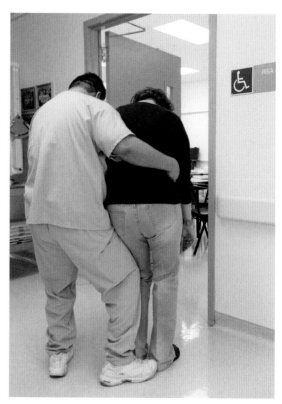

FIGURE 9-11 The radiographer places their knee behind the patient's knee to support them safely to the floor.

and then, when the procedure is over, made to sit up, then stand again. Patients that are in pain or ill often do not handle all this movement well. Be aware of the patient's appearance and watch for the clammy skin and complaints of dizziness. Not paying attention to the details of the patient's condition and the resulting legal action is demonstrated in the case study.

CASE STUDY

Just as the radiographer is responsible for the patient in the imaging department, there is also a responsibility for the patient who is in another area and is to be transported to the radiographic department for a study. In this particular case, the patient came into the ED around 11:30 PM, complaining of chest pain, dizziness, and nausea. The patient was connected to the monitor for blood pressure, heart leads, and pulse oximeter and had oxygen flowing through a cannula. A nurse practitioner ordered a posteroanterior and lateral chest. By the time the order was sent through to the radiographer, it was after 1 AM. The technologist came to the ED with a wheelchair to transport the patient to the radiology department. The technologist explained to the patient that he was going to the department for a chest radiograph. The patient was quite emphatic that he could not sit up in a wheelchair, nor could he stand long enough for the x-rays. He felt that he was too dizzy and nauseous to be moved.

The radiographer convinced the patient that he would be fine, removed all the monitors, and took the patient to the department without alerting nursing staff in the ED. The patient was made to stand up while the technologist set up the technical factors on the control panel. The patient was not able to stand that long, and fainted, falling backward, hitting his head on the corner of the radiographic table, which had not been moved out of the way. It was later found that the patient had sustained a skull fracture because of this fall.

The multiple ramifications illustrated by this true case could have been prevented.

ISSUES TO CONSIDER

1. Should the radiographer have questioned the nursing staff about the safety of taking the patient to the imaging department?
2. Could the patient have been transported by using the stretcher he was already on?
3. What are the ramifications of removing the monitors and not informing the nursing staff? Thinking about the technologist's actions and what could have been done differently, consider the following:
4. If the patient was able to stand and come down to the department, how could the room have been prepared more appropriately?
5. If the patient came down by stretcher, could a lateral image still have been taken?
6. Is it within the scope of practice for the radiographer to suggest that a mobile image be taken to avoid moving the patient at all? How could communication between the technologist and the ED staff have been improved?

If the technologist had used his critical thinking skills and training, this unfortunate situation could have been easily avoided. This case demonstrates how important it is to pay attention to the patient's appearance and what the patient is saying. It is much better to err on the safe side than to injure a patient in any manner.

OTHER MEDICAL CONDITIONS

There are other medical conditions that the radiographer may be exposed to. Many of the patients in the imaging department become nauseated, particularly after a contrast media injection. The radiographer must watch the patient carefully and be ready with an emesis basin if there is a possibility the patient may vomit. Also, be aware of the possibility of choking if the patient is supine. Patients with facial trauma may have bleeding from the nose, known as epistaxis. Other causes include prolonged inhalation of dry air or nasal irritation. Provide the patient with gauze to hold under the nose, but only if there is no trauma. Patients may experience vertigo in the imaging department after remaining supine on the imaging table for a prolonged time. Along with postural hypotension, vertigo can cause a patient to fall when getting off the table. It is extremely important that the patient is never allowed to get off a radiographic table without the radiographer standing alongside the patient. Finally, the radiographer must be aware that there are a great many patients that suffer from asthma. This is a condition in which the patient's airways narrow and swell and may produce extra mucus. This makes breathing difficult and triggers coughing, wheezing, and SOB. Asthma signs and symptoms include SOB, chest tightness or pain, and wheezing (particularly in children). If the radiographer notices the patient is suffering from any of these, the study must be stopped and the patient must be attended to.

Summary

1. Neurologic and cognitive function
   a. Assess the patient's levels of neurologic and cognitive functioning while preparing for the assigned procedure. It is at this time that changes in the patient's LOC and mental status can be observed if they occur.
   b. Rapid assessment can be done with the Glasgow Coma Scale, which addresses the following three areas of neurologic functions to give an overview of the patient's level of responsiveness:
      i. Eye opening
      ii. Motor response
      iii. Verbal response
   c. If the patient's score begins to drop after the initial assessment, notify the physician immediately.

2. Shock
   a. Shock is the failure of circulation to oxygenate the tissues and remove carbon dioxide because of inadequate blood pressure.
   b. It can be life-threatening and must be treated immediately.
   c. There are different types of shock:
      i. Hypovolemic: This means literally not enough blood. It follows the loss of large amount of blood or plasma.
      ii. Cardiogenic: This occurs when the heart fails to function, either from cardiac arrest or from some other interference.
      iii. Neurogenic: This occurs when the blood pools in the peripheral vessels and does not move to the body as it should.
      iv. Septic: This occurs during massive infection causing toxins to create a large drop in blood pressure.
      v. Anaphylactic
         1. Caused by an allergic reaction and is most often seen in the diagnostic imaging department because of contrast media injections
         2. Early signs of anaphylactic shock are nasal congestion, periorbital swelling, itching, dyspnea, tearing of eyes, and peripheral tingling, followed by flushing, urticaria, anxiety, and bronchospasm.
         3. If early symptoms of an anaphylactic reaction are suspected, the technologist must stop the administration of the contrast medium immediately and initiate emergency action. If symptoms are not relieved, the patient may have seizures and respiratory arrest.
   d. Symptoms of shock are basically all the same. The patient may experience some or all of the following:
      i. Fast pulse
      ii. Weakness
      iii. Pale skin color that is cool and clammy to the touch
      iv. Very low systolic blood pressure but a fast pulse rate
      v. Restlessness and a feeling of anxiety
   e. The radiographer must respond immediately to effectively stop the shock continuum.
      i. Stop the procedure and obtain help immediately—even to the point of calling a "CODE BLUE" if necessary.
      ii. Place the patient in a Trendelenburg position.

      iii. Be ready to give oxygen as prescribed by the physician.
      iv. Take a blood pressure reading and document the time and occurrence of the event along with the symptoms demonstrated and the response taken.

3. Pulmonary embolus
   a. PE is a medical emergency that may occur without warning.
   b. Patients who have had recent surgery should be watched more closely for this situation.
   c. PEs can be fatal if not treated immediately.
   d. Clinical manifestations include:
      i. Diaphoresis
      ii. Hypotension
      iii. Apprehension
      iv. Changing LOC
      v. Tachycardia and hyperventilation
   e. The response by the radiographer should be:
      i. Stop the procedure and call for assistance.
      ii. Get the crash cart if not already in the room.
      iii. Monitor vital signs.
      iv. Prepare to assist as needed with oxygen administration and IV fluids.

4. Diabetic emergencies
   a. Patients who have diabetes may come for procedures after having taken insulin or oral hypoglycemic medication and be without sufficient food intake to use the drug.
   b. Type 1
      i. Younger than 30
      ii. Insulin dependent
   c. Type 2
      i. Most common type
      ii. Patients are usually over 40
      iii. Insulin is made but the body does not use it properly
   d. Gestational
      i. Occurs in the later months of pregnancy
      ii. Goes away after delivery
   e. Clinical manifestation of all types:
      i. Tachycardia
      ii. Blurred vision
      iii. Thirst
      iv. Sweet smelling breath if the patient is in ketoacidosis
   f. Response to the manifestations include:
      i. Stop the procedure and notify a physician.
      ii. Monitor vital signs.

      iii. Prepare to give IV fluids, medication, and oxygen as requested by the physician.

5. Strokes

    a. CVAs are medical emergencies that must be recognized and dealt with immediately to prevent life-threatening consequences.

    b. The early signs and symptoms are often one-sided flaccidity of the face and limbs, difficult or absent speech, eye deviation, dizziness, ataxia, possible neck stiffness, nausea, vomiting, and loss of consciousness.

    c. The response to these signs and symptoms are:

      i. Stop the procedure and notify the physician.

      ii. Make sure to be able to assist in any manner required such as oxygen administration and IV fluids. The crash cart must be in the area to prevent loss of time hunting it down.

6. Cardiac arrest

    a. Cardiac failure results in an immediate cessation of the pulse and respiration and a loss of consciousness.

    b. The patient has loss of consciousness, pulse, and blood pressure. There is a possibility of seizures.

    c. The emergency medical team must be called immediately (CODE BLUE).

    d. After calling a "code" the radiographer must begin CPR until the team arrives to take over. The crash cart must be available for the team to use. Make sure that there is one in the same room as the patient.

7. Respiratory arrest

    a. Respiratory failure is recognized by a lack of chest movement, absence of breath sounds, a diminishing pulse rate, and loss of consciousness.

    b. There are several causes of respiratory arrest including:

      i. Edema of the upper airway

      ii. Edema of the tracheolaryngeal area secondary to allergic reaction to contrast media

      iii. Choking

      iv. Central nervous system failure

    c. If the arrest is caused by failure of the central nervous system, then a "code" for respiratory arrest must be called and the emergency team handles this event.

    d. If the arrest is caused by choking, the Heimlich maneuver may be necessary.

8. Airway obstruction

    a. Airway obstruction by a foreign object should be suspected:

      i. If a patient is feeling well and suddenly begins to demonstrate respiratory distress

    b. If the patient is found unconscious and, when ventilation is attempted, the chest cannot be made to rise and fall

    c. The Heimlich or the abdominal thrust maneuver must be performed in response to this emergency.

9. Seizures

    a. Seizures are an unsystematic discharge of neurons in the brain.

    b. There may be ALOC.

    c. Seizures are classified as generalized or partial, with partial being either complex or simple.

    d. If the radiographer suspects the patient is having a seizure, stay with the patient to prevent injury. Do not put anything in the patient's mouth.

    e. Do not try to move the patient to the floor, but after the seizure, make sure the patient is in a position to prevent aspiration of secretions or vomitus.

10. Syncope

    a. Fainting and convulsive seizures may occur with little or no warning.

    b. It is critical that the radiographer not leave the side of a patient that is dizzy or unable to stand without assistance.

    c. Elderly patients are more prone to fainting if they have been lying down for a period of time.

    d. If the patient feels dizzy or light-headed, sit or lie the patient down with feet elevated.

11. Other medical conditions

    a. Radiographers must be alert for patients exhibiting nausea as they may vomit.

    b. Epistaxis (nose bleeds) are not a common occurrence in the imaging department but the resourceful technologist must be able to help the patient.

    c. Vertigo and postural hypotension can cause a patient to fall.

    d. Asthma is a common condition shown as SOB and chest tightness or pain. If the patient exhibits any symptoms of an asthma attack, the radiographer must stop and attend to the patient's breathing.

CHAPTER 9 REVIEW QUESTIONS

1. List and describe the levels of neurologic functioning according to the Glasgow Coma Scale.

2. General signs and symptoms that the technologist must learn to recognize as probable indicators that the patient is in shock include: (Circle all that apply)
   a. Strong, irregular pulse
   b. Hypertension
   c. Flushed face
   d. Increased respiration
   e. Cold, clammy skin
   f. Acetone breath
   g. ALOC
   h. Decreased temperature
   i. Weak, thready pulse
   j. Rapid heartbeat, hypotension

3. Why is anaphylactic shock the most frequently seen type of shock in the diagnostic imaging department?
   a. Patients who come for diagnostic imaging procedures are weak and debilitated.
   b. Iodinated contrast media are frequently used.
   c. Patients here have more allergies.
   d. X-radiation causes this problem.

4. Early signs and symptoms of anaphylactic reaction are: (Circle all that apply)
   a. Itching at the site of the injection
   b. Tearing of eyes
   c. Feeling of warmth
   d. Anxiety
   e. Bronchospasm and edema of the airway
   f. Decreasing blood pressure
   g. Sneezing

5. Myrtle is a 43-year-old female who has come to diagnostic imaging this morning from her home for an upper gastrointestinal series. After she has been in the room for a short time, she complains of a severe headache. Shortly after, you notice that she has cold, clammy skin and speaks in a slurred manner. You suspect that she is:
   a. A diabetic and is having a hypoglycemic reaction
   b. Having a cardiac arrest
   c. An alcoholic and is drunk
   d. An epileptic and is having a seizure

6. The immediate emergency treatment of Myrtle's problem in Question 5 is imperative. What is the first action the radiographer should take?
   a. Prepare for oxygen administration and call the emergency team.
   b. Notify the physician in charge, check for an identification of the patient as a diabetic, and then give her some form of concentrated sugar as directed.
   c. Place the patient in a supine position, keep her warm, and call the emergency team.
   d. Continue with your work, but do not leave the patient alone.

7. Symptoms of a partially obstructed airway may include:
   a. Cold, clammy skin; pallor; weakness; anxiety
   b. Flushed, hot skin; hyperactivity; confusion; seizures
   c. Labored, noisy breathing; wheezing; use of neck muscles to assist with breathing
   d. Acetone breath, irregular pulse, noisy respiration, rapid heartbeat, flushed skin

8. A 16-year-old male patient comes to the diagnostic imaging department for a computed tomography (CT) scan. He is lying on the table in a supine position. He suddenly seems to lose consciousness and begins to move violently with jerking motions. You realize that he is having a generalized seizure. What is the most appropriate action to take?
   a. Go to the patient immediately and restrain him with immobilizers.
   b. Call for help and get the crash cart ready.
   c. Place the patient on the floor and begin CPR.
   d. Call for help and make sure that the patient does not injure himself.

9. Gertrude is a 35-year-old female who had an open reduction of her left femur 3 days earlier. She has been transported to the diagnostic imaging department by gurney from her hospital room for radiographs. As you prepare the patient for the radiograph, she suddenly begins to complain of pain in her mid-chest and appears to be out of breath. You stop your preparation and take her pulse and blood pressure. You find that her blood pressure is 120/80 but her radial pulse is 120 per minute and is very difficult to palpate because it is so weak and thready. You quickly notify the physician of the problem, and he directs you to call the emergency team (but not a CODE BLUE). You do this and make other emergency preparations. You believe that this patient may be having:
   a. A stroke
   b. A seizure
   c. A PE
   d. An episode of syncope

10. Fainting is a common medical emergency in the diagnostic imaging department. If a patient appears to be fainting, what is the first thing to do?
    a. Assist the patient to a safe position and then call for help
    b. Give smelling salts
    c. Get the emergency cart
    d. Prepare to administer oxygen

11. Match the different types of shock with the symptoms displayed:

    a. Hypovolemic shock   i. Difficult speech, severe headache, one-sided, drooping eye and face, loss of consciousness

    b. CVA   ii. Choking, inability to speak, eventual loss of consciousness

    c. Airway obstruction   iii. Itching of eyes, apprehensiveness, wheezing, choking

    d. Cardiogenic shock   iv. Loss of consciousness; decreased blood pressure; weak, rapid pulse

    e. Anaphylactic shock   v. Pallor; slow irregular pulse; cool, clammy skin; restlessness

Tubes, Lines, and Other Devices

10

OBJECTIVES

After studying this chapter, the student will be able to:

1. Define nasogastric and nasointestinal tubes and the radiographer's responsibilities regarding them.

2. Describe all considerations for patients with a central venous catheter.

3. Outline the steps in the operation and maintenance of suction equipment.

4. Explain the precautions necessary when working with a patient who has a tracheostomy.

5. Define precautions taken for patients with a chest tube.

6. Explain care considerations for patients with a tissue drain.

7. Describe precautions to be taken with patients undergoing retrograde pyelography or placement of a ureteral stent.

8. Identify specific types of tubes, lines, catheters, and devices seen on radiographic images.

KEY TERMS

Asphyxiation: Severe hypoxia leading to hypoxemia, hypercapnia, loss of consciousness, and death

Cannula: A tube used to allow fluids, gases, or other substances into or out of the body

Dyspneic: Having shortness of breath or difficulty breathing

Enteric: Occurring or relating to the intestines

Gastric: Relating or occurring to the stomach

Gastrostomy: Creation of an opening in the stomach to provide food and liquid administration

Hemostat: A clamp-like instrument used to control flow of fluids or blood

Lavage: The process of washing out an organ, usually the stomach, bladder, or bowel

Nasoenteric tube: A tube much like a nasogastric tube, but it is allowed to pass into the duodenum and small intestine by means of peristalsis

Nasogastric tube: A tube of soft rubber or plastic inserted through the nostril and into the stomach

Nasointestinal: Meaning from the nose to the intestine (put usually to the stomach)

Saline solution: A solution consisting of a percentage of sodium chloride and distilled water that has the same osmolarity as that of body fluids

INTRODUCTION

Nasogastric (NG) and **nasoenteric** (NE) **tubes** are inserted for therapeutic and diagnostic purposes. These tubes have a hollow lumen through which secretions and air may be evacuated or through which medications, nourishment, or diagnostic contrast agents may be instilled.

The radiographer must be able to care for and transport patients with these tubes in place. The purposes of **gastric** suction and the ability to attach or discontinue it when the physician's orders require it must also be understood to prevent any injury to the patient.

Abdominal images may be required before, during, or after the passage of NG or NE tubes. This image can be performed either in the diagnostic imaging department or with a bedside mobile x-ray machine. Although radiographers do not insert these tubes, preparation of the patient may be required if the tube is to be inserted in the diagnostic imaging department. What type of equipment to assemble and how to assist with the procedure are requisite knowledge.

Occasionally, a patient requiring a procedure has a gastrostomy tube in place. These tubes may be required for persons who are gravely debilitated and unable to obtain nutrition in a normal physiologic manner. These patients must be cared for in a safe and sensitive manner.

Patients who are unable to take in nutrients through the gastrointestinal (GI) system, either partially or completely, may be nourished intravenously. This can be accomplished in the short term parenterally by peripheral intravenous means and in the long term by reliance on central venous catheters.

Occasionally, it is necessary for the patient who has vomited or who has an accumulation of blood or secretions in the mouth or throat to be suctioned while under the care of the technologist. Although the technologist does not perform these procedures, a quick assessment of the patient is critical so that the procedure can be done quickly to prevent aspiration of the fluid into the lungs or cause respiratory failure.

Patients with the tracheostomy tubes in place may also need diagnostic imaging examinations. They must receive proper care to prevent injury and to keep them comfortable while the examination is in progress.

Patients who are unable to maintain adequate respiration may require mechanical ventilation to support life. Mobile chest imaging examination for these patients is a frequent occurrence; therefore, precautions when working with patients on a ventilator are required.

Chest tubes are inserted after surgical procedures, injury, or diseases of the lungs to permit drainage of fluid or air out of the pleural space. If air and fluid become trapped in the pleural space, pressure builds and creates what is called a tension pneumothorax. If this condition is not relieved, the resulting respiratory distress may produce a life-threatening situation. The precautions needed to care for patients with a chest tube must also be learned.

After surgical procedures, a variety of tissue drains are placed in the areas of the body that cannot tolerate an accumulation of fluid. The radiographer must be able to recognize these drains and direct patient care in a manner that prevents dislodging of the drains during the imaging process.

NG TUBES

NG tubes are made of polyurethane, silicone, or rubber. They are inserted through the nasopharynx into the stomach, the duodenum, or the jejunum. If a patient has an anatomic or physiologic reason why the nose cannot be used for passage, the tube may be inserted through the mouth over the tongue. NG tubes are used for diagnostic examinations, for administration of feedings or medications, to treat intestinal obstruction, and to control bleeding (Table 10-1). The two most commonly used tubes are the Levin and the Salem Sump tubes.

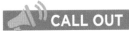 **CALL OUT**

The technologist is often asked to perform a mobile abdomen x-ray for NG tube placement at the patient's bedside.

TABLE 10-1	Common Nasogastric Tubes		
Name	**Number of Lumens**	**Description**	**Use**
Levin	1	Plastic tube that is passed through the nose into the stomach	Gastric decompression
Salem Sump	2	Radiopaque tube with a plug pigtail that lets airflow into the stomach	Drain fluid from the stomach
Nutriflex	1	Mercury-weighted tip; coated with a gastric secretion–activated lubricant	Feedings
Moss	3	Has a balloon to anchor into the stomach, whereas the second and third lumens are used for aspiration and feeding	Aspiration of fluid; duodenal feeding
Sengstaken-Blakemore	3	Thick catheter with two balloons used to exert pressure against the walls of the esophagus	Control of bleeding from esophageal varices

Two of the most common NG tubes are the Levin (Fig. 10-1) and the Salem Sump tubes (Fig. 10-2). Other NG tubes often seen are the Nutriflex, the Moss, and the Sengstaken-Blakemore (S-B) esophageal NG tube. The Levin tube is a single-lumen tube with holes near its tip. The Salem Sump tube is a radiopaque, double-lumen tube. The opening of the second lumen is a blue extension off the proximal end of the tube. This is the end

that remains outside and is called a "pigtail." This end is always left open to room air for the purpose of maintaining a continuous flow of atmospheric air into the stomach, thereby controlling the amount of suction pressure that may be placed on the gastric mucosa. This is a means of preventing injury and ulceration of these tissues.

The Nutriflex tube is used primarily for feeding. It has a mercury-weighted tip and is coated with a lubricant that becomes activated when moistened by gastric secretions. The Moss tube is a more complex triple-lumen tube. One lumen has an inflatable balloon to anchor it in the stomach. The second lumen is used for aspiration of fluid, and the third is for duodenal feeding.

The S-B tube is also a triple-lumen tube; two of the lumens have balloons. The balloons are inflated to exert pressure on bleeding esophageal varices. The third lumen is used for **lavage** and to monitor for hemorrhage. The balloon pressure must be maintained at all times, but if the patient becomes **dyspneic**, the balloon pressure must be relieved at once by cutting the balloon lumens with scissors. If the patient is in the imaging department for a lengthy period, the technologist should not attempt to care for a patient with an S-B tube in place without the patient's nurse on hand. **Asphyxiation** or aspiration of gastric contents into the lungs is possible without keen and continuous monitoring. The patient with an S-B tube in place is usually cared for in the intensive care unit (ICU), and portable images are ordered.

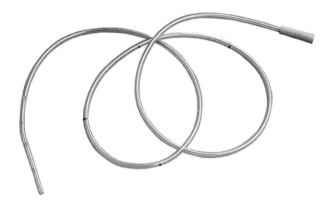

FIGURE 10-1 This NG tube is a Levin tube.

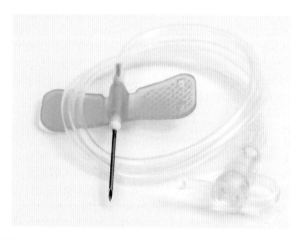

FIGURE 10-2 Another NG tube is the Salem Sump tube. Notice the blue pigtail that is put over the tube when it is disconnected from suction. (Courtesy of ShutterStock/zairiazmal.)

NE Tubes

NE tubes and nasointestinal tubes are different names for tubes that are allowed to proceed down the GI tract and into the small intestine. **Nasogastric** means the nose to the stomach. **Nasointestinal** or **enteric** means nose to the small intestine. NE tubes are made of the same materials as NG tubes and are inserted in much the same way as NG tubes; however, they are allowed to pass into the duodenum and small intestine by means of peristalsis. They are also used for decompression, diagnosis, and treatment purposes (Table 10-2).

Three of the most commonly used NE tubes are the Cantor, the Harris, and the Miller-Abbott. The Cantor

TABLE 10-2	Common Nasoenteric Tubes		
Name	Number of Lumens	Description	Use
Cantor	1	Long tube with a small mercury-filled bag at the end; contains drainage holes for aspiration	Relieves obstructions in the small intestine
Harris	1	Mercury-weighted tube passed through the nose and carried through the digestive tract by gravity	Gastric and intestinal decompression
Miller-Abbott	2	Long small-caliber catheter; one is a perforated metal tip, and the other has a collapsible balloon; radiopaque tube	Decompression

and Harris tubes have a single lumen, whereas the Miller-Abbott tube is a double-lumen tube. One lumen of the Miller-Abbott tube is used for intestinal decompression, and the other is for the introduction of mercury after insertion. Some single-lumen tubes are weighted with a metal tip. The progress of the tube may be observed in the diagnostic imaging department fluoroscopically. Radiographs are taken after passage of these tubes to establish correct placement (Figs. 10-3 and 10-4).

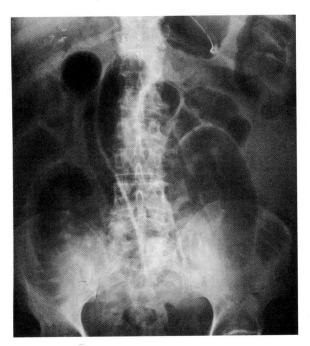

FIGURE 10-3 Radiograph showing a Levin tube in place in the stomach.

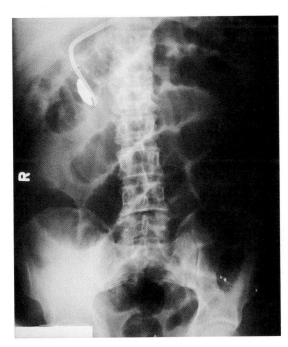

FIGURE 10-4 Radiograph of a small bowel obstruction with a Cantor tube in place.

Passage of Tubes

Technologists are not responsible for inserting NG or NE tubes. A registered nurse usually inserts an NG or NE tube, or a physician may insert the NE tube. Insertion of a tube is an uncomfortable and frightening procedure for the patient, who is often very ill. If this procedure is to take place in the imaging department, explain to the patient what is being done and for what purpose. If the patient can concentrate on swallowing and breathing as the tube is inserted, the procedure will go smoothly and quickly.

The patient is placed in a semi-Fowler position with pillows supporting the head and shoulders. When the physician or nurse is ready to insert the tube, the distal end is lubricated with a water-soluble lubricant, and the patient is instructed to swallow as it is passed. The tube should go down easily and with little force. When the tube is believed to be in the stomach, an initial radiographic image verifies its position. Radiographs in Figure 10-5A and B show different locations of the tube within the stomach. When it is certain that the tube has reached the stomach, make the patient comfortable and explain that the tube is in place. NG tubes are taped in place, but NE tubes are not taped because their position is achieved through peristaltic action. The Levin tube is securely taped so that it is not accidentally withdrawn. It should never be necessary to repeat passage of a gastric tube because of careless handling. There should be no pulling pressure on the tube. Patients with gastric tubes in place are not to eat or drink anything unless the physician specifically orders it. Patients who may accidentally pull their NG tubes out may have immobilizers on their wrists.

The placement of an NG tube must be ascertained before any medication, food, water, or contrast agent is administered into it. If this is not done, accidental administration of an agent into the pleural cavity may occur with adverse consequences for the patient.

The correct position of an NG or NE tube initially may be determined with a radiographic image or by fluoroscopy. Obviously, a radiographic image cannot be used each time it is necessary to know whether the tube is correctly positioned. The other means of determining the correct placement of an NG or NE tube is by aspirating the contents of the stomach or the bowel through the tube with a syringe. The aspirant is then tested with litmus paper to measure its acidity.

If there is any doubt concerning the position of either type of tube, nothing should be administered into it. If instillation of an agent has begun, discontinue it immediately. If the patient seems to have regurgitated gastric contents, the technologist must summon assistance immediately and prepare to assist with suctioning. To reduce the risk of aspiration, the patient with the tube should be placed in a semi-Fowler position during and for 30 minutes after administration of any medium into the tube.

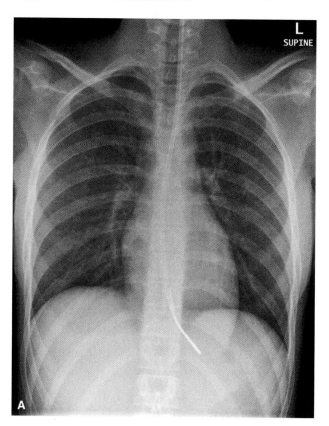
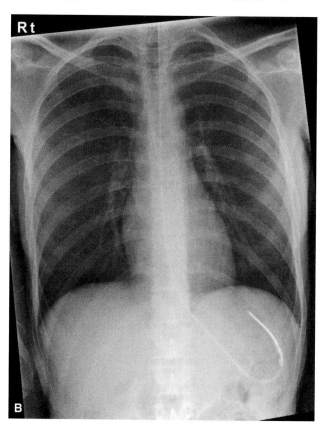

FIGURE 10-5 **(A)** Chest radiograph showing the tube in its entirety. The nasogastric (NG) tube ends just at the opening of the esophagus into the stomach. **(B)** Chest radiograph showing the tube farther advanced into the stomach of this patient.

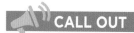 CALL OUT

A small bowel series examination may be ordered for patients with an NG tube or with an NE tube by the physician. The contrast media is instilled via the NG tube according to department protocols.

Removing Gastric Tubes

The Levin tube, the Salem Sump tube, and other tubes positioned in the stomach are easily removed; however, it must never be assumed that simply because an imaging examination that involved its use is complete, it is permissible to remove the tube. Unless ordered by the physician to remove the tube, it must be left in place.

Do not remove NE tubes. The physician or registered nurse may remove the tube, or it may be passed through the intestinal tract and removed rectally. Although it is not in the purview of the technologist to remove the NG tube, Table 10-3 identifies the equipment that will be necessary to have on hand and describes the procedure in the event the radiographer is required to assist in the procedure.

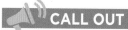 CALL OUT

Radiographers are never to remove an NE tube.

Transferring Patients with NG Suction

NG and NE tubes are used before or after surgical procedures that involve the digestive system, for illness of the GI system to keep the stomach and bowel free of gastric contents, and for gastric decompression. The tube may be attached to a suction apparatus that is either portable or piped into the room from a central hospital unit (Fig. 10-6). The suction is maintained either continuously or intermittently, as the patient's needs demand. When the technologist is responsible for transferring a patient who is having either continuous or intermittent gastric suctioning, the physicians' orders must be verified before making the transfer. If it is permissible to discontinue the suction, the length of time that it can be interrupted safely must be known. If it is for only a short time, be certain that suction can be reestablished in the diagnostic imaging department. This can be accomplished by taking the patient's portable

TABLE 10-3	Equipment and Procedure to Remove a Nasogastric Tube
Equipment	**Procedure**
Emesis basin	Identify the patient and explain the procedure.
Tissues and paper towels	Wash hands and put on the protective apparel.
Impermeable waste receptacle	Loosen tape, disconnect suction.
Clean disposable gloves	Instruct the patient to take in a deep breath.
Face shield	Gently withdraw the tube, wrap in paper toweling, and place in disposal bag.
Impermeable gown	Make the patient comfortable and dispose of items correctly.

suction machine or by using the suction available in the department. The amount of suction must also be known so that the pressure can be accurately adjusted. The amount of pressure that is ordered varies, and the correct level can be determined by reading the physician's orders or by asking the nurse in charge of the patient. The maximum amount of suction that can be used is a pressure equal to 25 mm Hg for an adult patient. More than this can damage the

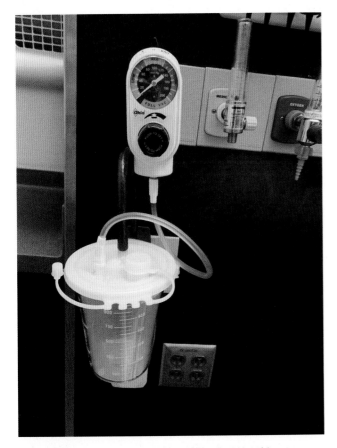

FIGURE 10-6 Suction equipment is often used in diagnostic imaging. It is piped to the department from a central area in the hospital. The vacuum-collecting canister is disposable.

gastric mucosa. If the suction must be disconnected for a period, the technologist is allowed to do this with the proper education.

If the NG tube is a double-lumen tube, never clamp it closed with a **hemostat** or regular clamping device because this may cause the lumens to adhere to each other and destroy the double-lumen effect. To prevent leakage from this type of tube, the barrel of the piston syringe may be inserted into the suction-drainage lumen (the blue pigtail). It is then pinned to the gown with the barrel upward to prevent reflux drainage.

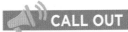
 CALL OUT

Never clamp a double-lumen NG tube because this may destroy the effect.

THE GASTROSTOMY TUBE

A **gastrostomy** is the surgical creation of an opening into the stomach. Through this opening, a tube is placed from the inside of the stomach to the external abdominal wall for the purpose of feeding a patient who cannot tolerate oral food intake (Figs. 10-7 and 10-8). This can be a temporary or permanent provision. The tube can be sutured in place or may be held in place with a crossbar that holds the tube against the wall of the stomach.

The patient with a newly applied gastrostomy tube has an unhealed surgical incision and have a dressing in place. An older gastrostomy may or may not have a dressing applied. The tube is closed off after feeding with a clamp or a plug-in adapter to prevent leakage of gastric fluid or food. The tube is then coiled and kept in place with tape or a small dressing.

While caring for a person with a gastrostomy tube in place, the radiographer must be aware of the potential for infection. If the operative area around the gastrostomy tube is not healed, sterile gloves must be worn if contact

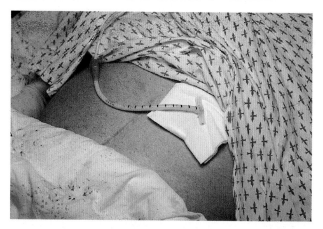

FIGURE 10-7 A percutaneous endoscopic gastrostomy tube with the site protected by a dressing that covers the exit site. (From Hinkle JL, Cheever KH. *Brunner & Suddarth's Textbook of Medical-Surgical Nursing.* 13th ed. Wolters Kluwer Health/Lippincott Williams & Wilkins; 2014.)

with the open area is possible. This is to prevent introduction of microorganisms that may result in infection. The potential for dislodging the tube is also present. Take care to prevent this. There must not be any tension placed on the tube.

The technologist must be sensitive to the feelings of the patient with a gastrostomy. The patient may be grieving owing to the change in their body image or because of a chronic illness. Sensitive and thoughtful communication is required, and the patient who is able to should be allowed to direct the care of the tube.

ENDOTRACHEAL TUBES

The endotracheal (ET) tube is made of polyvinyl chloride with a strip of radiopaque material running through the side. A cuff is located at the end of the tube that seals the tube against the walls of the trachea, preventing contents from the stomach entering into the trachea (Fig. 10-9). It is inserted through the mouth, between the vocal cords, and into the trachea. It is a means of establishing or opening an airway on patients that aren't able to breathe on their own because of a closed airway system. After being placed in the trachea, the cuff is inflated, which keeps the airway open. At the same time, the tube prevents aspiration of foreign objects into the bronchus.

A correct placement of the tube is approximately 5 to 7 cm above the tracheal bifurcation (carina). A

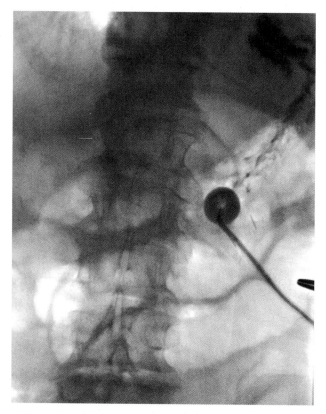

FIGURE 10-8 A radiographic image shows the gastrostomy tube in place. The image was made in the negative mode.

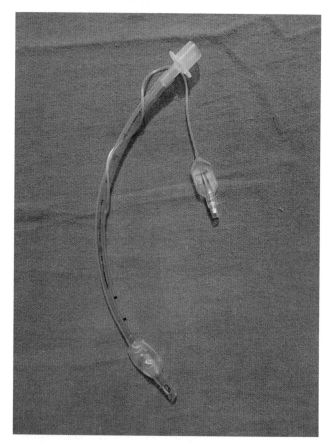

FIGURE 10-9 An endotracheal tube.

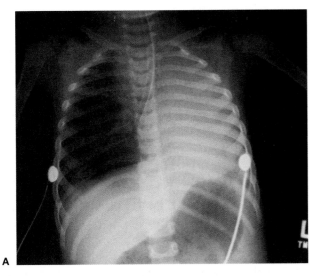 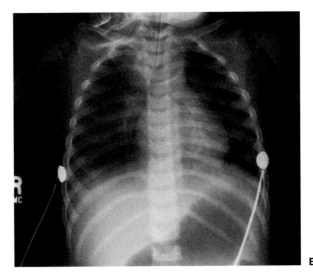

FIGURE 10-10 **(A)** Radiographic image demonstrating a collapsed left lung because of incorrect endotracheal tube placement. **(B)** An image showing that the left lung has now reinflated when the endotracheal tube was withdrawn and the tip of the tube is above the carina.

chest radiographic image should always be obtained after intubation to ascertain the proper placement of the tube. Up to 20% of all ET tubes require repositioning after initial insertion. Because of the anatomic position of the right main bronchus, tubes that are inserted too far usually enter the right bronchus. This causes collapse of the left lung (Fig. 10-10A and B). A tube positioned too high in the trachea may cause air to enter the stomach, causing the patient to regurgitate any gastric contents. This regurgitation may lead to aspiration pneumonia.

Radiographic images may be ordered on a daily basis to ensure that the tube has not accidentally shifted. The tube can be moved by the patient's coughing, the weight of the ventilator tubing, or the movement of the patient by a health care worker.

Although ET tubes are necessary, they are a concern as they have been associated with ventilator-associated pneumonia.

SUCTION

Rarely the radiographer may be left alone with patients that may need to be suctioned. Radiographs are often needed on the patient in the ICU who may need suctioning, or the patient may be in the emergency department following trauma and requires suctioning. The radiographer must be aware of the conditions that are present when the patient is unable to clear fluids from the airway by coughing or swallowing. If the airway is not cleared quickly, complications such as respiratory

arrest can occur. Signs that indicate that a patient may need to receive nasopharyngeal or oropharyngeal suctioning are:

1. Profuse vomiting in a patient who cannot voluntarily change position
2. Audible rattling or gurgling sounds coming from the patient's throat
3. Signs of respiratory distress
4. Profuse bleeding from facial wounds and the patient cannot clear their airway

Suctioning is an emergency procedure. It is not within the scope of practice for a radiographer to perform suctioning procedures as there are many instances in which suctioning may be contraindicated. Some contraindications for suctioning may be head and facial injuries, bleeding esophageal varices, nasal deformities, trauma, cerebral aneurysms, tight wheezing, bronchospasm, and croup.

The radiographer must be able to determine if the patient needs to be suctioned, to call for the physician or the registered nurse to do this if necessary, and to assist with the procedure. The scope of practice for radiographers does not include suctioning. However, the radiographer is responsible for checking the emergency suctioning equipment in the department each day to be certain that it is in good working order and that all necessary items are available.

Pediatric suctioning is different from that for adults. The pediatric patient has a smaller mouth and nasal passages and therefore requires a catheter with a smaller tip.

Their tissues are more delicate and the suction pressure for an adult could easily damage these tissues. Also, hypoxia occurs more rapidly in pediatric patients, so prolonged suctioning can be detrimental. Adult patients may need suctioning through the tracheostomy tube, as discussed in the next section.

TRACHEOSTOMY

A tracheostomy is an opening into the trachea created surgically either to relieve respiratory distress caused by an obstruction of the upper airway or to improve respiratory function by permitting better access of air to the lower respiratory tract. This may be done as either a temporary or a permanent measure. Patients who require this procedure may have suffered traumatic injury or may be paralyzed, unconscious, or suffering from a disease that interferes with respiration.

After the surgical incision is made and the opening exists, a tracheostomy tube is inserted into the opening, as seen in Figure 10-11. Tracheostomy tubes are equipped with an obturator to ensure safe insertion; the obturator is removed as soon as the tube is in place.

There are several types of tracheostomy tubes. They are usually made of plastic but sometimes may be of metal. They have a cuff located near the end of the

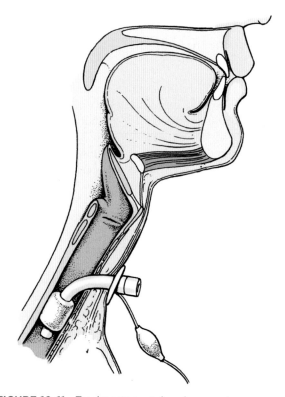

FIGURE 10-11 Tracheostomy tube placement.

portion of the tube that is located in the trachea that helps seal the trachea to prevent air leaks and aspiration of gastric contents. The fenestrated tracheostomy tube has an opening above the cuff that allows air to flow through the openings and over the vocal cords, thus allowing some voice action. The double-cuff tube has two low-pressure cuffs that are inflated to prevent air and gastric contents from passing into the trachea. The use of a single-cuff tube has shown that the mucosa of the trachea becomes irritated because of the high pressure necessary to avoid material passing into the trachea. The use of a double-cuff tube allows lower pressure to be placed on the walls of the trachea, but with two cuffs in place, the contents are prohibited from advancing. Figure 10-12A and B shows both types of tubes. Most tracheostomy tubes have an inner **cannula** that is locked into place. The tracheostomy tube is held in place at the back of the neck with ties or tapes, as seen in Figure 10-13. The tubes that are used for infants and small children do not usually have the cuff because they fit tightly enough without one.

Patients with newly inserted tracheostomy tubes are unable to speak because the opening in the windpipe prevents air from being forced from the lungs past the vocal cords and into the larynx. They may be afraid of choking because they are unable to remove secretions that accumulate in the tracheostomy tube. These secretions must be suctioned out by a registered nurse. If a patient with a new tracheostomy is brought to the diagnostic imaging department, a nurse qualified to care for this patient should accompany them. Sterile suction catheters, suctioning equipment, and oxygen administration equipment must be prepared before the patient arrives in the department. The semi-Fowler position is usually most comfortable for these patients, and bolsters or pillows should be provided so that the best position for the patient can be maintained.

While caring for the patient with a tracheostomy, plan the care with the patient's nurse and the patient before any diagnostic imaging procedure is begun. The tracheostomy tube must not be removed, and the tapes holding it in place must not be untied for any reason, because the tracheostomy tube may be dislodged and may not be able to be replaced immediately. All procedures must be explained to the patient in order to alleviate anxiety. If the patient appears to be breathing noisily or with difficulty, immediately stop working and allow the nurse to suction the patient or otherwise relieve the discomfort. The radiographer should not perform the suction as fenestrated tubes require a non-fenestrated inner cannula to be placed first.

In the event the patient goes into a respiratory or cardiac arrest and should need cardiopulmonary resuscitation (CPR), an Ambu bag is attached to the outside of the tracheostomy tube and compressed to give the

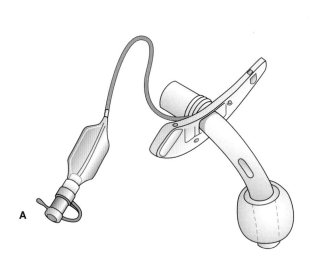
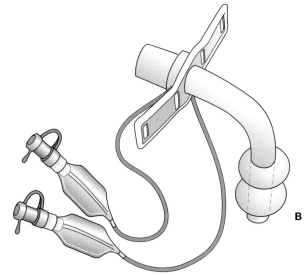

FIGURE 10-12 **(A)** Fenestrated tube. **(B)** Double-cuff tube.

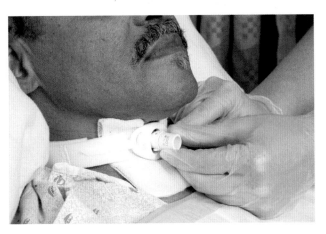

FIGURE 10-13 Tracheostomy tube is held in place by ties that are around the neck. (From Springhouse. *Lippincott's Visual Encyclopedia of Clinical Skills*. Wolters Kluwer Health; 2009.)

breaths as would normally be done. Figure 10-14 shows the top of an Ambu bag equipped with a face mask that would cover the nose and mouth of the patient, and the blue cap covering the tracheostomy attachment. If the bag is to be used on a tube, the mask is rotated away, which closes off the air valve to it, allowing air to flow through the tracheostomy. The blue cap is removed and the bag is attached to the tube with gentle but firm pressure to make sure that it does not pop off during compression of the bag.

THE MECHANICAL VENTILATOR

The radiographer may be frequently called to the ICU of the acute care hospital to take radiographic images

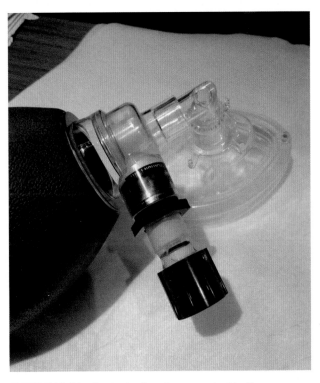

FIGURE 10-14 An Ambu bag is connected to the tracheostomy tube when manual breaths must be given through the tube.

of patients who are being ventilated mechanically. Because mechanical ventilators support life, it is of great importance that all precautions be understood when taking care of a patient whose breathing is supported by mechanical means.

The need for mechanical ventilation may be the result of a disease process that affects the mechanics of breathing by interfering with the neurologic or neuromuscular functions related to breathing. These are called extrapulmonary disorders. Other disorders may be of the gas exchange type such as pulmonary emboli or respiratory distress syndrome (RDS).

There are two general classifications of mechanical ventilators: negative-pressure ventilators and positive-pressure ventilators. Positive-pressure ventilators are the more commonly used type. There are three general categories of positive-pressure ventilators: pressure cycled, time cycled, and volume cycled. They inflate the lungs by exerting positive pressure on the lungs, stopping inspiration when a preset pressure is attained. The lungs are then allowed to expire passively. All positive-pressure ventilators require an artificial airway, either an ET tube or a tracheostomy. When imaging a patient who is on a positive-pressure ventilator, consult the nurse assigned to care for the patient before beginning the radiographic imaging procedure.

The following precautions must be taken for a patient who is being ventilated by positive pressure:

1. Obtain as much assistance as necessary to move the patient safely.
2. Do not place tension on any intravenous tubing or on the tube to the ventilator.
3. Do not displace the ET tube or tracheostomy tube.
4. Do not disconnect the power to the ventilator.
5. Do not disconnect the spirometer.
6. If the patient becomes suddenly restless or confused or seems to be fighting the respirator, stop and notify the nurse immediately.
7. Use meticulous medical aseptic technique when working with the patient to prevent infection. Put on gloves if there is any possibility of being in contact with blood or body fluids.

If displacement or malfunction of any part of the equipment occurs, an alarm will sound on the machine. This may indicate a life-threatening problem that must be attended to immediately. The potential complications caused by a positive-pressure ventilator equipment displacement or malfunction include cardiovascular compromise related to inadequate oxygenation, pneumothorax resulting from excessive ventilator pressure, or infection resulting from exposure to microorganisms introduced into the pulmonary system.

The patient who is on a positive-pressure ventilator is unable to communicate because of the ET tube or a newly acquired tracheostomy. This is extremely frustrating for the patient. An explanation of what is about to happen goes a long way toward relieving this frustration, as does providing the patient with a means to give written feedback.

CHEST (THORACOSTOMY) TUBES

The pressure in the pleural cavity is normally lower than atmospheric pressure, but disease or injury can alter this. Air in the pleural cavity, known as a pneumothorax, causes a collapse of the lung. A condition caused by a collection of blood in the pleural cavity that prevents the lungs from expanding normally is called a *hemothorax*, whereas fluid other than blood that builds up in the pleural cavity is called *pleural effusion*. In any case, the lung is unable to expand and get enough oxygen necessary to fulfill the body's requirements.

A thoracotomy, the surgical creation of an opening into the chest cavity, is performed to diagnose or treat diseases or injury to the lungs or pleura. Conditions such as these require the placement of one or more chest tubes inserted into the pleural cavity. The chest tube is attached to a water-sealed drainage unit to remove any air or fluid from the pleural cavity. This is done to reestablish the correct intrapleural pressure and to allow the lungs to expand normally. A patient with a complete pneumothorax on the left is seen in Figure 10-15. The chest tube can be seen inserted into the pleural cavity to reexpand the lung capacity on the right side of the image.

A water-sealed drainage system is established by connecting the chest tube that originates in the pleural cavity to a clear tube that ends in a chamber containing sterile water or sterile normal **saline solution**. The tube leading from the chest tube remains below chest level at all times to maintain the seal. When the patient inhales, air and fluid from the intrapleural spaces are drawn into the drainage tube and emptied into a chamber prepared to receive them (chamber 1 in Fig . 10-16). Because

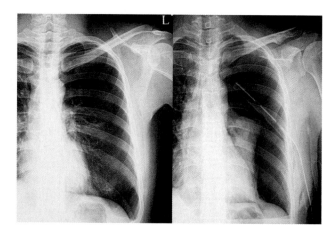

FIGURE 10-15 The image on the left shows a large pneumothorax of the left lung. The image on the right shows the chest tube that has been inserted into the pleural cavity to suck the air out so that the lung reexpands.

the fluid in the drainage chamber is heavier than air, it cannot be drawn back into the tube on inspiration nor can air from the atmosphere enter because of the water seal.

There are several variations of the water-sealed systems. There may be one, two, or three chambers. Additional chambers, also with water seals, are needed for drainage from the patient's pleural cavity and for suction regulation (chamber 3 in Fig. 10-16) if suction is also attached to the chest tube. If two chest tubes come from the pleural cavity, a Y connector joins the two tubes near the patient's body and continues to the water-sealed drainage apparatus. Several commercial water-sealed drainage systems are on the market; most are disposable.

The following items are important to remember when caring for a patient with a chest tube with water-sealed drainage:

1. Keep the tubing from the pleural cavity to the drainage chamber as straight as possible. If it is long, loosely coil it on the patient's bed, and do not allow it to fall below the level of the patient's chest.
2. All connections must be tightly taped to the tubing, and stoppers must fit tightly into receptacles.
3. A heavy sterile dressing and tape are kept at the patient's bedside so that if the tubing is accidentally dislodged from the pleural cavity, the dressing can be taped to the open area immediately.

4. Do not empty water-sealed chambers or raise them. The water seal must remain below the patient's chest at all times.
5. Do not clamp chest tubes.
6. If a water-seal chamber is continuously bubbling, notify the patient's nurse immediately, because this may indicate a leak in the system. There should be a steady rise and fall of the water as the patient breathes.
7. Immediately report to the patient's nurse rapid, shallow breathing, cyanosis, or a complaint from the patient of a feeling of pressure on their chest.
8. The drainage tube from the chest should be long enough to allow free patient movement. If the patient must be moved for images, do not allow tension to be placed on the chest tube or the patient to be positioned in a way that causes the tubing to be kinked or sealed off.

CALL OUT

Always ascertain whether the patient has a chest tube before moving and placing the image receptor (IR) behind the back, as these tubes are often hidden under blankets.

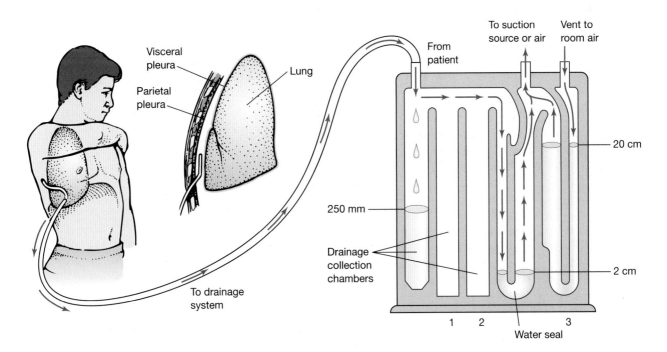

FIGURE 10-16 An example of a disposable chest drainage system.

VENOUS CATHETERS AND IMPLANTED DEVICES

Central venous catheters and implanted ports are being used more frequently for patients who must have long-term medication administration, frequent blood transfusion, hyperosmolar solutions, or total parenteral nutrition (TPN).

When a patient does not have an adequate nutritional intake and cannot tolerate nourishment by means of the GI tract, the physician may order partial or total nutrition to be given by an intravenous route. Partial parenteral nutrition is used when the patient is able to supply a part of the nutritional requirements by natural means. A large-gauge catheter is inserted into a large peripheral vein in the arm, and a parenteral solution containing a combination of lipid emulsion and amino acid/dextrose solution is administered as needed to satisfy the patient's nutritional needs. Vitamins and minerals are often added to these solutions.

When the patient requires total nutritional support by the parenteral method, it is delivered through a central vein. TPN solutions are hyperosmotic. This means that they are highly concentrated and would damage the intima of a peripheral vein; therefore, a large vein in the central venous system is used. Because fluid imbalance may result if TPN is administered too rapidly, administration is controlled by a pump or an infusion controller.

Central venous catheters are used for measuring the central venous pressure (CVP) as well as allowing nutrients and other fluid to be instilled into the patient. To obtain a true CVP measurement, the catheter must be correctly placed in the patient. The best location for a CVP line would be the brachiocephalic vein at the junction of the superior vena cava (SVC) or actually within the SVC itself. The location of the catheter must be confirmed either by a mobile chest radiographic image or by C-arm fluoroscopy imaging during the actual insertion of the catheter. The line should be seen just medial to the anterior border of the first rib on the image (Fig. 10-17A).

There are several types of central venous catheters. The tunneled type of catheter is inserted into the subclavian or internal jugular vein and then advanced into the SVC or the right atrium. The exit site is on the anterior chest. Most central venous catheters have more than one lumen and several access ports at the exit site (Fig. 10-17B).

The Hickman and Broviac catheters are two commonly used tunnel-type central venous catheters. Other commonly used central venous catheters are the peripherally inserted central catheter (PICC; Fig. 10-18) and the Groshong. The PICC may be inserted into the patient's arm and advanced until its tip lies in a central vein. Radiographers are often called on to operate the C-arm mobile fluoroscopy unit in the ICU or operating suite during the placement of one of these catheters.

Another alternative central venous catheter is an implanted port (also known as a port-a-cath). These are meant for patients who have long-term illnesses that require frequent intravenous medications or transfusions. The purpose of a port is to allow the physician to give

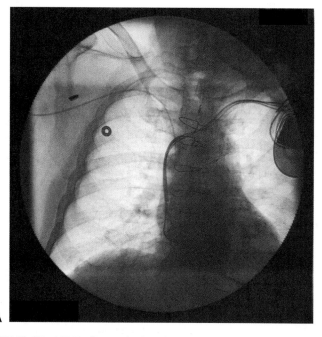
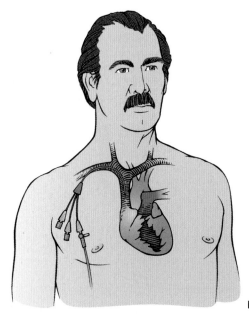

FIGURE 10-17 **(A)** Radiograph showing not only the central venous catheter in place on the patient's right side but also a pacemaker on the left side. The image is made in the negative mode. **(B)** Subclavian triple-lumen catheter for total parenteral nutrition and other adjunct therapy. The catheter is threaded through the subclavian vein and placed into the vena cava.

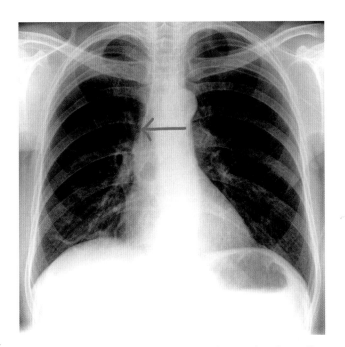

FIGURE 10-18 A peripherally inserted central catheter line can be seen at the blue arrow on this chest radiograph.

intravenous fluids, blood transfusions, chemotherapy, and other drugs. Blood samples can be taken through the port.

The port is made of plastic, titanium, or stainless steel. It is implanted into the subcutaneous tissue, usually in the chest under the clavicle, and sutured in place. The port is not visible but can be felt as a small, hard surface under the subcutaneous tissue. The radiographer should recognize this as a port and not apply pressure to this area. A catheter from the port is then inserted into the subclavian or internal jugular vein. A needle, called the Huber needle, is inserted to access the central vein through the port. A port can remain in the chest for years and does not require as much care as a PICC. This reduces the number of needlesticks that patients may need over the course of a prescribed treatment.

While caring for a patient with a central venous catheter or port in place, great care must be taken to prevent infection at the insertion site. If a dressing around the catheter must be removed, a physician's order to do so must be received first. Medical aseptic technique is used to remove the dressing. If the dressing is in the upper thoracic region, both the health care worker and the patient should wear a mask to prevent breathing on the area. The dressing must be removed carefully to avoid dislodging or moving the needle.

Implanted cardiac devices include both pacemakers and implantable cardioverter defibrillators (ICDs). A pacemaker is a device used to control an irregular heart rhythm. The flexible leads run from the pacer to the chambers of the heart to deliver electrical pulses. These pulses happen when the heart rate needs to be adjusted. There are newer pacemakers available that don't require leads. The ICD is placed just under the skin near the

clavicle and has leads that run through the SVC and into the chambers of the heart, very much like a pacemaker. ICDs keep track of the heart rate, and if an abnormal rhythm is detected, the device "shocks" the heart to restore it to a normal rhythm. The difference between the two devices is that the ICD can work like a pacemaker if the heart is beating too slowly. If the heart is beating too fast, it is a defibrillator to shock the heart, stopping the abnormal rhythm and restoring normal rhythm. The American Heart Association recommends that ICDs only be used after all other correctable measures have been taken and the arrhythmia is life-threatening. The chest radiographs seen in Figure 10-19A and B show two different patients. The lateral image (Fig. 10-19B) shows how anterior the pacemaker is within the chest.

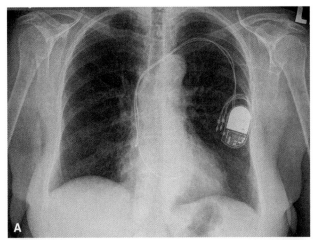

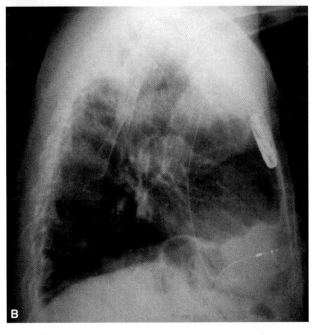

FIGURE 10-19 **(A)** Posteroanterior chest image shows placement of the cardiac pacemaker and the leads going into the chamber of the heart. **(B)** Lateral chest image of a different patient shows the anterior location of a cardiac pacemaker and the leads in the heart.

Display 10-1 provides a summary of the different tubes and catheters seen in radiographic images.

DISPLAY 10-1

Tubes and Catheters Displayed by Chest Radiography

1. Tracheotomy tube is a curved tube used to keep the opening free after tracheotomy to provide or protect an airway.
2. Swan-Ganz catheter is inserted into the subclavian vein, the internal or external jugular vein, or in a large peripheral vein to provide an accurate and convenient means of hemodynamic assessment, and to obtain blood pressure readings to introduce medications and intravenous fluids (Fig. 10-20).
3. CVP catheter is inserted into the subclavian, basilic, jugular, or femoral vein and advanced to the right atrium by way of the inferior vena cava or SVC, depending on the site of insertion to monitor the amount of blood returning to the heart.
4. Hickman catheter is inserted into the SVC and is used for monitoring, providing nutrition, administering medications, and drawing blood.
5. PICC is inserted into the subclavian vein to the SVC; it is commonly used for prolonged antibiotic therapy, nutrition, and to draw blood.
6. Temporary or permanent pacemakers are artificial devices that can trigger mechanical contractions of the heart by emitting periodic electrical discharges, which regulate the heart rate by assisting or taking over for the heart's natural pacemaker.
7. Chest tubes are large catheters placed in the pleural cavity to evacuate fluid and air; these are commonly inserted in the sixth intercostal space in the midaxillary line or posterior axillary line.

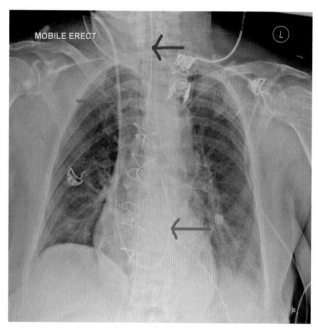

FIGURE 10-20 Chest image shows a Swan-Ganz line at the blue arrows and an endotracheal tube at the red arrow. In addition, heart monitor leads can be seen on the patient's chest.

TISSUE DRAINS

Tissue drains are placed at or near wound sites or operative sites when large amounts of drainage are expected. The use of these drains was a well-established practice for many years in both orthopedic and abdominal surgeries.

Although many surgeons continue to use these drains to decompress or drain either fluid or air from the area of surgery, there are other surgeons that are abandoning the use of these drains as they consider them unnecessary, particularly after an uncomplicated total joint arthroplasty. Research indicates that drains used after laparoscopic surgeries can increase wound infection rates, which delays discharge from the hospital.

Table 10-4 lists the drains that may be seen over the course of the radiographer's career. The student radiographer should be familiar with the different drains and take care not to put pressure on them or dislodge them while imaging the patient. Figures 10-21 through 10-24 are discussed within Table 10-4.

Other types of drains are placed into the hollow organs of the body and may be sutured in place and attached to a collection bag. Some of these are the T tube, which may be placed into the common bile duct; the cecostomy tube, which is placed in the cecum; and the nephrostomy tube, which is placed in the kidney.

All these drains must be identified during the assessment of the patient, and care must be taken to avoid any tension on these drains, which might dislodge them partially or completely. Infection control must also be a concern. The presence of a tissue drain indicates that the patient has an opening directly into the body where infection may be easily introduced. If radiographing the patient includes touching an area in which a drain is inserted, surgical aseptic technique must be used to prevent introduction of new microorganisms into the wound. Always wear gloves and perform a 30-second handwash when coming into contact with drainage from these areas.

TABLE 10-4	Tissue Drains and Their Use		
Name	**Use**	**Location**	**Figure**
Penrose	Soft rubber tube, looks like a tourniquet. Drainage is allowed to flow freely out of tube.	Superficial wounds or abscesses	10-22
Jackson-Pratt	Constant low pressure by means of a small bulb that acts as suction. Drainage goes into bulb, causing it to expand.	Abdominal surgery	10-23
Hemovac	Constant low pressure expands an accordion-style container as fluid is suctioned out.	Most often seen after hip replacement	10-24
ConstaVac, Stryker	Drainage and blood conservation system. Blood can be reinfused back into the body without disconnecting system.	Total joint replacement	10-25

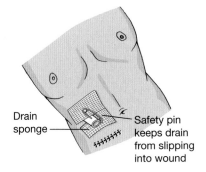

FIGURE 10-21 A Penrose tissue drain.

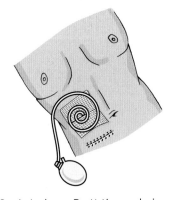

FIGURE 10-22 A Jackson-Pratt tissue drain.

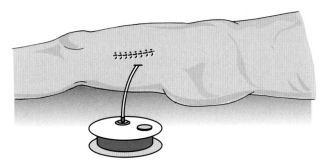

FIGURE 10-23 A Hemovac tissue drain.

URINARY DEVICES

Urinary tract infections (UTIs) are the most common nosocomial infections. A common cause of these infections is poor infection control practices by health care workers during placement of catheters in the urinary bladder or during care for patients who have indwelling catheters in place. Radiographers frequently work with patients who have urinary catheters in place.

Catheterization of the urinary bladder refers to the insertion of a plastic, silicone, or rubber tube through the urethral meatus into the urinary bladder. Catheters are inserted into the urinary bladder for a number of reasons: to keep the bladder empty while the surrounding tissues heal after surgical procedures; to drain, irrigate, or instill medication into the bladder; to assist the incontinent patient to control urinary flow; to begin bladder retraining; or to diagnose disease, malformation, or injury of the bladder.

Cystography, retrograde pyelography, and placement of ureteral stents all involve radiographic imaging. These procedures are performed frequently in the special procedures area of the radiographic imaging department or in the cystoscopy laboratory. As part of the health care team, radiographers actively participate in these diagnostic examinations and treatments because fluoroscopy and radiographic images are required while they are in progress.

Preparation for Catheterization

The urinary bladder is sterile; therefore, urinary catheterization requires sterile technique. Because the urinary bladder is easily infected, any object or solution that is inserted into it must be free of bacteria and their spores. Infection or injury may result when the technique used in the performance of the catheterization of the urinary bladder is poor or when caring for a patient.

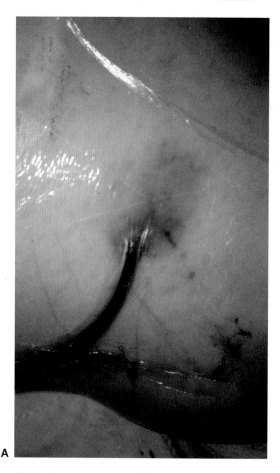

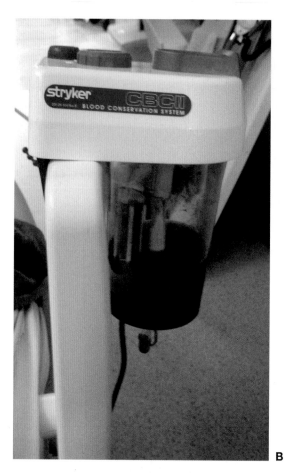

FIGURE 10-24 The ConstaVac (CBCII) is a drainage reservoir or a reinfusion system. **(A)** The drain comes from the patient's joint (in this case, a right knee). **(B)** The drainage reservoir hangs from the side rail of the bed, thereby making measurement reading easy.

Catheterization is not performed without a specific order from the physician in charge of the patient. Although there is probably a radiology nurse available in the imaging department to perform catheterization, or the patient may come from the floor with a catheter already in place, it is important for the technologist to understand the procedure in the event it becomes necessary to perform it.

When a physician requests catheterization of a patient, it must be established which type of catheter is to be used. Depending on the reason for the radiographic procedure, a straight catheter or an indwelling catheter (usually a Foley) is chosen. A straight catheter is used to obtain a specimen or to empty the bladder and is then removed. An indwelling catheter is inserted and left in place to allow for continuous drainage of urine. Most hospitals provide prepared sterile trays for catheterization with the desired type and size of catheter and the necessary equipment included. A tray set is chosen according to the type of catheter to be inserted.

A straight catheter is a single-lumen tube (Fig. 10-25). Indwelling catheters have a double lumen with an inflatable balloon at one end. One lumen is attached to a urinary bag to allow for continuous urinary drainage; the other

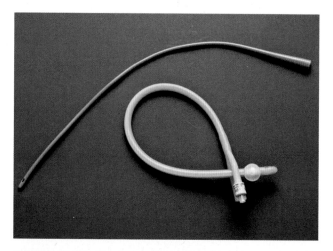

FIGURE 10-25 The top catheter is a single-lumen straight catheter that is not meant to stay in the patient except for the length of the procedure.

lumen is a passageway controlled by a valve that serves as a portal for instilling sterile water into the balloon. The balloon holds the catheter in place after it is inserted into the bladder (Fig. 10-26).

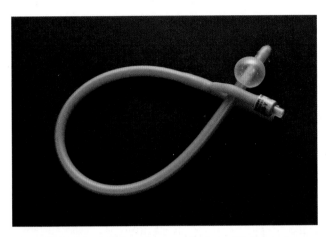

FIGURE 10-26 A Foley urinary catheter with the balloon cuff inflated.

CATHETER CARE IN THE DEPARTMENT

Often, patients must be transported to the diagnostic imaging department with indwelling catheters in place. If this is the case, the drainage bag must be kept below the level of the urinary bladder (Fig. 10-27). This maintains gravity flow and prevents contamination because of backflow of urine. If urine is allowed to flow back into the bladder or if drainage is obstructed, a UTI may result. The drainage tubing must be placed over the patient's leg and coiled on the gurney or tabletop, not below the level of the patient's hips. If the drainage bag is to be lifted above the patient during a move, the drainage tubing should be clamped to prevent backflow of urine into the bladder.

If the patient with an indwelling catheter is transported by wheelchair, attach the drainage bag to the underside of the wheelchair. The tubing must be coiled at the level of the patient's hips. Take care not to allow the tubing or drainage bag to become entangled in the wheels of the chair or to touch the floor. Never place a drainage bag on the patient's lap or abdomen during transport because this may cause a reflux of urine into the bladder.

Avoid disconnecting the catheter from its closed drainage system. Maintenance of a closed urinary drainage system is essential if infection is to be prevented. Once the closed drainage system has been invaded, it should not be reconnected. The patient must have a new catheter with new closed drainage system reinserted if catheter drainage of the bladder is to be continued. The technologist should never disconnect the catheter from the drainage system, nor should the technologist empty the drainage bag without a physician's request to do so. If this becomes necessary, a nurse should be consulted to determine whether urinary output is being monitored or whether the urine is being saved for laboratory testing purposes.

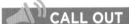
CALL OUT

The radiographer should never disconnect a catheter from the closed drainage system, nor should the drainage bag be emptied.

ALTERNATIVE METHODS OF URINARY DRAINAGE

There are two common methods of dealing with urinary drainage on a temporary or permanent basis, the suprapubic catheter (also called a cystocatheter) and the condom, or Texas, catheter. The *suprapubic catheter* (Fig. 10-28) is placed directly into the bladder by means of

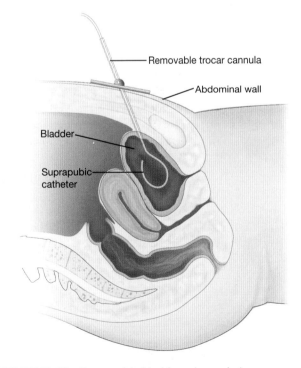

FIGURE 10-28 Suprapubic bladder urinary drainage system. (From Russel S. Management of patients with urinary disorders. In: *Brunner & Suddarth's Textbook of Medical-Surgical Nursing*. 15th ed. Wolters Kluwer; 2022, with permission.)

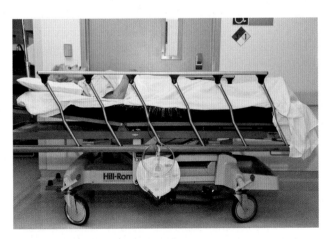

FIGURE 10-27 The urinary drainage bag from an indwelling catheter must be placed below the level of the urinary bladder when transporting a patient.

an abdominal incision. This method is sometimes chosen to divert the flow of urine from the urethral route after gynecologic surgery, urethral injuries, or prostatic obstructions or for chronic incontinence or loss of bladder control. Suprapubic catheters are believed to reduce the risk of infection as a long-term method of bladder drainage and to facilitate normal urination after surgical procedures. The catheter is attached to a closed urinary drainage system and is secured with sutures, tape, or a body seal system.

When caring for the patient with a suprapubic catheter, the radiographer must be careful not to put any tension on the catheter. The same rules of asepsis as for patients with other closed urinary drainage system, such as keeping the bag below the patient's bladder level at all times, must be followed.

The *condom catheter* is an externally applied drainage device used for male patients who are susceptible to UTIs or are incontinent or comatose and whose bladder continues to empty spontaneously (Fig. 10-29). If the patient is not prone to UTIs, a Foley indwelling catheter is most likely to be used.

The condom catheter is a soft rubber sheath that is placed over the penis and secured with a special type of adhesive material. The distal end of the condom has an

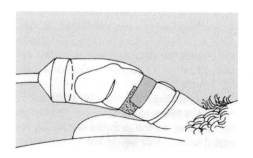

FIGURE 10-29 A condom catheter.

opening that fits onto a drainage tube and terminates in a drainage bag that attaches to the patient's thigh. The drainage bag can be emptied easily when necessary.

The condom catheter is changed every 24 to 48 hours. This helps to reduce the possibility of acquiring a UTI. This is not usually a task that the technologist needs to perform unless the catheter must be removed for an examination. When caring for patients who have condom catheters in place, the technologist must guard against dislodging the catheter from the drainage tube or twisting the condom and causing pain or skin irritation.

 ## Cultural Considerations

Cultural differences are an important aspect in radiography that must be considered at all times by the radiographer. Treating the patient with the respect and dignity that is due them as a human being is accomplished by understanding the beliefs and traditions of their culture. Because of the very nature of the procedures of catheterization of the urinary bladder, culture is an extremely important consideration that needs to be taken into account when assessing the patient for understanding and cooperation. The age of

the patient plays a critical role in females from other cultures. Younger women may be more accepting of the procedure than the elderly. Religious beliefs may dictate what is acceptable in the performance of catheterization, and it is the technologist who must help the patient and the family, if necessary, understand the importance of the procedure in order to perform the diagnostic test. Every catheterization is different, and the technologists must be extremely professional and understanding of the patient's beliefs and fears.

Retrograde Pyelography

Retrograde pyelography is a radiographic technique performed to visualize the proximal ureters and the kidneys after injection of an iodinated contrast medium (Fig. 10-30). This procedure is usually performed in a cystoscopy suite, routinely located in the surgery area under the direction of a urologist. The technologist must be present to take the necessary images and to provide fluoroscopic images of the patient as ordered. Retrograde pyelography is performed to assess the ureters for obstruction resulting from strictures, tumors, stones, scarring, or other pathologic processes when other methods are contraindicated. Because this procedure is a filling of the renal collecting system through a catheter, renal function is not studied.

A contrast medium is injected through a catheter inserted into the ureter (ureteral catheter) from the

bladder by means of a cystoscope. Retrograde pyelography is normally performed on one side. However, it is possible that both the kidneys must be studied. When this is the case, each side is catheterized and examined independently of the other. Images are taken to demonstrate the proximal ureters and the structure of the renal pelvis. The catheter is withdrawn, and more contrast agent is injected to visualize the remaining portion of the ureter. The procedure takes approximately 1 hour.

Ureteral Stents

If the patient has an obstructed ureter because of a stricture, edema, or an advanced malignant tumor, a stent may be inserted into the ureter on a temporary or permanent basis to relieve the problem (Fig. 10-31). Stents are made of soft, pliable silicone and may be placed surgically or during a retrograde pyelogram.

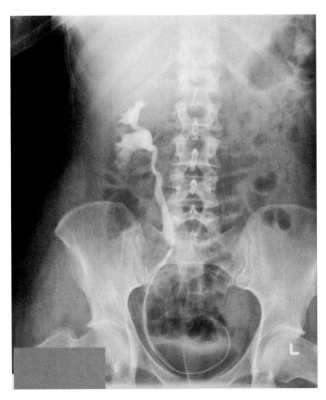

FIGURE 10-30 A retrograde pyelogram. The catheter can be seen coiled in the bladder then extending into the right ureter.

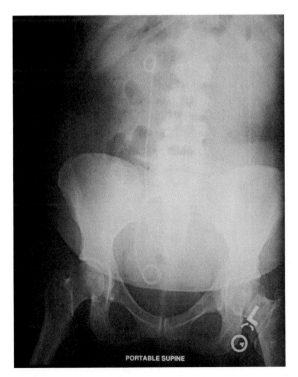

PORTABLE SUPINE

FIGURE 10-31 Ureteral stent. Although the image is light because of the patient's size, the double pigtail on the patient's right can be seen in the renal pelvis, and the distal curled end of the stent is in the bladder.

There are complications associated with the presence of any foreign body in the ureter, including stents. Complications are infection and obstruction from encrustation and clot formation. The technologist is responsible for the imaging aspects of this procedure, and patient care and instruction are the responsibility of the physician and the nurse. The patient usually receives a general anesthetic for this procedure and is allowed to recover in the recovery suite.

OSTOMIES

Several conditions of the lower GI tract require the creation of a stoma through which the contents of the bowel can be eliminated. A stoma is created by bringing a loop of bowel to the skin surface of the abdomen. Some diseases that are treated in this manner are cancer, diverticulitis, and ulcerative colitis. Traumatic injuries of the bowel may also require this type of treatment.

The surgical procedure to repair the bowel and create the ostomy is named by the area of bowel on which the operation is done. For instance, if the opening is from the colon, it is called a colostomy; if it is from the ileum, it is known as an ileostomy (Fig. 10-32). The stoma may be temporary, performed to rest and heal a diseased portion of the bowel, or it may be permanent, done to remove a diseased or traumatized portion of the bowel.

The stoma may have either one or two openings, depending on the type of surgery that was performed. When two openings are surgically created, one opening is located toward the rectum and the other toward the small bowel. One opening, called the proximal stoma, emits fecal material. The other opening, the distal stoma, is relatively nonfunctioning and emits only mucus. Some stoma patients (also called ostomy patients) have had their rectum and lower bowel removed, whereas others have not. A patient who has an ostomy may require barium studies for further diagnosis or further study of the progression of the disease.

Ostomy causes a major change in a patient's body image, and many persons with a new colostomy or ileostomy stoma are going through a grieving process. This is particularly true of younger patients. They may be angry, depressed, in a stage of denial, or just beginning to accept the fact that they must learn to live with this physical change.

Caring for the patient with a new ostomy requires sensitivity and a matter-of-fact attitude. It is suggested that the radiography student who has never seen an ostomy should observe the diagnostic studies being performed for these patients until care for them easily be provided.

The ostomy patient will have a dressing or drainage pouch in place over the area of the stoma (Fig. 10-33). The dressing is removed while wearing clean gloves. Remove the drainage pouch and put it aside in a safe place

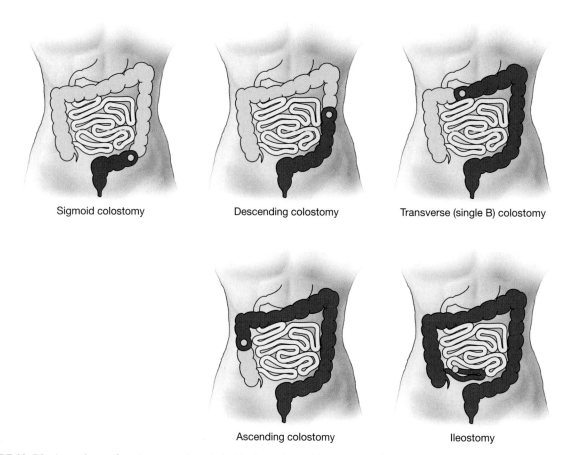

Sigmoid colostomy   Descending colostomy   Transverse (single B) colostomy

Ascending colostomy   Ileostomy

FIGURE 10-32 Locations of various openings into the large bowel known as colostomies or ileostomy.

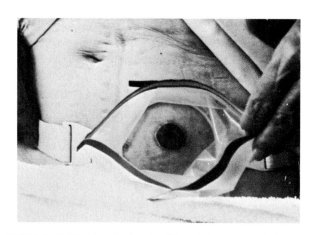

FIGURE 10-33 A colostomy with a drainage pouch in place.

to be reused. The patient may want to do this procedure without assistance. The pouch must be kept dry in order for it to be reused.

A patient who has a colostomy or ileostomy and is going to have a barium study of the lower GI tract needs special instructions to be adequately prepared. The radiologist and the patient's physician should give the instruction before and after the procedure. All ostomy

patients should be instructed to bring an extra pouch with them if they are coming from outside the hospital.

Administering a Barium Enema to an Ostomy Patient

Ostomy patients have barium studies for diagnostic purposes, and the procedure is somewhat different from that performed on a person with normally functioning bowels. The radiographer must plan the procedure with the radiologist before beginning in order to ensure the patient's comfort and safety. A cone-shaped tip with a long drainage bag that attaches to it after the procedure is frequently the instillation instrument of choice (Fig. 10-34A and B). Occasionally, a small catheter with an inflatable cuff is used. Other ostomy tips may be used, depending on the patient's situation and the preference of the physician. Examples are the nipple tip and the double-barrel tip. The patient who has had the ostomy for some time may prefer to insert the tip without assistance from the radiographer.

Never place a stoma patient in the prone position because this may cause damage to the patient's ostomy site.

When the examination is complete, attach the drainage bag to the cone and drain the barium into it. When

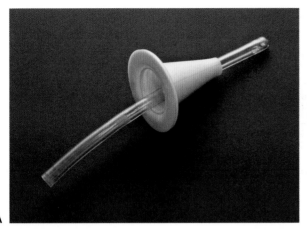
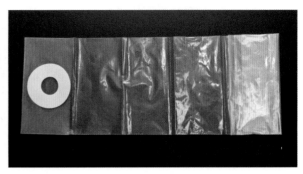

FIGURE 10-34 **(A)** Cone tip used for colostomy patients undergoing a lower gastrointestinal (GI) procedure. **(B)** Drainage bag used for emptying out barium from a stoma after a lower GI procedure.

the drainage is complete, the patient whose physical condition permits may be taken to the lavatory with the drainage bag still in place; there the drainage bag may be cleaned and the ostomy pouch replaced. Give the patient as much assistance as needed and offer towels, washcloths, and any other articles that may be needed. Allow the patient privacy to provide for independent care of the area.

Summary

1. NG tubes are inserted into the stomach, whereas nasointestinal (NE) tubes are allowed to travel into the small intestine.
   a. They are used for gastric decompression, diagnosis of diseases of the GI tract, treatment of diseases of the GI tract, and feeding persons who are unable to swallow food in the normal manner.
   b. The patient should be moved carefully so that the tubes are not dislodged.
   c. It may be necessary to reconnect the patient to suction if they are in the department for a long period of time.
2. Gastrostomy tubes are surgically inserted directly into the stomach.
   a. These tubes provide nourishment to a person unable to take food or fluids by mouth.
   b. When caring for a patient with a gastrostomy tube in place, take precautions not to dislodge the tube or to introduce infection at the insertion site.
3. ET tubes are inserted into the trachea through the mouth when a patient is unable to breathe on their own.
   a. The position is often verified with a chest radiograph.
   b. Patients will be attached to a mechanical ventilator.
4. Radiographers do not perform suction; however, they are responsible for having equipment prepared and for assisting with the procedure.

   a. Audible rattling or gurgling is a sign of needing suction.
   b. Suction equipment is disposable.
5. Tracheostomies are openings into the trachea to relieve respiratory distress.
   a. They may be permanent or temporary.
   b. Patients are not able to speak.
   c. Do not put pressure or pull on the tube attaching the tracheostomy to the ventilator.
6. Mechanical ventilators are used to support respiratory function.
   a. Never disconnect the ventilator from its power source.
   b. Obtain adequate assistance to prevent dislodging of the tubing connected to the tracheostomy.
7. Chest tubes may be connected to water-sealed drainage systems.
   a. It is used to remove fluid or air from the pleural space.
   b. Keep the tubing coiled at the patient's chest level.
   c. Keep all connections tightly sealed to maintain the water seal.
   d. Do not lift the water-sealed bottle higher than the patient's chest level.
   e. Do not clamp or kink the drainage tube.
8. Venous catheters may be kept in place for long periods of time.
   a. They are used for nutrition or chemotherapy.
   b. Care must be taken not to pull or push on these catheters in any way.

c. Radiographers must learn the different types of tubes and their location in order to provide quality radiographic images when verifying the locations of these lines.

9. Tissue drains are used to remove fluid from an operative site.

   a. They are not as common as they once were.

   b. Do not allow tension to be placed on the drain that might dislodge it.

10. Urinary catheters such as a Foley or suprapubic catheter drain the urinary bladder when a patient is unable to void naturally.

    a. When transporting patients with a urinary catheter in place, do not lift it above the level of the patient's bladder.

    b. UTIs are possible if urine is allowed to flow back into the bladder from the drainage bag.

    c. Be careful that the tubing is not clamped off, which would stop the flow of the urine.

11. Ostomies are openings into the large bowel (stomas).

    a. Location of the opening determines the name of the ostomy.

    b. It is performed in cases of cancer, colitis, or diverticulitis.

    c. Lower GI imaging is done through the opening with a cone tip.

CASE STUDY

You are working the evening shift at the community hospital. It has been a rather quiet evening until you get a call for a STAT mobile chest radiograph in the ICU. You gather the IR cover, the IR, two aprons, and the mobile unit and head off to the ICU. When you enter the unit, you see that the room you are about to enter is quite busy with nursing personnel. You review the radiology request and realize that the patient is a friend who has been having heart problems off and on over the past several years. You also know this patient has a pacemaker and a port-a-cath implanted on the opposite side as the pacemaker. She has just been intubated and attached to a ventilator. She appears to be unconscious. As the room clears of nursing staff, the physician asks you to take a chest image to show all the lines and tubes.

ISSUES TO CONSIDER

1. What must you assess as you get ready to take your image?

2. Knowing what has just been done and what the patient already had in place, what is your main concern to image?

CHAPTER 10 REVIEW QUESTIONS

1. What should the radiographer do while caring for a patient who has an NG tube in place? (Circle all that apply)

   a. Find out if the tube is to be reconnected to suction and, if so, what is the amount of pressure.

   b. Take care not to dislodge the tube.

   c. Remove the tube before the patient leaves the department.

   d. Wrap the end of the tube with gauze while it is not connected to suction.

2. In what position should an alert patient whose swallowing reflex is intact be placed in preparation for suctioning?

   a. Prone

   b. Sims

   c. Semi-Fowler

   d. Lateral

3. What are two points to remember when caring for patients with a new tracheostomy in place?

   a. They may be talkative and may need to be suctioned.

   b. They are anxious and unable to speak.

   c. They are in the stage of denial and will express anger.

   d. They are unconscious and will be accompanied by a nurse.

4. When caring for a patient who has a chest tube with water-sealed drainage, what must be remembered? (Circle all that apply)

   a. The water seal must be maintained at all times.

b. Continuous bubbling into the water-sealed chamber is an indication that all is well.

c. The tubing may be clamped if necessary.

d. Most patients with chest tubes complain of respiratory distress.

e. Never lift the drainage system above the patient's chest.

5. Signs and symptoms that indicate a patient needs to be suctioned are: (Circle all that apply)

a. Audible rattling and gurgling sounds from the patient's throat

b. Gagging

c. Signs of respiratory distress

d. Profuse vomiting in a patient who cannot voluntarily change positions

6. When caring for a patient who has a tissue drain in place, the following precautions must be taken:

a. Disregard these drains because they are not the technologist's concern.

b. Prevent tension on the drain and use surgical aseptic technique if in direct contact with the drain.

c. Measure intake and output from the drain.

d. Remove the drain because it impedes the success of the radiograph.

7. List two types of NG tubes commonly seen in the imaging department.

8. Name three types of tissue drains.

9. List the precautions taken when imaging a patient who has a central venous catheter in place.

10. Describe why a chest radiographic image is taken when a patient has been intubated.

11. If the patient has the large bowel removed at the sigmoid area and the opening is made on the anterior surface of the abdomen, the patient is said to have a(n):

a. Colostomy

b. Ileostomy

c. Sigmoidostomy

d. Colonostomy

Infection Control

OBJECTIVES

After studying this chapter, the student will be able to:

1. Define terminology related to infection control.

2. Describe Standard Precautions and isolation procedures to include their importance and purpose.

3. Explain the mode of transmission of infection and diseases.

4. List the regulatory agencies that set and maintain the guidelines for safety in health care and the community at large.

5. Demonstrate the various sterile procedures and maintain the sterile process.

KEY TERMS

Antibiotics: Soluble substances derived from a mold or bacterium that kills or inhibits growth of other microorganisms

Antifungal: Kills or inhibits fungi or their growth or reproduction

Antimicrobial drugs: Drugs that tend to destroy microbes or prevent their multiplication

Aseptic technique: Use of methods that totally exclude microorganisms as one works

Bacteria: Colorless, minute, one-celled organisms with a typical nucleus

Bloodborne Pathogens Standards: A set of regulations complied by the Occupational Safety and Health Administration (OSHA) that requires employers to provide infection control to all health care workers

Broad-spectrum antimicrobial drug: A drug effective against a wide variety of microorganisms

Carrier: A person or an animal that harbors a particular infectious agent and does not have clinical disease but is able to transmit the disease to others

Chemical sterilization: Low-temperature sterilization

Contamination: The presence of an infectious agent on a body surface or on inanimate objects

Disinfectant: A chemical capable of destroying microorganisms or inhibiting their growth; same as antiseptic

Disinfection: The destruction of pathogenic microbes, toxins, vectors, and other pathogens by use of chemical agents or by physical means; that is, scrubbing

Fenestrated drape: A drape with one or more openings

Fomites: Objects, such as used dressings, used needles, or other objects that have been contaminated by an infected person

Fungi: Cells that require an oxygenated environment to live; may be either yeasts or molds

Genetic predisposition: Inherited potential through the genetic transmission for a particular illness or characteristic

Immune: Free from acquiring a particular infectious disease

Immunosuppressed persons: Persons whose immunity is prohibited for physiologic reasons

Infectious disease: A disease capable of being passed from one person to another

Medical asepsis: Microorganisms have been removed through the use of soap, water, friction, and various chemical disinfectants

Nucleoid: A part of a nucleolus (a nuclear inclusion body)

Parasite: An organism that lives in or on another and draws its nourishment from that on which it lives

Pathogenicity: The ability to cause disease

Personal protective equipment (PPE): A variety of barriers used alone or in combination to protect mucous membranes, skin, and clothing from contact with infectious agents

Prion: An infectious particle of non-nucleic acid composition; must mutate to become infectious

Pseudomembranous colitis: (SYN pseudomembranous enterocolitis) formation and passage of pseudomembranous material due to infection by *Clostridium difficile*

Retention urinary catheters: Tubes that are placed in the urinary bladder and fixed in place for a period of time

Sepsis: The presence of pus-forming and other pathogenic organisms

Skin prep: The removal of as many microorganisms as possible by mechanical and chemical means to reduce the chances of infection

Standard Precaution: A group of infection prevention practices that apply to all patients, regardless of suspected or confirmed diagnosis

Sterile: Free of all living microorganisms

Sterilization: Destruction of microbes by steam under pressure or other means, both chemical and physical

Surgical asepsis: Complete removal of microorganisms and their spores from the surface of an object

Transmission-Based Precautions: The second tier of basic infection control precautions that are used in addition to Standard Precautions to prevent the spread of certain types of infectious agents

Universal Precautions: A set of infection control guidelines published in the 1980s by the Centers for Disease Control and Prevention (CDC). They have been replaced by the Standard Precautions.

Vascular access devices: Catheters or needles that are able to enter the blood vessels

Virulent: Extremely toxic Virulence refers to the causative organism's ability to grow and multiply with speed.

Viruses: Minute microbes that cannot be visualized under an ordinary microscope; the smallest microorganism known to produce disease

INTRODUCTION

All health care workers must be vigilant in the practice of infection control to protect themselves and others from acquiring **infectious diseases**. The practice of infection control measures is a necessity for all who are working in, being treated in, or visiting health care settings.

Radiographers must understand the methods of isolating body substances (called **Standard Precautions**) and be able to correctly perform all Transmission-Based Precautions as they work with patients. Correct cleaning of equipment, correct hand hygiene, and correct disposal of contaminated waste must be part of every procedure in imaging to guard against the spread of infection.

INFECTIOUS PATHOGENS

A pathogen is a microorganism that can cause a disease in a host. Another name for a pathogen is an infectious agent because they cause infections. When a person is healthy, the body is usually able to defend against pathogens and the diseases they cause. However, individuals can be susceptible to diseases caused by different types of pathogens depending on the type and how they are transmitted.

Types

Infectious diseases are caused by pathogenic microorganisms, or pathogens. Microorganisms known to produce diseases are **bacteria**, **fungi**, **viruses**, and **prions**. There are also believed to be unidentified pathogens that produce newly recognized disease. Within the known groups of microorganisms, many different species may produce infections in humans, and many are useful or, at least, not harmful. Microorganisms are used in a variety of ways including as a means of effecting a positive change in the environment.

Bacteria

Bacteria are colorless, minute, one-celled organisms with a typical nucleus. They contain both DNA and RNA. DNA carries the inherited characteristics of a cell, and RNA constructs cell protein in response to the direction of DNA.

Bacteria may be spherical in shape (*cocci*), oblong (*bacilli*), comma shaped (*vibrio*), spiral (*spirilla*), or tightly coiled (*spirochetes*). A small number of bacteria are cuboidal in shape. They may also be classified according to their divisional grouping as diplococcic (groups of two), streptococci (chains), or staphylococci (grapelike bunches; Fig. 11-1). Bacteria must be stained to be seen under a microscope and are classified according to their reaction to various staining processes in the laboratory.

Gram-positive bacteria are able to form a highly resistant structure called an *endospore*. This endospore encases the genetic material in the cell and allows the bacteria to survive for many years in most unfavorable conditions. When conditions for survival are again favorable, the endospore germinates and the bacterial cell grows again and replicates. Endospores are more difficult to destroy than are vegetating bacteria; therefore, many methods of destroying pathogenic bacteria do not affect endospores.

There are bacteria that survive only in an oxygen environment and are called *aerobes*. Others are unable to live in the presence of oxygen and are called *anaerobes*. Many bacteria are opportunists and learn to adapt or thrive in any environment. They may also learn to live in the presence of antimicrobial drugs or disinfectants.

Some diseases caused by bacteria include tuberculosis (TB), streptococcal infections of the throat, staphylococcal infections in many parts of the body, *Salmonella* poisoning, gonorrhea, syphilis, and tetanus.

Fungi

Fungi require an aerobic environment to live and reproduce. Fungi include yeasts and molds that can be harmful and cause a number of infectious diseases. However, molds

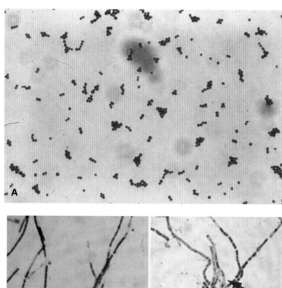
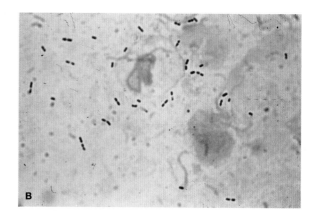
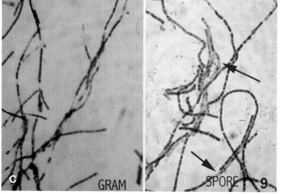

FIGURE 11-1 Forms of bacteria. **(A)** *Staphylococcus aureus*; **(B)** *Streptococcus pneumoniae*; **(C)** *Bacillus anthracis*. (From Winn W Jr, Allen S, Janda W, et al. *Doneman's Color Atlas and Textbook of Diagnostic Microbiology*. 6th ed. Lippincott Williams & Wilkins; 2006.)

are often extremely useful. They are a primary source of material for the production of antibiotic drugs; they produce enzymes for medical use and are used in the production of foods to flavor various cheeses. Yeasts are used commercially to produce beer and wine and to leaven bread. They are also a source of vitamins and minerals; however, some yeasts are pathogens that produce diseases in humans and animals. A commonly seen disease caused by yeast infection is thrush (caused by *Candida albicans*).

Viruses

Viruses are minute microorganisms that cannot be visualized under an ordinary microscope. They are the smallest microorganisms known to produce disease in humans. The genetic material of a virus is either DNA or RNA, but never both. A *virion* is a complete infectious particle with a central **nucleoid**. The genetic material is protected by a capsid or protein coat that is composed of minute protein units called *capsomeres*. The complete nucleocapsid with a nucleic acid core constitutes a complete virus. Some viruses are surrounded by an envelope that is composed of a lipoprotein. Viruses must invade a host cell to survive and reproduce.

Whatever its structure, the virus is transported by way of its capsid to a host cell that has receptor sites on its surface that are suitable to a particular virus that it invades. A virus does not invade a cell at will. It must attach itself at a membrane receptor site for which it has a specificity; that is, specific for that particular type of host cell and no others.

To reproduce, the virus uses the genetic machinery of the host cell. When reproduction is complete, new viruses

leave the original host cell. As some types of viruses leave the host cell, they destroy the cell by the rapid release of new viruses. This is called *lysis*. The second type of viral replication produces viruses that lie dormant, but very much alive and destructive, within the host cell.

Some viruses have the capacity to invade nerve ganglia and leave their genetic material in the ganglia in a latent phase after an acute infective period. The virus remains there until the body is under some type of stress such as an emotional life event or illness or until it is exposed to sunlight for a period of time. This will often induce the virus to take over nearby cells and produce more viruses, as in the case of herpes simplex (fever blisters) or herpes zoster (shingles). Such viral infections may occur repeatedly.

A virus may be classified on the basis of its genetic composition; the shape or size of the capsid; the number of capsomeres or the absence of an envelope; the host it infects; the type of disease it produces; or its target cell and **immune** properties.

Viruses are capable of infecting plants, animals, and humans. Some common viral diseases that affect humans are influenza, the common cold; mumps; measles; HIV (AIDS); and hepatitis A, B, C, D, and E.

Prions

Prion proteins exist in all mammals and are abundant in brain cells. When they fold in a particular manner, the malformed prion proteins proceed to convert normal proteins to become infectious disease. A mutant prion may be present by **genetic predisposition** or may be the result of infection. Acquiring an infectious prion is the result of transmission from an infected animal or person. Because the misfolded prion proteins destroy brain cells, the prion diseases cause dementia.

Growth Requirements for Microorganisms

Microorganisms have the ability to grow and form a population. For this to be accomplished, there must be a supply of water, oxygen, nitrogen, and phosphorous. Elements such as iron, copper, and zinc are used for the synthesis of enzymes. Certain bacteria cannot grow without the presence of vitamins! Temperature of the environment is important. There is a minimum and a maximum temperature for each type of microorganism that will allow the best growth to occur. Osmotic pressure and the pH of a solution in which the microorganism is residing are important for growth. For example, neutrophilic bacteria grow well in the body because of the pH of 7.0. However, acidophilic bacteria would not be able to thrive in the body because it requires a pH of 6.0 or lower.

Hospital-Acquired Infections

Despite increasing use of infection control measures and the control or elimination of many diseases, infections in patients while they are receiving health care have increased. This is the result of the increase in organisms becoming resistant to anti-infective drugs. Anti-infective drugs include **antimicrobial**, **antibiotic**, and **antifungal drugs**. Infections acquired in the course of medical care are called *nosocomial infections*. This term is most often applied to infections contracted in an acute care hospital; however, it also applies to infections patients receive while in extended care facilities, outpatient clinics, and behavioral health institutions. Infections contracted at birth by infants of infected mothers are also classified as nosocomial. A nosocomial infection that results from a particular treatment or therapeutic procedure is called an *iatrogenic infection*. Although a patient acquires a particular infection while in a health care unit, symptoms of the illness may not develop until leaving the health care environment. This is still considered to be a nosocomial infection. A person who enters a health care facility with an infection is said to have a *community-acquired infection*.

Everyone has microorganisms in their body at all times. These microorganisms are called *normal flora*. Infections that are caused by microorganisms that are not normal flora are called *exogenous* infections. When a person acquires an infection in the health care setting as a result of an overgrowth of normal flora, it is called an *endogenous* nosocomial infection.

Endogenous infections are often the result of the alteration in the number of normal flora present in the body or the alteration in placement of normal flora into another body cavity. Endogenous infections may also be the result of treatment with a **broad-spectrum antimicrobial drug** that alters the number of normal flora. Many factors in health care facilities, as listed in Display 11-1, encourage nosocomial infections.

Individuals who present themselves for health care come from many social and economic environments. A variety of factors in the social and economic environment may render a person more susceptible to acquiring a nosocomial infection, as Display 11-2 shows.

DISPLAY 11-1

Factors That Encourage Nosocomial Infections

Factor	Reasons for Increased Incidence
Environment	Air contaminated with infectious agents; other patients who have infectious diseases; visitors; contaminated food; contaminated instruments; hospital personnel
Therapeutic regimen	Immunosuppressive and cytotoxic drugs used to treat malignant or chronic diseases, which decrease the patient's resistance to infection; antimicrobial therapy, which may alter the normal flora of the body and encourage growth of resistant strains of microbes sometimes called hospital bacteria
Equipment	Instruments such as catheters, intravenous tubing, cannulas, respiratory therapy equipment, and gastrointestinal tubes that have not been adequately cleaned and sterilized
Contamination during medical procedures	Microbes transmitted during dressing changes, catheter insertion, or any invasive procedure may introduce infective organisms if correct technique is not used.

DISPLAY 11-2

Factors That Increase the Potential for Nosocomial Infection

Factor	Reasons for Susceptibility
Age	The very young have immature immune systems and are more susceptible to nosocomial infections. Also, as one ages, the immune system becomes less efficient and organ function declines, making infections more difficult to resist.
Heredity	Congenital and genetic factors passed on from birth make individuals more or less resistant to disease.
Nutritional status	Inadequate nutritional intake, obesity, or malnourishment as a result of illness renders one increasingly susceptible to nosocomial infections.
Stress	Work-related or other stress factors increase the potential for infection as levels of cortisone in the body increase related to constant tension.
Inadequate rest and exercise	Efficient elimination and circulation decline as a result of inadequate rest or exercise.
Personal habits	Smoking, excessive use of drugs and alcohol, and/or dangerous sexual practices contribute to lowering the body's defenses against nosocomial infections.
Health history	Persons with a history of poor health such as diabetes, heart disease, or chronic lung disease, or children who have not been immunized against diseases of childhood are at increased risk for acquiring a nosocomial infection.
Inadequate defenses	Broken skin; burns or trauma; or immunocompromised persons related to a medical regimen are at increased risk for acquiring a nosocomial infection.

The bloodstream and the urinary tract are common sites of nosocomial infections. These are often the result of long-term use of **vascular access devices** (VADs) and **retention urinary catheters**. Infections in wounds following surgical procedures and respiratory tract infections also occur frequently. Early removal of urinary catheters, intravenous catheters, and other types of invasive treatment devices is recommended whenever possible to reduce the incidents of nosocomial infections. Meticulous care of VADs and retention catheters while they are inserted is of great importance.

Communicable Diseases

Communicable diseases are ones that are spread from one person to another through a variety of ways that include contact with blood and body fluids, airborne viruses that were breathed in, or even insect bites. Preventing and controlling the spread of disease is much of what public health is about. From the coronavirus (COVID-19) and its variants to the flu, malaria and Ebola, outbreaks of infectious diseases have an extraordinary impact on human health. Childhood diseases such as chickenpox, mumps, and measles are very contagious and are easily passed from child to child, partly because of children not understanding proper hand hygiene or covering their mouths when they sneeze or cough. Every fall season, influenza becomes an issue for many people; however, with the precautions taken with COVID-19, there has been a recent drop in the number of cases of the flu being reported.

The World Health Organization (WHO) has been continuing to support countries with infection control measures and to ship and vaccinate nearly 11,000 high-risk individuals. Vaccination is the key to controlling and even ending certain infections. Polio was a communicable disease that was eradicated in the United States because of a vaccine. However, poliovirus continues to affect children and adults in parts of Asia and Africa. The last case of naturally occurring polio was in 1979.

Multidrug-Resistant Organisms

Multidrug-resistant organisms (MDROs) are microorganisms that are resistant to more than one antibiotic. This means that certain treatments will not work or may be less effective. These organisms are found mainly in hospitals and long-term care facilities and often affect people who are older or very ill, causing infections that are hard to treat.

Each year there are new microbes that become resistant to treatment with antibiotics. They are as follows:

1. **Methicillin-resistant *Staphylococcus aureus* (MRSA):** Shortly after penicillin was used to treat *S. aureus*, it became resistant to it. The newer semisynthetic penicillin (methicillin) was used successfully for a time to treat these infections, but the war against *S. aureus* is being lost because it becomes resistant to this drug.

   Some diseases produced by MRSA are decubitus ulcers, pneumonia, endocarditis, bacteremia, osteomyelitis, and septic thrombophlebitis. MRSA is transmitted by direct contact or contact with infected objects or surfaces.

2. **Vancomycin-resistant *S. aureus* (VRSA):** Vancomycin was used successfully for a time to treat MRSA; however, it is feared that *S. aureus* becomes resistant to this drug.

3. **Vancomycin-resistant *Enterococcus* (VRE):** *Enterococcus* is a part of the normal flora in the gastrointestinal tract; however, it is capable of causing disease when it affects blood, urine, or wounds. It is able to reproduce in large numbers in areas of the body thought to be protected by normal body fluids and enzymes and has become resistant to many antibiotics. VRE is thought to be the second most causative microbe for nosocomial infections.

4. **Bacteremia and fungemia:** Bacteremia is the result of bacteria in the bloodstream. Fungemia is the result of fungi in the bloodstream. Both are usually the result of microbes entering the blood by way of VAD. Most persons admitted to the hospital at present receive some type of VAD during their stay.

5. ***C. difficile:*** Most hospitalized patients receive antibiotics that may predispose them to infection with *C. difficile* by disrupting the normal flora of the intestinal tract. This organism is emerging as a frequent cause of nosocomial infections. *C. difficile* is a spore-forming bacterium that releases toxins into the bowel that are resistant to disinfectants and so can be easily spread from the hands of health care providers. The disease process resulting from *C. difficile* is a **pseudomembranous colitis** and can produce profound **sepsis**.

6. **Extended-spectrum beta-lactamase (ESBL):** An ever-increasing threat to treatment by antibiotic therapy is beta-lactamase infections. Beta-Lactamase is a type of enzyme produced by some bacteria that is responsible for their resistance to beta-lactam antibiotics such as penicillin, cephalosporins, cephamycin, and carbapenems. *Escherichia coli* and many gram-negative bacteria are resistant to treatment by most antibiotics that are the result of ESBLs.

CENTERS FOR DISEASE CONTROL AND PREVENTION

There are international, federal, state, and local agencies that control safe practices for the general public and for all accredited health care institutions, including the various extended care facilities. As health care in the United States changes, more emphasis is being placed on transferring patients from acute care institutions to extended care facilities and into their own homes for care as soon as it is safe to do so. This increases the burden of overseeing the safety of both the patient and the health care worker. Institutions now being overseen by some or all of the regulatory agencies are acute care hospitals, skilled and intermediate care nursing facilities, inpatient rehabilitation centers, inpatient chemical dependency centers, inpatient behavioral health hospitals, and home health care agencies. Display 11-3 lists the agencies that control institutional, patient, and workplace safety in the United States and throughout the world.

The agency that has been in the forefront as of 2020 (due to COVID-19) is the Centers for Disease Control and Prevention (CDC). The CDC is a major component of the Department of Health and Human Services. It creates the information and tools that people and communities need to protect themselves and to be prepared for new health threats. According to the CDC website, the organization uses advanced computing and lab analysis to track diseases and bring that knowledge to individual health care and community health systems. It uses science to understand and predict the threat of dangerous health issues that can affect a population. This allows the CDC, through various means, to inform the public on how to stay healthy.

Information is available through publications and bulletins that are available through the CDC's website, *www.cdc.gov*. Publications on any health-related issue are available through a search engine, for example, publications on health in the United States, life table, national health statistics, national immunizations, studies on aging, and even publications on health hygiene and how to wash hands to prevent the spread of disease.

CYCLE OF INFECTION

Infection cannot be transmitted unless the following elements, shown and described in Display 11-4, are present.

A human host can be any susceptible person. Persons particularly susceptible to infection are those who are poorly nourished or are fatigued. Those at greater risk are persons with chronic diseases, such as diabetes mellitus or cancer. **Immunosuppressed persons** are at great risk for acquiring infections. Previous infection with

DISPLAY 11-3

Agencies That Control the Safety of Patients, Workers, and the General Public

- *The Joint Commission:* Sets requirements for hospital safety, infection control practices, and patient care standards (quality assurance [QA]) that must be met if the institution or agency is to receive accreditation

- *The Occupational Safety and Health Administration (OSHA):* A federal agency that protects workers and students from work-related injuries and illnesses, inspects work sites, and makes and enforces regulations concerning workplace safety

- *Centers for Disease Control and Prevention (CDC):* Performs research and compiles statistical data concerning infectious diseases; develops immunization guidelines and administers OSHA and OSHA's research institute, the National Institute of Occupational Safety Health (NIOSH)

- *U.S. Public Health Service:* Investigates and controls communicable diseases, controls carriers of communicable diseases from foreign countries, prevents spread of endemic diseases, and controls manufacture and sale of biologic products

- *Food and Drug Administration (FDA):* The U.S. Public Health Service branch responsible for protecting the public from false drug claims and regulates the manufacture and sale of medications; requires preclinical tests for toxicity of new drugs on animals and the testing of medications clinically on humans in three phases before marketing

- *World Health Organization (WHO):* Works under the auspices of the United Nations to reduce famine and disease throughout the world; compiles information concerning infectious diseases from all countries and compiles this information into reports for every country

- *United Nations Children's Fund:* Helps children, especially children in developing countries, to avoid malnutrition and disease; also assists with educational programs for deprived children

- *The U.S. Department of Health and Human Services (DHHS):* Specifies and notifies agents to destroy various types of medical waste

- *The U.S. Environmental Protection Agency (EPA):* Specifies destruction practices for waste from patients with contagious highly communicable diseases

- *Nuclear Control Agency (NCA):* Controls disposal of nuclear waste

a particular disease or vaccination against a particular disease can render an individual immune to infection.

Socioeconomic status and culture also play a role in host susceptibility. Persons living in poor environments are more likely to contact some diseases because of poor hygienic conditions and the poor diets that they are forced to endure. Some diseases have a strong hereditary aspect, which makes them more likely to occur in particular races or families who are genetic carriers of the disease.

PREVENTING DISEASE TRANSMISSION

People who are ill are particularly susceptible to infection. Preventing infection or breaking the cycle of infection is the duty of all health care workers. Medical aseptic practices

and use of Standard Precautions must become routine for the radiographer. It is the duty of the radiographer to practice strict medical asepsis at all times in their practice. There is a difference between medical asepsis and surgical asepsis. **Medical asepsis** means, insofar as possible, microorganisms have been eliminated through the use of soap, water, friction, and various chemical disinfectants. *Surgical asepsis* means that microorganisms and their spores have been completely destroyed by means of heat or by a chemical process. It is not practical or necessary to practice surgical asepsis at all times but one must always adhere to the practice of strict medical asepsis.

Dress in the Workplace

Fingernails must be short. Cracked or broken nails and chipped nail polish harbor microorganisms that

DISPLAY 11-4

The Cycle of Infection

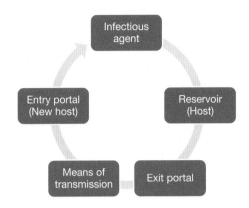

1. *An infectious agent, which may be a bacterium, fungus, virus, prion, or* **parasite**. Infectious agents vary in their ability to cause disease. These characteristics are **pathogenicity**, **virulence,** invasiveness, and specificity.
   Invasiveness is the term used to describe the organism's ability to enter tissues.
   Specificity characterizes the organism's attraction to a particular host.
2. *A reservoir or an environment in which the pathogenic microbes can live and multiply*. The reservoir can be a human being, an animal, a plant, water, food, earth, or any combination of organic materials that support the life of a particular pathogen.
3. *A portal of exit from the reservoir*. In the case of a human reservoir, the portals of exit might be the nose, mouth, urinary tract, intestines, or an open wound from which blood or purulent exudate can escape. There can be more than one portal of exit.
4. *A means of transmission*. A person who transmits disease-causing organisms but has no apparent signs or symptoms of that disease is called a **carrier**. Particular organisms require specific routes of transmission for infection to occur. Infection is transmitted by
   • Direct contact: contact that occurs when the blood or body fluids of a person with a disease is touched by someone who has an opening that allows the microorganisms to enter
   • Indirect contact: the transfer of pathogenic microbes by touching **fomites** such as dressings, instruments, or other items containing live infectious microorganisms
   • Droplet: involves contact with infectious secretions that come from the conjunctiva, nose, or mouth of a host or disease carrier as the person coughs, sneezes, or talks. Droplets can travel from approximately 3 to 5 ft and should not be equated with the airborne route of transmission.
   • Vehicle: transmission is through food, water, drugs, or blood contaminated with infectious microorganisms.
   • Vector: transmission comes from insect or animal carriers of disease. They deposit the diseased microbes by stinging or biting the human host.
   • Airborne: residue from evaporated droplets of diseased microorganisms is suspended in air for long periods. This residue is infectious if inhaled by a susceptible host.
5. *A portal of entry into a new host*. Entry of pathogenic microorganisms into a new host can be by ingestion, by inhalation, by injection, across mucous membranes, or, in the case of a pregnant woman, across the placenta.

are difficult to remove. Shoes must have closed, hard toes. Jewelry, such as rings with stones, should not be worn. All individuals working in acute care areas, such as the emergency department (ED) or the operating room (OR), must keep in mind that bacteria cannot be easily removed from the crevices of intricate jewelry and these may possibly be the source of a nosocomial infection.

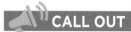

CALL OUT

Acrylic fingernails must not be worn in the workplace. They often harbor infectious microorganisms!

Always wear freshly laundered, washable clothing when working with patients. Uniforms or scrubs are recommended because they will not be worn for other purposes. Short sleeves are recommended because cuffs of uniforms are easily contaminated. If a laboratory coat is worn to protect clothing, button or zip it closed and remove it when not in the work area.

Laboratory coats, scrubs, and uniforms should be washed after one wearing with hot water and detergent. Chlorine bleach is recommended for clothes that have become heavily contaminated. A protective gown must be worn when working with any patient who may soil one's clothing or if it is possible that blood or body fluids will contaminate clothing. In some situations, the radiographer may need to wear **personal protective equipment (PPE)**.

Hair follicles and filaments also harbor microorganisms. Hair is a major source of staphylococcal **contamination**. For these reasons, hair must be worn short or in a style that keeps it up and away from your clothing and the patient. Hair should be shampooed frequently.

Eye Protection

If the radiographer is in a patient care situation in which a spattering of blood or body fluids is possible, they must wear goggles to protect the eyes from becoming contaminated. These goggles must have side protectors. If eyeglasses are worn for vision enhancement, the goggles must fit over the glasses (Fig. 11-2). Keep hands away from eyes during the course of work so that infection is not introduced into them. Another alternative to the goggles is a face shield that can fit over the head while a clear plastic shield covers the eyes, nose, and mouth (Fig. 11-3).

Gloves

It is possible that a patient's blood or body secretions may be touched any time; disposable, single-use gloves must be worn. These gloves should be readily available in containers in each room (Fig. 11-4). Because these gloves are to be used for medical aseptic purposes and not for surgically aseptic purposes, the radiographer may simply pull them on after handwashing.

When they are no longer needed, remove the gloves using the following techniques to prevent contamination of the radiographer's hands or clothing:

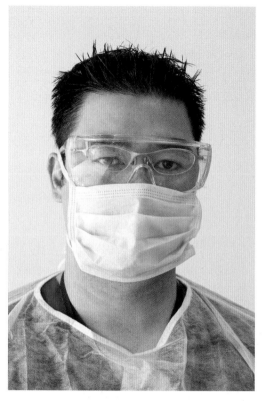

FIGURE 11-2 Clear plastic goggles can be worn over regular eye glasses to protect the eyes from the sides.

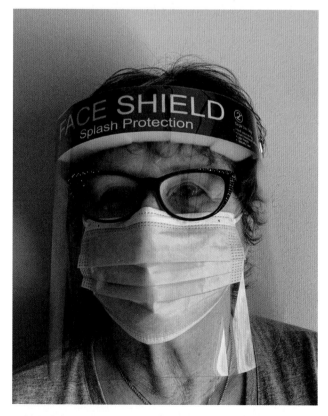

FIGURE 11-3 The use of a face shield is effective in preventing blood and fluids from getting into the eyes, nose, or mouth.

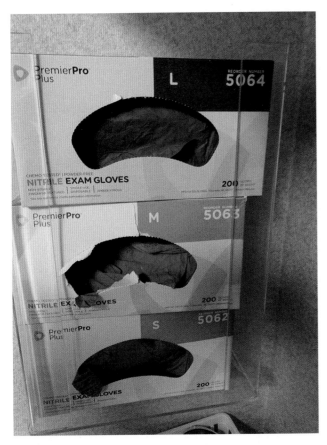

FIGURE 11-4 Gloves are located in easy-to-reach containers on the wall of each imaging area.

1. With the gloved right hand, take hold of the upper, outside portion of the left glove and pull it off, turning it inside out as you do so (Fig. 11-5A).
2. Hold the glove that was just removed in the palm of the gloved hand.
3. With the clean, bare index and middle fingers, reach inside the top of the soiled glove and pull it off, turning it inside out and folding the first glove inside it. Be careful to touch only the inside of the glove (Fig. 11-5B).
4. Drop the soiled gloves into a receptacle for contaminated waste (Fig. 11-5C).
5. Wash hands.

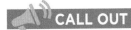

CALL OUT

If exposure to blood or body fluids is possible, wear PPE, which includes gloves, masks, respirators, goggles, face shields, and gowns.

Cleaning and Disposal of Contaminated Waste

Visual inspection is a simple method for evaluating the cleanliness of the work area; however, this is not adequate because pathogenic microorganisms cannot be seen if they are not harbored in blood or body fluid that is left on the radiographic table or the floor. Radiographic equipment should be cleaned with a disinfectant such as ethanol 75% or a diluted bleach solution, or the disinfectant that the manufacturer suggests. A separate cloth should be used for each piece of equipment if it is heavily contaminated with fluids. Mobile units should be wiped down starting with the tube and collimator housing, then the exposure switch and control area, and then the entire stand.

The following are guidelines for the disposal of waste or the cleaning of equipment after each patient in the imaging department.

1. Pillow coverings should be changed after each use by a patient. Linens used for drapes or blankets for patients should be handled in such a way that they do not raise dust. Dispose of linens after each use by a patient.
2. The radiographic table or other imaging or treatment equipment should be cleaned with a disposable disinfectant towelette or sprayed with disinfectant and wiped clean and dried from top to bottom with paper towels after each patient use.
3. When cleaning an article such as an imaging table, start with the least soiled area and progress to the most soiled area. This prevents the cleaner areas from becoming more heavily contaminated. Use a good disinfectant cleaning agent and disposable paper cloths.
4. Floors are heavily contaminated. If an item to be used for patient care falls to the floor, discard it or send it to the proper department to be recleaned.
5. Use equipment and supplies for one patient only. After the patient leaves the area, supplies must be destroyed or resterilized before being used again.
6. Flush away the contents of bedpans and urinals promptly unless they are being saved for a diagnostic specimen.
7. Dispose of the disposable urinals and bedpans properly, according to the department protocols.
8. Place dampened or wet items such as dressings and bandages into waterproof bags, and close the bags tightly before discarding them to prevent workers handling these materials from coming in contact with bodily discharges. Place in containers meant for contaminated waste.
9. Pour liquids to be discarded directly into drains or toilets. Avoid splashing or spilling on clothing.
10. If in doubt about the cleanliness or sterility of an item, do not use it.
11. When an article that is known to be contaminated with **virulent** microorganisms is to be sent to a central

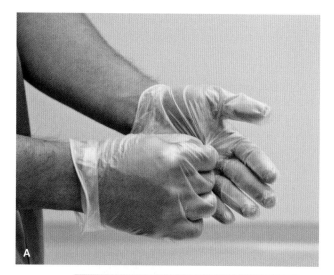

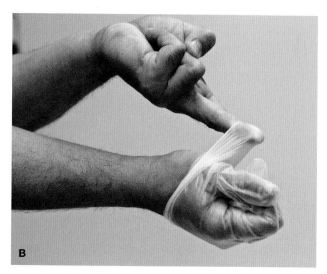

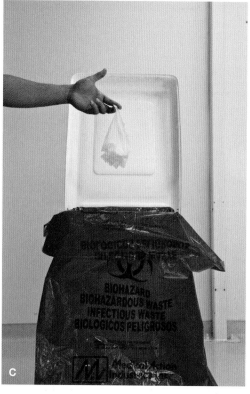

FIGURE 11-5 **(A)** Pull the first glove off by grasping it on the outside with the other gloved hand. Ball the removed glove into the palm of the hand that is still gloved. **(B)** With the bare finger, reach inside the top of the remaining soiled glove and pull it off, turning it inside out, encasing the other glove inside it. **(C)** Drop the soiled gloves into a designated waste receptacle.

supply area for cleaning and resterilizing, place it in a sealed, impermeable bag marked "BIOHAZARD." If the outside of the bag becomes contaminated while the article is being placed in the bag, place a second bag over it (Fig. 11-6).

12. Always treat needles and syringes used in the diagnostic imaging department as if they are contaminated with virulent microbes. Do not recap needles or touch them after use. Place them immediately (needle first) in a puncture-proof container labeled for this purpose (Fig. 11-7). Do not attempt to bend or break used needles because they may stick or spray you in the process.

13. Place specimens to be sent to the laboratory in solid containers with secure caps. If the specimen

is from a patient with a known communicable disease, label the outside of the container as such. Avoid contaminating the outside of the container and place the container in a clean bag. If a container becomes contaminated, clean it with a disinfectant before placing it in the bag. Specimens must be sent to the laboratory immediately after collection for examination (Fig. 11-8).

Infection Control in the Neonatal Intensive Care Unit (NICU)

The radiographer is often called to a nursery to take images on infants in the NICU. Before entering the newborn or intensive care nursery, the radiographer must carefully

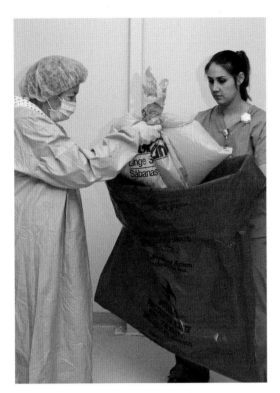

FIGURE 11-6 Place the contaminated bag into a second bag that is not contaminated.

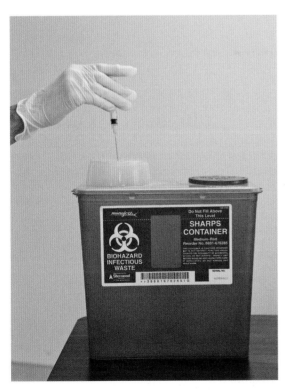

FIGURE 11-7 Place used syringe and uncapped needle into a puncture-resistant container.

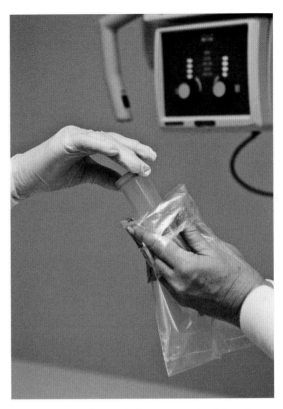

FIGURE 11-8 Specimens being sent to the laboratory must be placed into an outer clean bag.

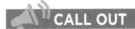 **CALL OUT**

The radiographer must never enter a nursery if an infection of any type is suspected.

Hands must be scrubbed for 3 minutes with an antibacterial soap before working with all infants. If the infant has or is suspected of having an infectious disease such as MRSA, VRSA, or ESBL, Transmission-Based Precautions are to be used as specified.

Transferring the Patient with a Communicable Disease

Occasionally, it is necessary for a patient with a communicable disease to come to the diagnostic imaging department. The following precautions must be taken to prevent infecting anyone else.

1. Place a mask properly on the patient's face. The radiographer also wears a gown, gloves, and mask as appropriate.
2. Place a sheet on the gurney or wheelchair and then cover it completely with another blanket. Wrap the blanket around the patient and then complete the transfer (Fig. 11-9).

clean the mobile unit with disinfectant wipes. Some facilities have a dedicated mobile unit that does not leave the nursery area. Be sure to cover image receptors (IRs) if they will be placed in contact with the infant.

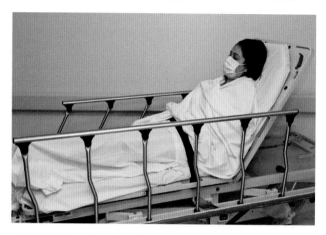

FIGURE 11-9 Place a cotton blanket on the wheel chair or gurney, then wrap the patient in the blanket. Make sure the patient is wearing a mask.

3. When the patient arrives in the department, open the blanket without touching the inside.
4. Place a protective sheet on the radiographic table, transfer the patient to the table, and then cover the patient with a sheet. Make the necessary exposures. Arrange work so that the patient does not have to spend more time than is necessary in the department.

Health Care Worker Protection

Most health care institutions now require all students and staff involved in patient care to be immunized or to show proof of immunization—for hepatitis B, rubella, rubeola, poliomyelitis, diphtheria, TB, and the coronavirus. Some institutions require varicella titers for health care workers. There may be wavier in place for those who, for personal or religious beliefs, do not want the vaccine. The health care worker must follow the facilities' protocols and procedures following exposure to any of these infectious diseases.

Recently, the COVID-19 pandemic made vaccinations a political issue when the Centers for Medicare and Medicaid Services (CMS), which is a part of the Department of Health and Human Services (HHS), made it mandatory for all staff working in facilities that are certified by Medicare and Medicaid to get vaccinated against COVID-19. Guidelines were issued by OSHA that all employers with more than 100 employees be vaccinated or be tested weekly for the virus before coming to work. Immunizations, vaccines, and boosters are put into place to protect the worker and the patient. Every individual must think carefully about the matter of receiving any type of vaccine, regardless whether it is for pneumonia, the flu, or COVID-19 and be aware of the employer's requirements.

PRECAUTIONS AND ISOLATION

Back in the 1980s, the CDC published two sets of guidelines that were meant to protect patients and health care workers alike in different instances. The first section was called "Blood and Body Fluid Precautions" and was used only when a patient was known to have a blood-borne infection, such as HIV. The second section was written in the late 1980s to reflect those precautions that should be used for all patients, regardless of any known infection status. With the additional set of guidelines, the precautions became known as **Universal Precautions**.

Moving forward to the 1990s, the CDC adapted the term **Standard Precautions**, which increased the focus on how to prevent the spread of infection. Standard Precautions are the minimum actions that all individuals involved in patient care must perform to prevent the spread of infections between patients and health care workers.

The CDC published the updated and expanded Standard Precautions (Display 11-5) to prevent the transmission of infection when the threat of infection with HIV, hepatitis A to E, MRSA, VRE, VRSA, ESBLs, TB, and other new pathogens emerged. Standard Precautions are effective because they are based on the assumption that every patient has the potential for having an infectious disease. Strict adherence to these principles greatly reduces the threat of infection.

Transmission-Based Precautions

When the use of the Standard Precautions is not sufficient to adequately protect and prevent the spread of infection-causing pathogens, a second tier of infection control is put into place. Known as **Transmission-Based Precautions** (Display 11-6), these are used in addition to the Standard Precautions for patients with certain types of infectious agents that are transmitted in ways that the standard means in not sufficient for containment.

DISPLAY 11-5

CDC Standard Precautions

1. Hand hygiene
2. Use of PPE when possible exposure is expected
3. Respiratory hygiene/cough and sneeze etiquette
4. Sharps safety to include injection and disposal
5. Sterile instruments and devices
6. Clean and disinfected environmental surfaces
7. Ensures appropriate patient placement

DISPLAY 11-6

Transmission-Based Precautions

Contact Precautions

1. Patient should be placed in a private room.
2. Use PPE appropriately. If available, the use of disposable equipment is best. If not available, the equipment should be dedicated to this patient only.
3. Limit the transport and movement of patients from outside the room to other locations.
4. Daily cleaning and **disinfection** of the room, especially those items that are frequently touched by the patient
5. Careful handling of any dressing materials, linens, or clothing to prevent cross contamination
6. Hand hygiene immediately after removing PPE

Droplet Precautions

1. A private room where the door may be left open
2. The patient must wear a mask.
3. A mask must be worn when entering the patient's room, particularly if the procedure requires less than 3 ft between the radiographer and the patient.
4. Limit the transport and movement of patients from outside the room to other locations.
5. Hand hygiene immediately after removing PPE

Airborne Precautions

1. Ensure appropriate patient placement in an airborne infection isolation room (AIIR) and the door must remain closed.
2. The patient must wear a surgical mask, and so must any visitors.
3. PPE must include a fit-tested National Institute for Occupational Safety and Health (NIOSH)-approved N95 or higher level respirator (Fig. 11-10A, B).
4. Restrict personnel from entering the room who may be susceptible to the patient's infection. If unprotected contact occurs, immunize susceptible persons as soon as possible.
5. Limit the transport and movement of patients from outside the room to other locations.
6. Use hand hygiene immediately after removing PPE.

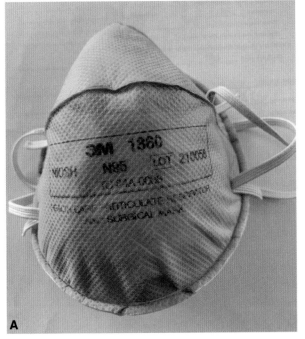
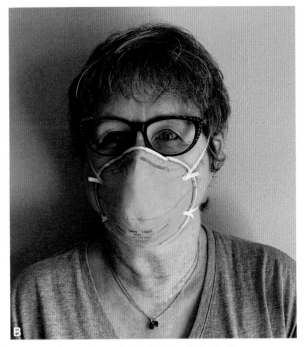

FIGURE 11-10 (A, B) An N95 respirator is used to prevent pathogens such as tuberculosis (TB) or COVID-19.

It is believed that there are three specific routes or modes of disease transmission, which may differ with each disease. These routes are by contact, airborne, and by droplet. Isolation precautions are meant to separate the patient who has a contagious illness from other hospitalized patients and from the health care workers. In institutions, there are card(s) posted on the patient's door with instructions informing the staff and visitors of the isolation requirements to be observed (Fig. 11-11A-C). These figures are example signs for each type of

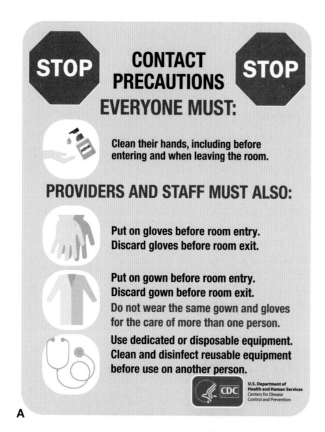

A

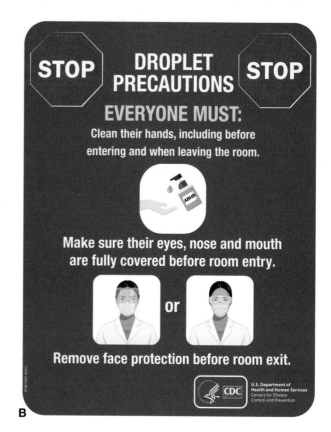

B

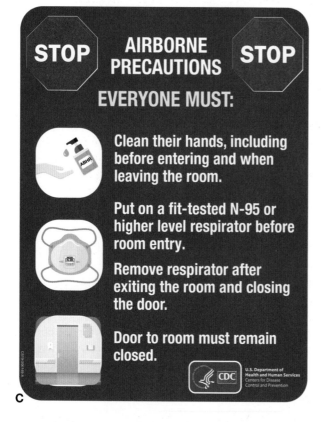

C

FIGURE 11-11 (A-C) These are transmission-based specific precautions that are mounted outside a patient's door. All visitors and health care workers must adhere to the guidelines.

Transmission-Based Precaution that can be posted outside the patient's room. Although these signs are from the CDC, the health care facility may use variations of these. However, some form of notification of transmission isolation must be posted for all those who enter the room to see and adhere to.

Contact Precautions

There are two types of contact spread of infection, *direct contact* and *indirect contact*. As described earlier, direct contact occurs when a susceptible person actually touches an infected or a colonized person's body surface in an area where infectious microbes are present.

Indirect contact occurs when a susceptible person touches or comes into contact with an object that has been contaminated with infectious microorganisms.

Droplet Precautions

Droplets from a sneeze, cough, or even talking, may be contaminated with pathogenic microorganisms. Usually, droplets are not spread for more than 3 ft by coughing, sneezing, or talking. Diseases spread by this route are influenza, rubella, mumps, pertussis (whooping cough), most pneumonias, diphtheria, pharyngitis, scarlet fever, and meningococcal meningitis.

Airborne Precautions

Microbes are spread on evaporated droplets that remain suspended in air or are carried on dust particles in the air and may be inhaled by persons in that room or air space. In some instances, air currents carry microorganisms, and special air handling and ventilation are required to prevent infectious microbes from circulating.

The OSHA amended federal regulations concerning infection control in the workplace. OSHA states that all workplaces in which employees may be exposed to human blood or body substances shall formulate a plan to prevent employee exposure to pathogenic microorganisms borne by these substances. These are known as the **Bloodborne Pathogens Standards** and require employers to do the following:

- Establish an infection exposure control plan.
- Implement and enforce the use of Standard Precautions by all health care workers.
- Provide PPE such as gloves, gowns, eye protection, and masks.
- Provide hepatitis B vaccination to workers with occupational exposure to blood-borne pathogens within 10 days of job assignment that involves occupational exposure.
- Provide a no-cost postexposure evaluation to any worker who experiences an exposure incident.

Protective Isolation

In some situations, if a patient is highly susceptible to becoming infected because of a particular treatment or condition, isolation precautions are used to protect them from becoming infected. Other names for practices designed to protect the patient from contracting infections include expanded isolation, strict isolation, or reverse isolation. Patients susceptible are those with neutropenia, pronounced immune compromise, transplant recipients who may be rejecting the transplanted organ, burn patients, and others designated by the physician or infection control officer.

In these situations, the health care workers are required to wear additional PPE for airborne infection isolation and droplet and contact precautions, which were previously addressed. The procedures for protective precautions are as follows:

1. Wash hands using the procedure described later in this chapter before entering and after providing care to patient.
2. Gown and gloves are required at all times while in patient's room.
3. Regular face mask may be required in select cases.
4. Equipment such as stethoscopes, blood pressure cuffs, and thermometers stay in the room.
5. No flowers, plants, fresh fruits, or vegetables are allowed for immunocompromised patients.
6. No visitors or staff with signs or symptoms of infection (colds, rashes, etc.) must go into the room.

To enter and leave a unit with expanded precautions, the radiographer needs the assistance of another radiographer or member of the nursing team who is caring for the patient in the unit. At the entrance to the room, there is a stack of disposable gowns, a container for masks and caps, and a box filled with clean, disposable gloves. The PPE item must be disposed of in the isolation unit waste receptacle.

Before entering the isolation room, the radiographer must have the mobile imaging unit prepared with as many IRs and other supplies on hand as needed. Make sure that they are covered with protective plastic bags to keep them from becoming contaminated. In addition, place an extra pair of clean gloves on the machine before placing it in the patient's room. Have an assistant available and then use the following procedures (Display 11-7).

The procedure for removing the contaminated PPE after leaving the isolation unit is described in Display 11-8.

PSYCHOLOGICAL CONSIDERATIONS

Patients in isolation may not be familiar with the requirements dictated for infection control and may feel that the radiographer, or others, are questioning their hygiene practices. Seeing a health care worker approach wearing gloves, a mask, and a protective gown may give the patient a sense of unworthiness. Explain that the precautions are to protect both the worker and the patient from infection.

DISPLAY 11-7

Isolation Procedures

1. Assemble the supplies and equipment needed (Fig. 11-12A).
2. Follow the type of isolation PPE requirements posted on the patient's door.
3. Make sure that the gown is tied at the back so as not to flap open and get contaminated.
4. Put gloves on, making certain that the cuffs of the gloves cover the cuffs of the gown.
5. Push unit into the room, verify and identify the patient, and explain the procedure. Make necessary adjustments to the mobile unit at this time. Do not touch the patient until the unit is positioned correctly. Once the patient has been touched, the gloves are contaminated and cannot touch any imaging equipment.
6. Position the IR for the exposure.
7. Remove contaminated gloves and discard them in a waste receptacle.
8. Make the exposure. Put on clean gloves that were placed on the mobile unit before entering the room.
9. If additional exposures are necessary, change gloves again. Place IR in contaminated plastic covers at the end near the patient's door.
10. When imaging exposures are completed and before gloves are contaminated, push the unit out of the room.
11. Remove the still covered IRs to the door of the unit, where the assistant is waiting. Slide the plastic bag covering back from the IR and allow the assistant to remove the IR (Fig. 11-12B). Discard the contaminated IR bag in the waste receptacle in the patient's room.
12. To provide for patient safety and comfort, return to the patient. Place the bed in the low (closest to the floor) position; put the side rails up and the call button within the patient's reach. Leave the patient's room, and return to the area prepared to dispose of your contaminated PPE.

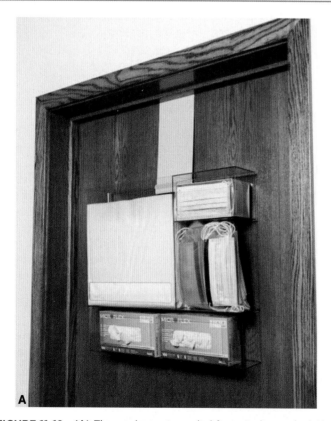

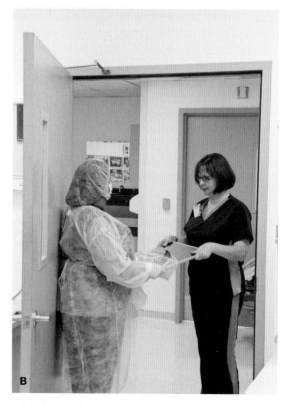

FIGURE 11-12 (A) The equipment needed for entering an isolation unit is located outside the patient's door. **(B)** Slide the image receptor from its covering, allowing the assistant to take it.

DISPLAY 11-8

Procedure for Removing Contaminated PPE

1. Untie waist ties of the gown (Fig. 11-13A).
2. Remove gloves and place in waste receptacle (Fig. 11-13B).
3. Untie the top gown ties (Fig. 11-13C).
4. Remove the first sleeve of the gown by placing fingers under the cuff of the sleeve and pulling it over the hand (Fig. 11-13D).
5. Remove the other sleeve with the hand being protected inside the gown (Fig. 11-13E).
6. Pull the gown off, hold it by the inside shoulders, and fold the sleeves forward so that the inside of the gown is facing out (Fig. 11-13F).
7. Roll the gown from top to bottom and place it in the receptacle provided for this purpose (Fig. 11-13G).
8. Remove the cap and mask and place them in the waste receptacle (Fig. 11-13H).
9. Wash hands or use an alcohol-based sanitizer.

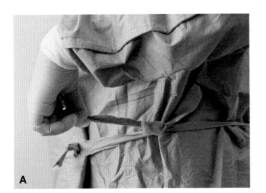

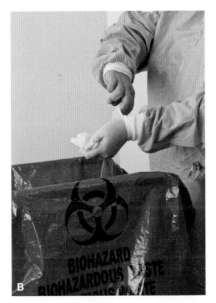

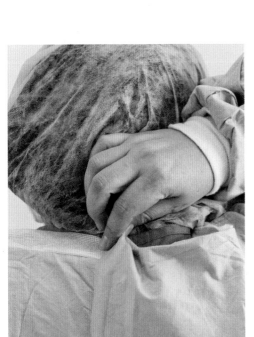

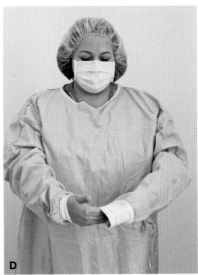

FIGURE 11-13 **(A)** Untie waist ties of gown. **(B)** Remove gloves and place in waste receptacle. **(C)** Untie the top gown ties. **(D)** Remove the first sleeve.

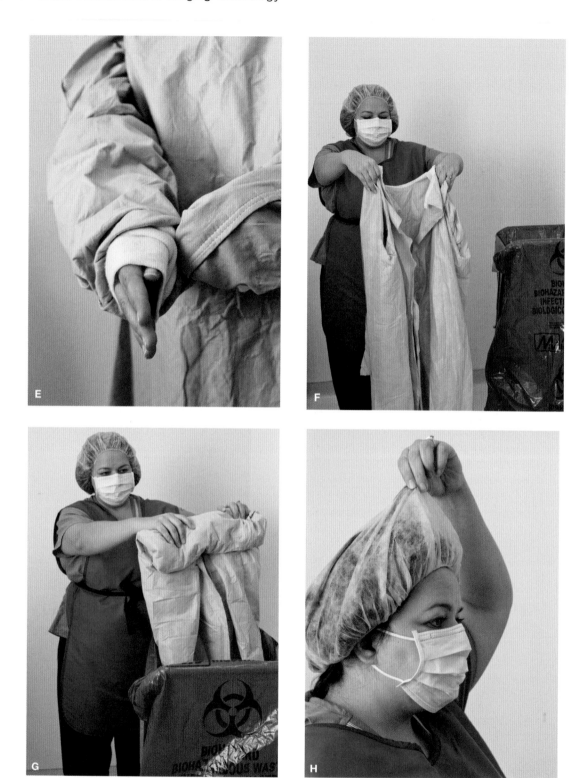

FIGURE 11-13 (*continued*) **(D)** Remove the first sleeve. **(E)** Remove the other sleeve. **(F)** Fold the gown forward. **(G)** Place the gown in the proper receptacle. **(H)** Remove the cap and mask and place them in the waste receptacle.

Strict isolation may create a sense of loneliness and rejection because of the lack of visitors being allowed into the room. These patients are forced to remain in solitude for long periods and are often treated by workers in a perfunctory manner. It is important to remember that the patient is a human being and

needs to be treated with dignity and worth. Spend a few moments explaining the procedure. Afterwards, ask the patient if there are any questions before leaving the room. A few moments spent with the patient conversing about what is happening is what quality patient care is about.

ASEPSIS

The term asepsis means that there are no disease-causing microorganisms on the surface of the skin or other material. There are two categories of asepsis that differ in their ability to remove the microorganism. **Medical asepsis** is defined as any practice that helps reduce the number and spread of microorganisms. **Surgical asepsis** is defined as the complete removal of microorganisms and their spores from the surface of an object. The practice of surgical asepsis begins with cleaning the object in question using the principles of medical asepsis followed by a **sterilization** process.

Medical Handwashing

Microbes are most commonly spread from one person to another by human hands. It follows that the best means of preventing the spread of microorganisms continues to be hand hygiene. According to the CDC guidelines, the term *hand hygiene* applies to handwashing with a nonantimicrobial soap and water or an antimicrobial soap and water and the use of antiseptic hand rubs, including alcohol-based (gels, rinses, and foams) products that do not require the use of water.

Correct handwashing procedure before and after handling supplies used for patient care and before and after each patient contact is required. Hand hygiene is required even if gloves have been worn for a procedure because there may be small punctures in the gloves. Treat all blood and body substances as if they contain disease-producing microorganisms and dispose of them correctly followed by hand hygiene. Cover any exposed break in the skin with a waterproof protective covering. If there is an open or weeping wound on the hands, the radiographer must not work with patients until it has healed.

Because of the high degree of noncompliance with handwashing before and after each patient contact, waterless antiseptic products, most often alcohol-based hand rubs (Fig. 11-14), are now used effectively in place of many handwashing situations. A small amount is applied to the hands and the hands are rubbed together rapidly making sure that all surfaces of the hands, fingers, and between the fingers are covered. Rub vigorously until the solution dries. If hands have been heavily contaminated, first wash them as described earlier and then use antiseptic rub.

The radiographer should follow a specific handwashing technique that is accepted as medically aseptic when working with patients (Fig. 11-15A-C).

1. Approach the sink. Do not lean against the sink or allow clothing to touch the sink because it is considered contaminated. Remove any jewelry except for a wedding band.
2. Turn on the water and regulate it to a comfortable warm temperature. Do not allow the water to splash onto clothing.
3. During the entire procedure, keep hands and forearms lower than the elbows. The water will drain

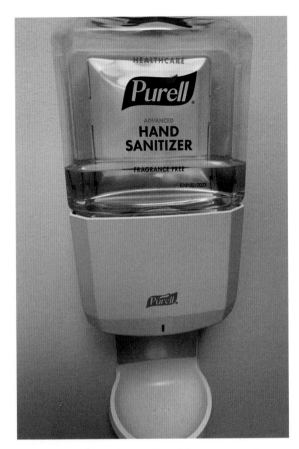

FIGURE 11-14 Alcohol-based hand sanitizer can be used between patients.

by gravity from the area of least contamination to the area of greatest contamination.

4. Wet hands and soap them well. A liquid soap is the most convenient.
5. With a firm, circular, scrubbing motion, wash palms, backs, each finger, between the fingers, and finally the knuckles. Wash to at least 1 in above the area of contamination. If hands are not contaminated, wash to 1 in above the wrists. Fifteen seconds should be the minimum time allotted for this.
6. Rinse hands well. If hands have been heavily contaminated, repeat the process.
7. Clean fingernails with a brush or an orange stick carefully once each day before beginning work and again if hands become heavily contaminated. Scrubbing heavily contaminated nails with a brush is recommended.
8. Turn off the water. If the handles are hand operated, use a paper towel to turn the water off to avoid contamination.
9. Dry arms and hands using as many paper towels as necessary to do the job well.
10. Use lotion on hands and forearms frequently. It helps keep the skin from cracking and thereby prevents infection.

Perform the foregoing procedure at the beginning of each workday, when in contact with a patient's blood or

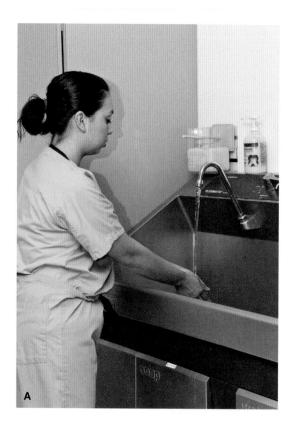

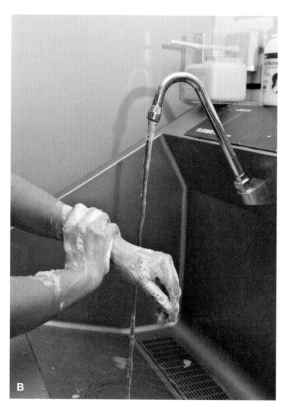

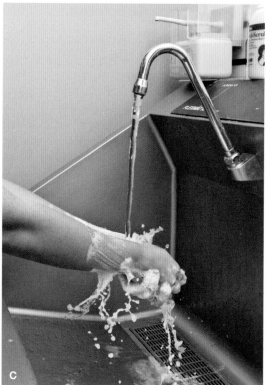

FIGURE 11-15 **(A)** Approach the sink and turn on the water. Do not allow clothing to touch the sink. **(B)** Apply soap. Clean the hands, knuckles, and areas between the fingers with a firm, rubbing motion. Clean the fingernails with running water to flush away dirt and microorganisms. **(C)** Clean the wrists and forearms with a firm circular motion.

body substances, when preparing for invasive procedures, before touching patients at greatest risk for infection, and after caring for patients with known communicable diseases. This is the case even if gloves are worn. A 15-second hand-washing should precede and follow each patient contact.

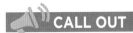

Remove gloves after each patient care situation and then wash hands. Do not wear gloves to another area or touch other items with gloves worn and used when attending to a patient!

Chemical Disinfectants

Disinfectants are categorized as high level, intermediate level, or low level. This classification depends on their disinfecting ability. Items to be sterilized or disinfected are classified as critical, semi-critical, and noncritical based on the risk of infection for the patient. This classification is called the Spaulding classification system named for its developer, Earle Spaulding. Display 11-9 lists the disinfectants and their status.

Many chemical disinfectants such as glutaraldehyde are used in the health care setting. Other disinfectants include alcohols, chlorine or its compounds, glutaraldehyde, iodophors, and ammonium compounds. These commercial formulas must be registered with the Environmental Protection Agency (EPA) or the U.S. Food and Drug Administration (FDA). The compounds are designed for a specific use and in a specific way. If the radiographer is going to use a disinfectant, the label must be read carefully because there are compounds that cannot be mixed with other types of disinfectants. For example, ammonium and bleach should not be mixed because they create a toxic smell that is harmful.

Disinfection

Disinfection is a term used to describe the removal, by mechanical and chemical processes, of pathogenic microorganisms, but frequently not their spores, from objects or body surfaces. Usually in reference to body surfaces, the term *antisepsis* or *antiseptic* is used rather than disinfect or disinfectant. Items are disinfected when they cannot withstand the process necessary to sterilize them or when it is not practical to sterilize. This is often the case with objects leaving an isolation unit.

DISPLAY 11-9

Commonly Used Disinfectants

Disinfectant	Status	Use
Alcohols (70% or 90%) (intermediate level)	Bactericidal, tuberculocidal, fungicidal, and virucidal	To disinfect thermometers, medication vials, etc.
Glutaraldehyde (high level)	Broad antimicrobial range, fungicidal, and virucidal	To disinfect endoscopes, thermometers, and rubber items
Chlorine compounds (dilution of 1:50 is high level)	Concentrations of 1,000 ppm inactivate bacterial spores	To disinfect countertops, floors, and other surfaces
Orthophthalaldehyde (high level)	Bactericidal, virucidal, fungicidal, and tuberculocidal in 12 min at room temperature	To clean and process endoscopes
Hydrogen peroxide (low level)	6% solutions effective against some bacteria, fungi, and viruses	May be used to clean work surfaces, not widely used in health care settings
Iodine and iodophors (intermediate level)	Vegetative bactericidal, *Mycobacterium tuberculosis,* most viruses and fungi, no sporicidal capability	May be used as disinfectant or antiseptic
Phenolics (intermediate or low level)	Most formulations are tuberculocidal, bactericidal, virucidal, and fungicidal	Have toxic effects, used as environmental not sporicidal disinfectants
Quaternary ammonium compounds	Not recommended for high-, intermediate-, or low-level disinfection	Cleaning agents for noncritical surfaces

If an object leaving an examining room or isolation unit has been contaminated, it is cleaned first by vigorous scrubbing (mechanical means) and then disinfected by wiping it with, or soaking it in, a chemical selected by the institution for this purpose.

Physical methods of disinfecting are boiling in water and ultraviolet irradiation. Boiling may be used as a means of disinfection if no other method is available; however, many spores are able to resist the heat of boiling (212° F or 100° C) for many hours. To increase the effectiveness of boiling, sodium carbonate may be added to the water in quantity to make a 2% solution. If an object is to be disinfected by boiling and sodium carbonate is added to the water, it should be boiled for 15 minutes. If sodium carbonate is not added, boiling time should be 30 minutes. Ultraviolet light is not a practical means of disinfecting for hospital use because there is no assurance that the ultraviolet has actually come into contact with the microbes, which are constantly in a mobile state because of air currents.

Not all disinfectants are equally effective. Before a disinfectant is chosen for the diagnostic imaging department, it should be thoroughly studied by an infection control consultant. The following are guidelines for the disposal of waste or the cleaning of equipment after each patient use in the diagnostic imaging department.

When a patient enters the diagnostic imaging department with a known or suspected contagious disease, it is the radiographer's responsibility to prevent the spread of infection. If the patient is coughing and sneezing, the patient must be provided with tissues and a place to dispose of them. The patient should be cared for and returned to the hospital room or discharged as quickly as possible.

After the patient has been cared for and leaves the imaging department, disinfect the imaging table and anything in the room that the patient has touched. This can be accomplished with a disinfectant solution designated by the infection control department to be acceptable for this use. The radiographer must use proper hand hygiene once again.

Surgical Asepsis

Any medical procedure that involves penetration of body tissues (an invasive procedure) requires the use of surgical **aseptic technique**. This includes major and minor surgical procedures, administration of parenteral medications, invasive imaging procedures, catheterization of the urinary bladder, tracheostomy care, and dressing changes. Skin preparation, including scrubbing and, at times, hair removal, precedes invasive procedures. This prevents **contamination** of the operative site, thereby reducing the chances of infection. The radiographer may be responsible for the skin preparation in the department and must learn to perform this procedure effectively.

Rules for Surgical Asepsis

The basic rules for surgical aseptic technique apply whenever and wherever the sterile procedure is performed. The radiographer must use these everywhere as necessary.

1. Know which areas and objects are sterile and which are not.
2. If the sterility of an object is questionable, it is *not* to be considered **sterile**.
3. Sterile objects and persons must be kept separate from those that are nonsterile.
4. When any item that must be sterile becomes contaminated, the contamination must be remedied immediately.
5. When tabletops are to be used as areas for creating a sterile field, they must be clean and a sterile drape must be placed over them.
6. Personnel must be clothed in a sterile gown and sterile gloves if they are to be considered sterile.
7. Any sterile instrument or sterile area that is touched by a nonsterile object or person is considered contaminated by microorganisms.
8. A contaminated area on a sterile field must be covered by a folded sterile towel or drape of double thickness.
9. If a sterile person's gown or gloves become contaminated, they must be changed.
10. A sterile field must be created just before use.
11. Once a sterile field has been prepared, it must not be left unattended because it may become contaminated and presumed to be sterile.
12. An unsterile person does not reach across a sterile field.
13. A sterile person does not lean over an unsterile area.
14. A sterile field ends at the level of the tabletop or at the waist of the sterile person's gown.
15. Anything that drops below the tabletop or sterile person's waistline is no longer sterile and may not be brought up to the sterile tabletop. The only parts of the sterile gown considered sterile are the areas from the waist to the shoulders in front and the sleeves from 2 in above the elbow to the cuffs.
16. The cuffs of the sterile gown are considered nonsterile because they collect moisture. Cuffs must always be covered by sterile gloves.
17. The edges of a sterile wrapper are not considered sterile and must not touch a sterile object.
18. Sterile drapes are placed by a sterile person. The sterile person places the drapes on the area closest first to protect the sterile gown.
19. A sterile person must remain within the sterile area. Do not lean on tables or against the wall.
20. If one sterile person must pass another, they must pass back-to-back.

21. The sterile person faces the sterile field and keeps sterile gloves above the waist in front of the chest. The sterile person must avoid touching any area of the body.

22. Any sterile material or pack that becomes damp or wet is considered unsterile.

23. Any objects that are wet with disinfectant solution and are to be placed on a sterile field must be placed on a folded sterile towel for the moisture to be absorbed.

24. A wet area on a sterile field must be covered with several thicknesses of sterile toweling or an impervious drape.

25. When pouring sterile solution, place the lid face upward and do not touch the inside of the lid or the lip of the flask. Pour off a small amount of solution before the remainder is poured into the sterile container.

26. When a sterile solution is to be poured into a container on a sterile field, the container is placed at the edge of the sterile field by the sterile person (Fig. 11-16).

CALL OUT

If the sterility of an item is questionable, it is not to be considered sterile.

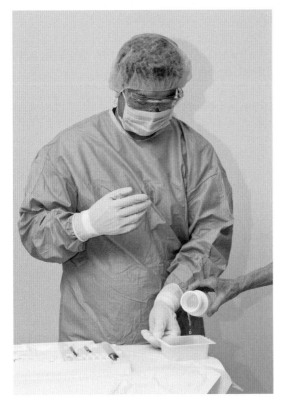

FIGURE 11-16 Place container at the edge of the sterile field so the field will not be crossed by the unsterile person.

Methods of Sterilization

Removal of microorganisms and their spores must be complete or the article is not sterile. Methods used to attain sterilization depend on the nature of the item to be sterilized. Display 11-10 lists the common methods used, with a brief description of each.

All effective methods of sterilization have advantages and disadvantages. The packaging systems and sterilizing of items used for medical purposes have become a highly specialized field and are described only briefly in this chapter because it is not within the scope of the radiographer's practice to perform these tasks.

There are various packaging systems with specific sterilization methods. Whichever sterilization system is

DISPLAY 11-10

Methods of Sterilization

Steam Under Pressure (Moist Heat): Items are double wrapped and placed in an autoclave.

Autoclaves are manufactured to sterilize by *gravity displacement and dynamic air removal*.

High-speed sterilizer or *flash sterilization* is an abbreviated gravity displacement method.

Dry Heat: Medical equipment that cannot undergo moist heat (steam) are sterilized through infrared heat. However, because of its lower wavelength (lower energy), it cannot penetrate and is only good for sterilizing the surface of the object.

Chemical Sterilization: Referred to as *low-temperature sterilization*. A maximum temperature of 54° C to 60° C of gaseous sterilization is used. An antimicrobial and sporicidal agent must be used, such as hydrogen peroxide, glutaraldehyde and formaldehyde, and bleach.

Ethylene Oxide (Gas): Used for items that cannot withstand moisture and high temperatures.

All items sterilized in this manner must be cleansed and dried because water united with ethylene oxide forms ethylene glycol, which cannot be eliminated by aeration and is toxic.

Radiation: Gamma radiation is used for wrapping products to ensure that the equipment inside the wrapper is safe and free of harmful organisms. Most products being sterilized by radiation include disposable gowns, surgical gloves, and sutures.

used, the radiographer must learn to evaluate the specific sterile packaging system to ensure the sterilization integrity of the contents.

STERILE PROCEDURES

There are procedures that radiographers perform within the scope of their employment that require sterile technique. Some of these duties may become common practice, such as opening a sterile pack, whereas others require careful thought and strict attention to detail because the task may not be performed often enough that it becomes routine. Whether it is drawing up contrast media to be used later or performing a sterile scrub with gowning and gloving, the radiographer must always keep the rules of sterile technique in mind by knowing what is sterile and what is not. If sterile touches clean, the sterility is broken. Sterile items can only touch other sterile items.

Opening Packs

The radiographer is called upon to open commercially packaged sterile packs and place sterile objects on sterile fields. The technologist must be able to do this without contaminating the sterile object or the sterile field. Commercial packs are usually wrapped in paper or plastic wrappers. They are frequently sealed in plastic to ensure prolonged sterility. Directions for opening the containers to avoid contamination are usually printed on the pack by the manufacturer and should be read before opening. Never cut packs open or pierce them with a knife or sharp object. Do not tear packs open and do not allow the contents to slide over the edges of the

pack. Follow the procedure listed for opening a sterile pack to keep it sterile.

Skin Preparation

The radiographer may be called upon to prepare a patient's skin for an invasive procedure. This is referred to as a **skin prep**. The purpose of the skin prep is to remove as many microorganisms as possible by mechanical and chemical means to reduce the chances of infection. The antimicrobial agents used for this purpose may vary; however, it must prevent tissue irritation and the rebound growth of microbes. Items the radiographer must have on hand include the following:

1. Commercial skin preparation package that includes a sterile drape, two small basins, and a set of large sponges with handles to distance the operator's hand from the site. The sponges are permeated with antiseptic soap.
2. Sterile gloves if they are not included in the commercial pack
3. A flask of sterile water and a flask of antiseptic solution as recommended by the physician
4. A sterile towel

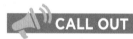
CALL OUT

The technologist must use at least two patient identifiers to verify the correct patient and verify the order to confirm the correct examination will be performed.

PROCEDURE

Opening Sterile Packs

1. Place the pack on a clean tabletop with the sealed end toward the radiographer.
2. Remove the outer plastic as directed and place the sealed end toward the radiographer (Fig. 11-17A).
3. Open the first corner back and away from the pack (Fig. 11-17B).
4. Next, open the second and third corners (Fig. 11-17C).
5. Then, open the fourth corner and drop it toward the radiographer (Fig. 11-17D).

To move a sterile object to another sterile field or to pass a sterile object to a sterile person:

1. Open the package as directed in Figure 11-17A-D.
2. Grasp the underside of the wrapper and let the edges fall over the hand (Fig. 11-18A).
3. Take the item to the next sterile field and, from a distance, drop or flip it onto the field (Fig. 11-18B). Do not allow the edges of the wrapper to touch the sterile field.
4. A sterile forceps may be used to pick up a sterile object and move it to a second field

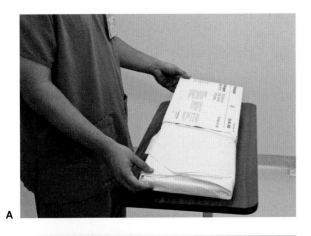
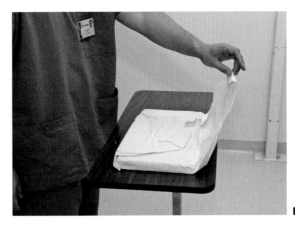
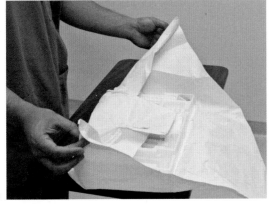
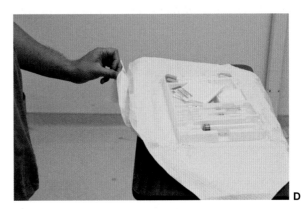

FIGURE 11-17 **(A)** Place the sealed end of the sterile pack toward the radiographer. **(B)** Open the flap farthest from the body making sure it stays down. **(C)** Open the two-sided flaps next. **(D)** Open the last flap closet to the body last.

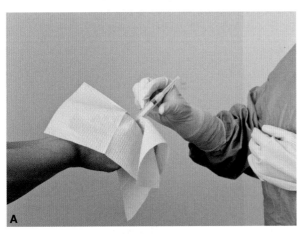
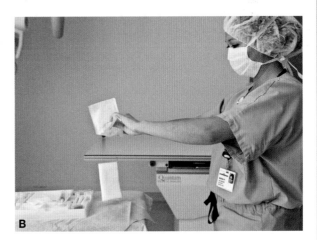

FIGURE 11-18 **(A)** Grasp the underside of the sterile wrapper and let the edges over the hands. **(B)** Take the item to the sterile field and drop it without crossing the sterile field.

(Fig. 11-18C). The forceps may be used for one transfer only.

5. To pass a sterile object to a sterile person, grasp the underside of the wrapper as in

Figure 11-18A and hold it forward to the sterile person so that he may take it (Fig. 11-18D). Do this away from the sterile field.

(continued)

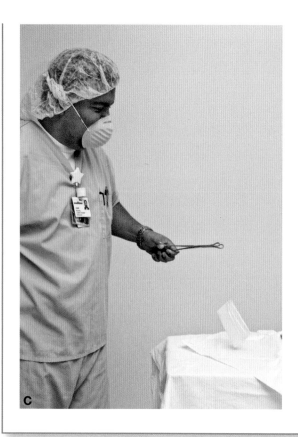

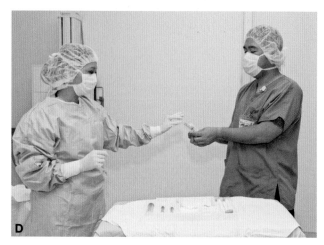

FIGURE 11-18 *(continued)* **(C)** Sterile forceps may be used to transfer an object to a sterile field without contamination of the existing field. **(D)** While protecting the hands as in Figure 11-17A, extend the item forward for the sterile person to take it.

PROCEDURE

Skin Preparation

1. Approach, identify, and assess the patient. Explain the procedure, and ascertain allergies to the antiseptic to be used. Open the sterile pack as described earlier.

2. Pour sterile water into one small basin and antiseptic solution into the other.

3. Put on sterile gloves.

4. Pick up one sponge permeated with antiseptic soap and dampen it in the sterile water. Then, begin scrubbing in the center of the area to be prepared. The physician will explain how large an area must be prepped; usually, an area approximately 6 to 10 in in diameter is prepped. Work outward in a circular motion using a firm stroke because friction is as important in the removal of microorganisms as the antiseptic soap (Fig. 11-19A).

5. Do not go back over the skin that has already been scrubbed with this sponge. When the edges of the area being scrubbed are reached, drop the sponge off the sterile field and repeat the procedure with a second sponge.

6. Following the scrub, rinse the skin well with sterile water or wipe away the lather without rinsing if that is the institution's procedure.

7. Blot the skin dry with the sterile towel.

8. Inspect the patient's skin during the skin prep. If the skin shows signs of irritation, stop the procedure and thoroughly rinse off the soap with sterile water and notify the physician.

9. Do not allow solution to drain off the area being prepped or to pool under the patient during the procedure because this may burn the skin.

10. Following the initial scrub, the skin around the area to be penetrated is often painted with an antiseptic solution. This destroys some of the remaining microbes and acts as a deterrent to further microbial growth

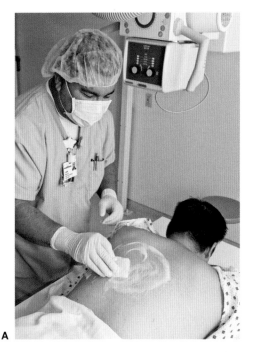 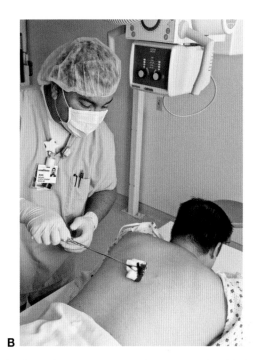

A   B

FIGURE 11-19 **(A)** Work in a circular motion using a firm stroke from the center outward. **(B)** Paint the skin in a circular motion from the inside out as was done with the cleaning.

for a brief period. Agents commonly used for skin prep are chlorhexidine and hexachlorophene. Alcohol is not used on mucous membranes or on open wounds because it may cause harm.

11. If the skin is to be painted after the scrub, it is performed in a circular motion beginning in the center of the area to be prepped and working outward (Fig. 11-19B). Allow the skin to dry.

12. If there are no long-handled sponges available, 4 × 4 sterile sponges may be folded and grasped with a sterile ring forceps and dipped into a container of antiseptic solution.

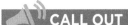 **CALL OUT**

Sterile technique is maintained during the skin prep for sterile procedures!

For invasive procedures, such as needle insertion into joints, a less complicated method of skin preparation is now used. A sponge applicator (Fig. 11-20A) contains antiseptic solution in the handle. When the area is ready to be cleaned, the sterile package is opened and the handle is squeezed slightly causing the solution to be distributed to the sponge (Fig. 11-20B). Now the area can be cleaned in the prescribed manner because the sponge provides the friction and physical means and the solution provides the chemical means of aseptic skin preparation.

Students must use their critical thinking skills for this procedure because what will be seen in the "real world" is most likely not what is taught in the classroom. However, if it is realized that there is one spot that needs to be the "cleanest," it cannot be rescrubbed with an applicator that has gone over another area and picked up possible organisms. This will recontaminate the area that needs to be most clean.

Draping

Following the skin prep for a sterile procedure, sterile drapes may be applied. These are used to provide a barrier to infection and also to create a sterile field on which to place sterile instruments. Usually, single-use, single-thickness, impermeable drapes are used; however, some cloth drapes may be chosen. Whatever the material is on hand, the process is the same. A **fenestrated drape** is often used, and, if so, the drape should be applied in such a way that the opening leaves only the operative site exposed.

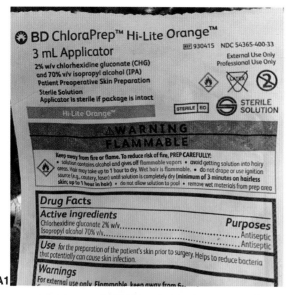

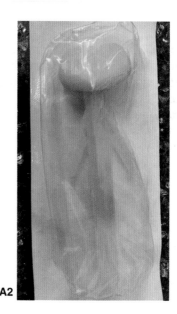

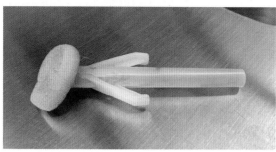

FIGURE 11-20 **(A)** A disposable sponge for skin preparation of sterile asepsis. **(B)** Once the handle is squeezed, the disinfectant flows through the sponge.

PROCEDURE

Draping the Skin

Sterile drapes must be handled as little as possible. If sterile towels are used, place them so that they are within the limits of the area prepared. They are folded so that they overlap and the folds face the operative site.

1. Place the pack of sterile drapes on the table on which they are to be opened.

2. Open a pack of sterile gloves and put them on.

3. Pick up the first drape, holding it in such a manner that the sterile gloves are protected (Fig. 11-21). Do not allow the drape to fall below the waist level or touch the uniform.

4. Place the drape on the patient and do not move it again because the underside is now contaminated. If the drape is a towel, it should be placed farthest away from the radiographer. In this manner, the sterile towel will not be "crossed over" while placing the other towel in position.

5. Add additional drapes as required. If a drape is contaminated during the draping process, it must be replaced.

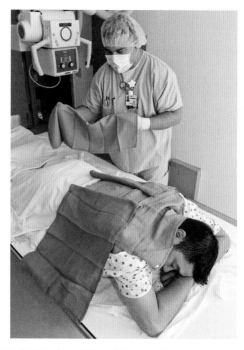

FIGURE 11-21 The folds of the sterile towel must face the open site. Cover the gloves with the drapes to protect sterility when placing the drape on the patient.

Dressing Changes

The radiographer is not likely going to need to change a dressing in the radiology department. However, it is possible that the patient may need to have a dressing removed for a procedure and then a clean one put on afterward. If this is the case, the dressing must be removed without contaminating the area in the process.

All dressings are to be treated as if they are contaminated because drainage from the area may contain pathogenic microorganisms. The procedure for removing and reapplying dressings must be followed for the protection of the patient as well as the radiographer.

PROCEDURE

Removing and Reapplying Dressings

Before removing a dressing, obtain a plastic bag for infectious waste, clean gloves, and a new bandage for reapplication. Turn the top of the bag inside out to form a protective cuff for the hands.

1. Perform a medical aseptic handwash.

2. Explain the procedure to the patient.

3. Place the patient in a comfortable position and provide for dignity.

4. Loosen the tape holding the patient's dressing in place. The tape will adhere to the gloves, so it is best to prepare it before putting on the gloves. Do not remove the dressing at this point.

5. Put on clean gloves and remove the dressing by pinching the top of it and pulling gently. If the dressing adheres to the wound, stop and determine the nature of the adhesion. If necessary, call for assistance. Do not forcefully remove a dressing because tissue may be damaged by doing so.

6. Fold the dressing in onto itself and place in the plastic bag. Remove the gloves placing them in the bag as well.

7. Place hands under the cuff of the bag, unfolding it upward to contain the contaminated material. Close the bag and place it in the receptacle for contaminated waste (Fig. 11-22).

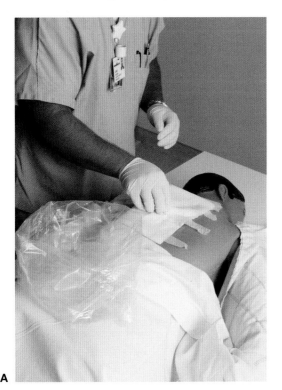
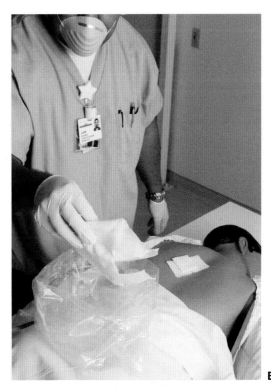

A   B

FIGURE 11-22 Place hands under the cuff of the waste receptacle and slowly unfold the cuff, keeping the contaminates in the bag.

(continued)

When the procedure has finished and a new dressing is to be applied, gather a new dressing of the appropriate size and tape.

1. Before beginning, determine whether the patient is allergic to the tape on hand. Then perform an aseptic handwash.

2. Tear off several pieces of tape and place them close at hand so that they may be applied to the dressing.

3. Open the dressing package, laying the wrapper flat to use as a sterile field. Do not remove the dressing at this point.

4. Put on a pair of clean gloves.

5. Pick up the dressing by handling only the top of the bandage (Fig. 11-23). This is not considered to be contaminated. Do not touch the other side of the bandage because this is still sterile.

6. Hold the bandage securely with both hands on the outside.

7. Carefully place the bandage over the wound area to be covered. Once it is in place, try not to readjust it repeatedly because the movement may damage or open the wound.

8. Remove the gloves in the proper manner. Secure the tape to the bandage and patient.

9. Perform a 30-second handwash.

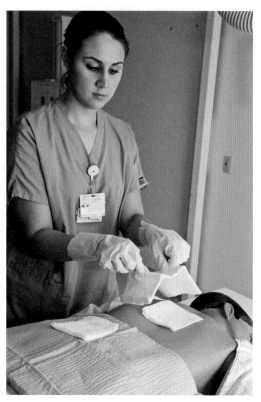

FIGURE 11-23 After putting on clean gloves, pick up the new dressing by touching only the top. The bottom will remain sterile and can be placed on the wound.

Packing and Storage of Medical Products

Aseptic packing of material uses ultrahigh temperatures that sterilize the product inside the package. Paper or plastic packaging material is used in the process of protecting products that must be sterile. Commercially packaged products are the most common types found in major hospital settings. However, an autoclave can be used to prepare cloth-wrapped packages in-house. If this is the case, two cloth wrappers are needed to place the material in that is to be sterilized. In addition, a color-changing strip of paper or tape is used to ensure that a certain temperature has been reached. When the correct temperature is reached, the tape turns from green to black (Fig. 11-24). This is placed inside the first wrapper with the product. After wrapping the product with both wrappers separately, the outside is closed with the color-changing tape and a date is then written on it so that an expiration date can be determined.

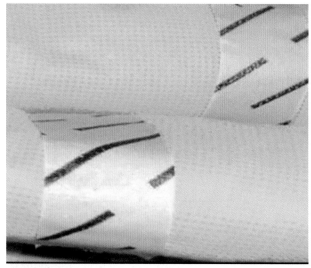

FIGURE 11-24 Temperature-indicating tape. Once the correct temperature has been reached, the green stripes will turn black.

Sterile instrument and supplies should be stored in covered or closed cabinets and never under sinks where they might become wet. Each facility has its own policies and procedures for storage and these must be followed at all times. The Joint Commission (TJC) checks how a facility, including the radiography department, stores its sterile equipment and issues citations if it is not properly done.

Shelf life is the period of time during which a sterile item is considered safe to use. Most packages are safe unless the package integrity has been broken or the expiration date on the package has been reached. If a package is outdated by even one day, it is no long considered to be sterile. Do not use it. Packages should not be stored against an outside wall because of the possible changes in temperature that might affect the inside of the package. High humidity will also affect sterility. Packages should not be packed tightly on a shelf or near a ceiling. Air must be allowed to flow through. Place packages that contain the same items in one area. Separate packages that contain different items. Figure 11-25 demonstrates what should not be done when storing sterile packs.

Linen

Linen in the imaging department must be handled with the same care as that used in the OR, ED, and in the patient's hospital rooms. The method with which linen is cleaned and stored is a criterion that TJC reviews when scoring a health care facility. This does include all areas within the department.

Although the cleaning of the linen is the duty of environmental services, how the linen gets from the radiology room to the laundry service area is important for review. The following steps should be carried out.

- Always wear gloves before handling obviously soiled linen.
- Never carry the linen against the body.
- Carefully roll up soiled linen to prevent contamination. Do not shake the linen.
- Place the soiled linen into a clearly labeled, leak-proof container in the room. The linen basket must have a lid.

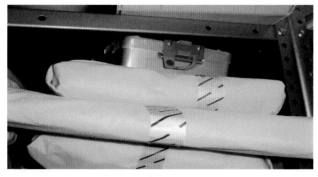

FIGURE 11-25 Sterile items should not be stored tightly on a shelf or with other types of items.

- Do not overfill the container, tie it securely, and remove it to the designated area for pickup.
- Hands should be washed thoroughly after handling the linen and removing gloves.

Clean linen should be stored in a designated room with a door that can be kept shut to prevent dust and other contaminates from settling on it. Nothing else should be stored in that area. If the linen is stored on a cart of some type, there must be a drape or closable screen that will protect the linen. Linen stored in a designated area must be a minimum of 8 inches from the floor, 18 in from the ceiling, and 2 inches away from the back wall. The door to the room must remain closed when not in use.

THE SURGICAL SCRUB

Although the radiographer is not often the "sterile person" in the OR, or in the special procedures rooms, they must be able to perform the surgical scrub if the situation calls for it. Before entering the surgical suite, the radiographer must change into a scrub suit, cover hair with a cap, cover shoes, and place a mask over the mouth and nose. Remove all jewelry. If ear studs are worn, they must be covered by the cap. If the radiographer is not to scrub, perform a 3-minute handwashing using an antiseptic soap.

The surgical scrub varies from institution to institution but the purpose is always the same—that is, to remove as many microorganisms as possible from the skin of the hands and lower arms by mechanical and chemical means and running water before a sterile procedure is begun. The procedures in this chapter are adequate for most cases.

1. Any person, including the radiographer, who will be present and unable to protect themselves from radiation, must don radiation-protective apparel before beginning the scrub. Arms should be bare to at least 4 in above the elbow.
2. Approach the sink. Adjust the water temperature and pressure. Most surgical scrub areas have either foot or knee pedals to regulate water flow.
3. Obtain a scrub brush. Brushes must be single use and disposable. Many have an antimicrobial agent permeated through them. The hands and forearms are wet to approximately 2 inches above the elbow. Hands must be held up to allow the water to drain downward toward the elbow from cleanest to dirtiest area. Apply the antimicrobial agent.
4. Scrub hands and arms using a firm, rotary motion. Fingers, hands, and arms should be considered to have four sides, all of which must be thoroughly cleansed. Follow an anatomic pattern, beginning with the thumb and proceeding to each finger. Next, do the dorsal surface of the hand, the palm, and up the wrist, ending 2 inches above the elbow. Wash all four sides of the arm. The surgical scrub always begins

with the hands because they are in direct contact with the sterile field (Fig. 11-26A-C). Rinse the soap from hands and arms and repeat the procedure.

5. When the scrub is completed, drop the brush into the sink or a receptacle prepared to receive used brushes. Do not touch the sink or the receptacle. Hold hands up above the waist and higher than the elbows during the surgical scrub.

6. Proceed to the area where a sterile towel, sterile gown, and sterile gloves have been prepared.

7. Pick up the towel, which is folded on top of the sterile gown, by one corner and let it drop and unfold in front of you at waist level. Do not let the towel touch the scrub suit or lead apron (Fig. 11-27A).

8. Dry one hand and one arm with each end of the towel. Do not go over areas already dried (Fig. 11-27B).

9. When hands and arms are dry, drop the towel to the floor or into a receptacle for this purpose. Do not let hands drop below the waist.

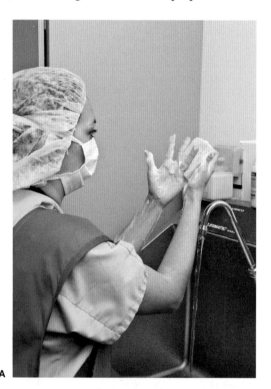

A

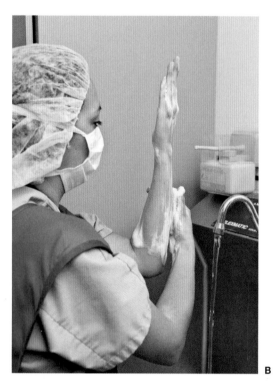

B

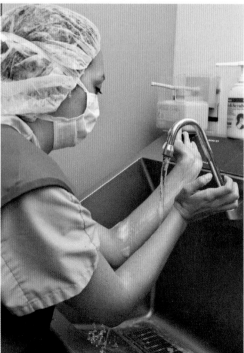

C

FIGURE 11-26 **(A)** Scrub the hand first because they are the dirtiest. **(B)** Next, scrub the wrists and forearms. Rinse and repeat. **(C)** For the final rinse, make sure the hands stay above the elbows so that dirty soap and water will not recontaminate the hands.

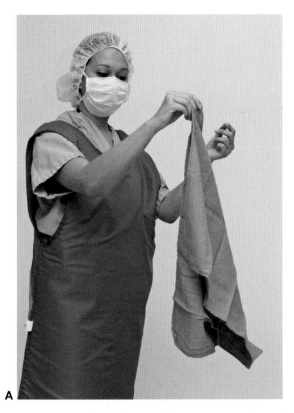 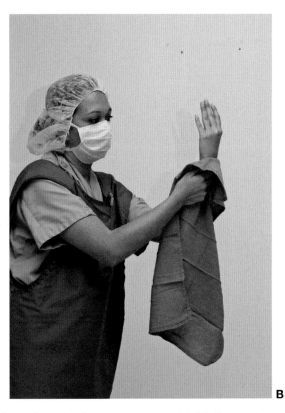

A   B

FIGURE 11-27 **(A)** Pick up the towel by one corner. Do not let it touch the body or below the waist. **(B)** Dry one hand and one arm with a corner of the towel. Use a separate corner for each part.

STERILE GOWNING AND GLOVING

If the radiographers must open their own sterile gown and towel pack, they must do this before they begin the surgical scrub. The gown is made of either a synthetic nonwoven material or cloth. To put it on, follow these steps:

1. Grasp the gown and remove it from the table.
2. Step away from the table. The gown is folded inside out.
3. Hold the gown away from the body and allow it to unfold lengthwise without touching the floor (Fig. 11-28A).
4. Open the gown and hold it by the shoulder seams. Place both arms into the armholes of the gown and wait for assistance (Fig. 11-28B). An assistant or the circulating nurse will place their hands inside the gown over your shoulders and pull the gown over the shoulders until your hands are exposed (Fig. 11-28C).

The radiographer is then ready to don sterile gloves. There are two methods of gloving—open and closed. For the radiographer's purposes, open gloving is most practical.

1. Open the wrapper as directed for opening sterile packs. Sterile gloves are always packaged folded down at the cuff and powdered so that they may be put on more easily.
2. Glove the dominant hand first. Assuming that the left hand is the dominant hand, pick up the left glove with the right hand at the folded cuff and slide the left hand into the glove, leaving the cuff folded down (Fig. 11-29A).
3. When the glove is over the hand, leave it and pick up the right glove with the gloved left hand under the fold (Fig. 11-29B).
4. Pull the glove over your hand and over the cuff of the gown (if you are wearing a sterile gown) in one motion (Fig. 11-29C).
5. Next, place the fingers of the gloved right hand under the cuff of the left glove and pull it over the cuff of the gown (Fig. 11-29D).

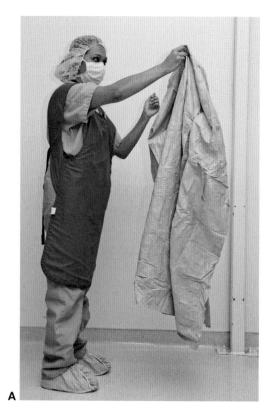

A

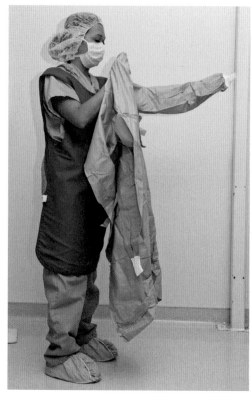

B

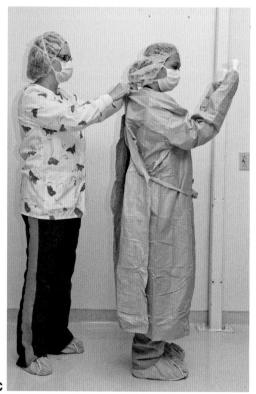

C

FIGURE 11-28 **(A)** Hold the gown away from the body and let it unfold. **(B)** Holding the shoulder inside seam, open the gown and place both arms inside the sleeves. **(C)** An assistant will pull the gown over the shoulders and tie the top tie.

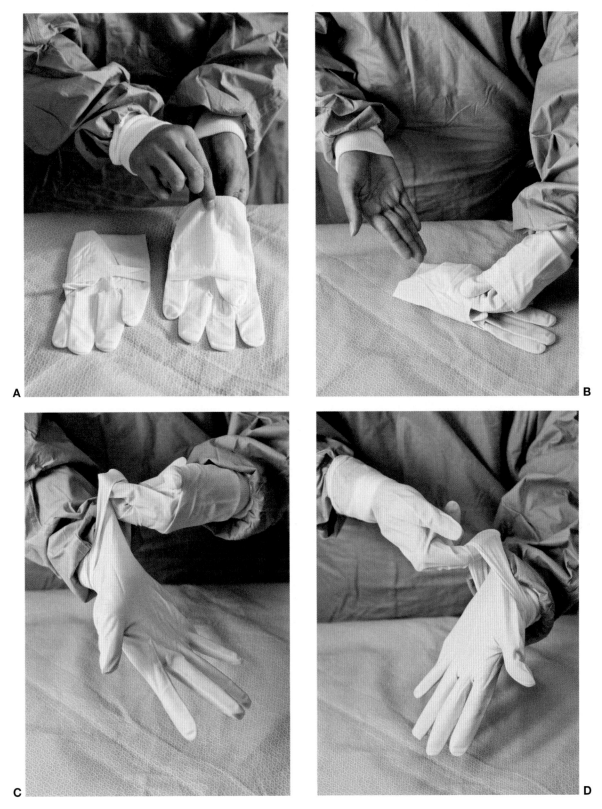

FIGURE 11-29 **(A)** Pick up the folded cuff with the nondominate hand. Be careful not to touch what is the outside of the glove. Pull the glove over the hand. **(B)** Once the dominate hand is covered, place the fingers inside the cuff of the remaining glove. **(C)** Pull that glove over the hand, unfolding the cuff over the sleeve of the gown. **(D)** Place the fingers of the nondominate hand under the cuff of the first glove, unfolding it over the sleeve of the gown.

Summary

1. Infections are caused by bacteria, fungi, and viruses.

   a. Bacteria contain both DNA and RNA. It is enclosed in an endospore that allows it to live in unfavorable conditions.

   b. Fungi require an aerobic environment to live and reproduce.

   c. Viruses are the smallest microorganisms. They are either RNA or DNA but not both, and must invade a host to live.

2. Growth requirements for microorganisms include water, oxygen, nitrogen, and phosphorous.

3. Nosocomial infections are acquired in the course of medical care either in an acute care hospital, long-term care facility, or in an outpatient clinic.

   a. Nosocomial infections are acquired through inadequately cleaned equipment.

      i. Urinary tract infections (UTIs) are most common because of the unsterile technique used when inserting the urinary catheter.

      ii. Bloodstream infections are also common because of the use of long-term use of VAD.

   b. Community-acquired infections are those that the individual has before entering a health care facility.

   c. Communicable diseases are spread from one person to another through a variety of ways.

      i. WHO and CDC support infection control measures.

   d. Multidrug-resistant organisms are resistant to more than one antibiotic, making treatment less effective.

      i. Those encountered in the hospital setting include MRSA, VRSA, and VRE.

4. The CDC has been creating tools and information for people to know what is needed to protect themselves.

   a. The CDC tracks diseases to understand and predict the threat of health issues affecting a population.

5. The cycle of infection includes a reservoir (environment), in which pathogenic microbes can live and multiply, an exit portal, a means of transmission, and an entry portal into a new host.

   a. Transmission includes the following:

      i. Direct: Infected patient touches a susceptible host.

      ii. Indirect: Inanimate object known as a fomite that contains infectious material touches a susceptible host.

      iii. Airborne: Droplets and dust are breathed in by a susceptible host.

      iv. Droplets: Water-based spray from a sneeze or cough

      v. Vectors: Animals that contain infectious material bite or otherwise transmit the infection to a susceptible host.

      vi. Vehicles: Food or water that contains infectious material is ingested by a new host.

6. Preventing Transmission

   a. Dress: Wear a clean uniform, long hair should be tied up, acrylic fingernails should not be worn, and nails should be kept short. Protect the eyes with the use of goggles or the use of a face shield.

   b. Gloves: Standard Precautions state that clean gloves should be worn with every patient that has any blood or body fluids that the radiographer may come into contact with.

      i. Remove gloves after each patient and wash hands.

      ii. Use a chemical hand sanitizer.

   c. Cleaning radiographic equipment after every patient is a must. This includes the mobile unit and IRs.

      i. Use ethanol 75% or a disinfectant that the manufacturer suggests.

   d. Transferring a patient with a communicable disease should only be done if absolutely necessary.

      i. Mask the patient and the transporter.

      ii. Wrap the patient in a cotton blanket that can be properly cleaned after the transfer.

      iii. Do not touch the inside of the blanket once it has been on the patient.

   e. Health institutions require staff to be vaccinated for hepatitis B, TB, the flu, and COVID-19.

      i. Waivers are available for some of the vaccinations depending on place of employment.

      ii. Boosters to the vaccines may also be required.

7. Precautions and Isolation

   a. Standard Precautions (originally called Universal Precautions) are the first level of transmission-based isolation precautions.

   b. It assumes that all body fluids are sources of infections and that all patients are infected.

   c. Always wear gloves if in contact with body substances.

   d. Wear a mask, gown, and/or eye protection if there is any possibility of blood or body fluid getting on clothes, or the mouth and nose.

   e. Because hands are the most common transmission of infection, hand hygiene is the most important means of stopping the spread.

   f. Transmission-Based Precautions

      i. Contact: Private room, appropriate PPE, hand hygiene

    ii. Droplet: Private room, masks must be worn, hand hygiene

    iii. Airborne: Private room with proper ventilation, N95 masks required, restricted entrance, hand hygiene

  g. Protective isolation protects the patient. Also called expanded, strict, or reverse isolation

    i. Appropriate PPE and hand hygiene

    ii. No flowers or plants allowed

    iii. Visitors are limited.

  h. Psychological effects of being in isolation should be considered.

    i. Treat the patient as a human with dignity.

    ii. Spend some time answering questions.

8. Asepsis: Two types are medical and surgical asepsis.

  a. Medical asepsis eliminates the microorganisms as much as possible through soap, water, and chemicals.

  b. Handwashing is the number one way to stop the spread of infection.

    i. Hand sanitizers can also be used between patients and after glove removal.

    ii. Fifteen seconds is minimum time to wash "clean" hands.

    iii. Three minutes should be minimum for contaminated hands.

  c. Chemical disinfectants are categorized as high, intermediate, or low level depending on their ability to disinfect.

    i. Glutaraldehyde (high level), iodine and iodophors (intermediate level), and hydrogen peroxide (low level) are some common disinfectants.

    ii. Skin cannot be sterilized, so it is disinfected using chemicals and scrubbing (physical).

  d. Surgical asepsis is defined as the complete removal of microorganisms and their spores.

    i. Rules for surgical asepsis must be followed.

    ii. Methods of sterilization include the following:

      1. Steam under pressure (autoclave) is best and the most often used type.

      2. Dry heat can only sterilize the surface of an object.

      3. Chemicals (low-temperature sterilization), using gas.

9. Sterile procedures

  a. Radiographers must follow the procedure to open a sterile pack to keep the inside of the pack sterile.

    i. This means not crossing over the open tray.

  b. Preparation of the skin involves removing as many microorganisms as possible to reduce the possibility of infection.

    i. Mechanical and chemical methods are used.

  c. Draping the skin with sterile drapes after it has been prepped will keep the area as free from microorganisms as possible.

    i. There is a proper method of placing sterile towels so that one does not cross the prepped field.

    ii. The use of a fenestrated drape protects the cleaned area.

  d. Dressing changes are not likely to be performed by the radiographer.

    i. May be done by others such as sonographers if dressing is in the way of a scan

    ii. Must be performed without contaminating anything with the contents on the dressing

  e. Most sterile packs are commercially wrapped and enclosed in a sealed outer bag.

    i. Storage of sterile packages must follow the guidelines of the hospital or clinic.

    ii. Must be kept dry

    iii. Shelf life must be adhered to for sterility purposes.

  f. Linen must be stored in a separate enclosed area if not in its own room.

    i. TJC mandates specific criteria to keep linen clean.

10. Surgical scrub is performed before a sterile gown and gloves are donned for a surgical aseptic procedure.

11. Surgical gowning and gloving procedures are specific to guarantee sterility of a person.

  a. Radiographers must know the procedure for gowning so as to be able to help in the OR if needed.

  b. The open gloving method for putting on sterile gloves is easiest and should be practiced until perfected.

CHAPTER 11 REVIEW QUESTIONS

1. Mr. Ryan has been a patient at the community hospital for 3 days. During his stay in the hospital, he was taken to the diagnostic imaging department several times where he was cared for by a radiographer who had an upper respiratory infection. Two days after he returned home from the hospital, he also developed an infection. It would be appropriate to say that Mr. Ryan had developed:
   a. An iatrogenic infection
   b. A nosocomial infection
   c. A community-acquired infection
   d. A blood-borne infection

2. Mary Mandura has been hospitalized for several weeks as a result of multiple injuries suffered in an automobile accident. She has been treated with a series of broad-spectrum antibiotics to discourage infection. She now has severe diarrhea and the stool culture has produced *C. difficile*. This would be called:
   a. A blood-borne infection
   b. A community-acquired infection
   c. A viral infection
   d. A superinfection

3. Hepatitis B and C are blood-borne viral infections. When caring for persons known to have either of these diseases, use the following infection control techniques. (Circle all that apply)
   a. Wear gloves if you are likely to come in contact with blood or body substances.
   b. Wear goggles if there is a possibility of your being splashed with blood or body substances.
   c. Wear a particulate mask at all times.
   d. Wear a waterproof gown or apron if there is a possibility that your clothing may be splashed by blood or body substances.

4. The radiographer should always dress for the workplace with infection control in mind. This means that:
   a. Clothing must be washable; fingernails must be kept short; and shoes must be comfortable and have closed toes.
   b. The radiographer must look unattractive because anything that looks good spreads infection.
   c. A scrub suit must be worn at all times.
   d. The rules are to be followed when TJC is inspecting the institution where you work.

5. Microorganisms that need a host cell to reproduce and are virtually unresponsive to antimicrobial drugs are:
   a. Bacteria
   b. Fungi
   c. Prions
   d. Viruses

6. The radiographer must use strict infection control measures that include blood and body substance precautions for:
   a. Every patient who enters the diagnostic imaging department
   b. Patients who have known communicable diseases
   c. Only patients who have AIDS and hepatitis B
   d. Patients who seem ill

7. Blood and body substance precautions include:
   a. Use of clean, disposable gloves for sick persons
   b. Use of clean, disposable gloves for contact of the hands with blood or body fluids; a mask and goggles if blood or body fluids may spray on your face; and a gown if the blood and body fluids may touch your clothing for any patient care that may involve contact with blood or body fluids
   c. Clean, disposable gloves as necessary
   d. Gown, gloves, mask, and goggles for all patient care

8. The most common means of spreading infection are:
   a. Soiled instruments
   b. Infected patients
   c. Human hands
   d. Domestic animals

9. The elements needed to produce an infection are a source, a host, and a means of transmission. An example of a source of infection might be:
   a. A visitor in the hospital who has a "fever blister" on the mouth
   b. A patient who develops pneumonia
   c. A radiography student who has a cold and comes to work
   d. All of these

10. A safety precaution that must be taken when disposing of used hypodermic needles and syringes is:
    a. To place the needles in the waste basket as soon as possible
    b. To recap the needle and dispose of it quickly
    c. To place the syringe immediately after use with the uncapped needle attached directly into the contaminated waste receptacle provided
    d. To detach the needle from the syringe and place only the needle in the contaminated waste receptacle

11. When sterile drapes are placed by the sterile person, the drape is placed:
    a. In the area farthest away from the sterile person first
    b. In the area nearest the sterile person first
    c. Over the operative site first
    d. It is not important which area is placed first

12. Hand hygiene is to be used in the following situations by radiographers in the workplace: (Circle all that apply)

    a. Before caring for a patient
    b. After caring for a patient
    c. When preparing for invasive procedures
    d. After eating or using the restroom

13. When opening a sterile wrapper, the fold closest to the radiographer is opened first.

    a. True
    b. False

14. The route of transmission of MRSA, VRE, VRSA, and ESBL is:

    a. Droplet contact
    b. Airborne contact
    c. Direct contact
    d. Vector contact

15. What must be done when the radiographer is to enter the newborn nursery? (Circle all that apply)

    a. Always wear a cap and mask.
    b. Always scrub hands for 3 minutes.
    c. Always clean the equipment with disinfectant solution.
    d. Ask the nurse to take the x-ray.

PART III

SPECIAL PROCEDURES

Pharmacology for Radiographers

12

OBJECTIVES

After studying this chapter, the student will be able to:

1. Describe the symptoms and medical interventions for a patient having a reaction to contrast media.

2. Distinguish between the chemical, generic, and trade names of various drugs.

3. Explain the uses and impact on the patient of different categories of drugs.

4. Define the categories of contrast agents and give examples for each category.

5. Describe general pharmacologic principles of radiologic contrast media.

6. Describe the pharmacokinetic, pharmacodynamic, and pharmacogenetic principles of drugs.

7. Identify and explain drug safety in the administration of contrast and other drugs.

8. Describe methods and techniques for administering various types of contrast media.

KEY TERMS

Adverse reaction: An effect produced by a drug that is severe or life-threatening

Affinity: The chemical force that impels particular atoms or molecules to unite

Alternative therapies: Natural plant extracts, herbs, vitamins, minerals, and therapeutic techniques, such as massage and acupuncture

Angina: A severe constricting pain or sensation in the chest that may radiate to shoulder or arm; related to coronary artery disease

Aqueous: Watery

Bioavailability: Physiologic availability of a given amount of a drug

Biologic: A medicine derived from living products and not chemicals

Biotransformation: The alteration of a substance (drug) within the body.

Clearance rate: The amount of time it takes for a drug to leave the body

Contraindication: A situation in which a drug should not be used because it may be harmful to the patient

Dependence: Reliance on a drug that may be physiologic or psychological in nature

Drug: Any substance, other than food, used to prevent, diagnose, treat, or cure a disease

Enteral: Within the gastrointestinal (GI) tract

First-pass effect: Partial metabolism of a drug before it reaches the systemic circulation

Half-life: The time it takes for the drug present in the body to be decreased by 50%

Hypertonic: The same as hyperosmolar; when a fluid is hypertonic, it creates dehydration.

Indication: The basis for initiation of treatment or use of a particular drug

Intra-arterial: Within the artery

Intra-articular: Into the cavity of the joint

Intraosseous: Contrast media can be injected into the humerus when normal intravenous (IV) access is not available.

Intrathecal: Route of drug administration into the spinal canal (subarachnoid space)

Lipoid: Pertaining to fat

Macromolecular: A molecule in a finely divided state dispersed in liquid or solid media

Medication: Treatment of a disease by giving drugs

Metabolism: Alteration of the chemical structure by the body

Narcotic: Any drug synthetic or naturally occurring that induces a state of stuporous analgesia

Parenterally: Refers to administration of a drug by penetrating the skin

Pharmacodynamics: The study of uptake, movement, binding, and interactions of drugs at the area of interaction in the tissue

Pharmacokinetics: The study of the movement of drugs within biologic systems and includes absorption, distribution, metabolism, and excretion

Pharmacology: The science concerned with drugs and their sources, appearance, chemistry, actions, and uses

Radiolucent: Classification of contrast agents that allow the photon energy to pass through it, creating a dark area on the image

Radiopaque: Classification of contrast media that absorb the photon energy, creating a white area on the image

Retrograde: Instillation of contrast in the direction opposite to that of the physiologic flow of fluids in the body

Side effect: An effect produced by a drug that is mild, common, unintended, and nontoxic

Sublingual: Under the tongue

Thrombosis: Clotting within a blood vessel

Tonicity: The osmotic pressure of a solution relative to that of blood

Topical: Designed for or involving local application and action (on the skin)

Toxic reaction: A life-threatening effect of a drug that may occur immediately or over a long period of the particular drug's administration

Vasovagal: A type of effect that occurs from high anxiety rather than from the actual examination or drug injection

INTRODUCTION

Pharmacology is the study of drug actions and interactions with living organisms. Drugs are chemical substances that are not required for normal maintenance of body function but produce a **biologic** effect in an organism. All drugs are, or can be if misused, poisons. If used correctly, they are meant to relieve human diseases and suffering.

There are three categories assigned to substances applied or administered for therapeutic purposes—drugs or medications, biologics, and alternative therapies. A **drug** is a chemical agent capable of producing biologic responses in the body. These responses may be desirable (therapeutic) or undesirable (adverse). After a drug is administered, it is called a **medication**. A biologic is an agent naturally produced in animal cells, microorganisms, or by the body itself, such as hormones, natural blood products, or vaccines. **Alternative therapies** include natural plant extracts, herbs, vitamins, minerals, dietary supplements, and therapeutic techniques that may be considered unconventional, such as acupuncture.

Pharmacology and its clinical application is a scientific discipline unto itself and cannot be covered adequately without combining theoretical knowledge and clinical coursework. Drug therapy is a complex and ever-changing aspect of patient care. The radiographer is not licensed to dispense drugs nor able to enter a hospital pharmacy and select a drug. Radiographers are held legally liable if any drug taken from a dispensary results in adverse effects. If a drug error is made by the radiographer, the incident must be completely documented and an institutional incident report must be completed according to the policy of the employer.

DRUG STANDARDS AND CONTROL

The federal government of the United States has standards for control of drug safety that are strictly enforced. These drugs must bear the legend "Caution: Federal law

prohibits dispensing without prescription." The drugs that must have this on the label are those that:

Must be administered **parenterally**

Are hypnotic or **narcotic**

May cause **dependence**

Contain derivatives of habit-forming substances

May be toxic if not administered under the supervision of a physician, dentist, or nurse practitioner

Are new and limited to investigational use and are not safe if used indiscriminately

Drugs that are considered safe for self-administration are called over-the-counter (OTC) drugs. Some drugs that must be prescribed may also be purchased as OTC drugs because they are marketed in a lesser potency when sold in this manner. OTC drugs must also be reviewed by the U.S. Food and Drug Administration (FDA) and deemed safe for self-administration. When taking a patient's drug history as part of an initial assessment, the patient's use of OTC drugs and alternative medications is important information because they may affect treatment.

Alternative dietary and herbal supplements are not regulated by the FDA in the United States. They are regulated and classified as foods, not drugs. There is no requirement to prove the efficacy, quality, or safety of these substances. These treatments are not part of standard medical care.

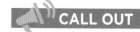 **CALL OUT**

Any alternative medicines, regardless of the type or use, must be included in a drug history of the patient, especially if one is about to undergo interventional radiography.

DRUG NOMENCLATURE

Drugs come from many natural and synthetic sources. Some are produced from animal sources, such as hormonal drugs. Many come from plant sources, such as digitalis and atropine. Others are produced from microorganisms, as are many antibiotics. Minerals are the source of calcium, iron, and other dietary supplements and herbal remedies. Drugs from synthetic materials are made in laboratories. Some drugs are genetically engineered and used to treat specific diseases. Learning drug names is complicated because most drugs have several names. The following list should help sort out the way drugs are named:

- *Proprietary* or *trade* names are assigned to a drug by a particular manufacturer of the drug.
- *Chemical name* presents the exact chemical formula of a drug and always remains the same.
- *Generic name* of a drug is the name given to a drug before its official approval for use. It is assigned by the U.S. Adopted Name Council. This is the name used to describe the drug. There is one generic name for each drug and, because it is often used, it must be learned by all persons who administer drugs. For instance, a drug frequently administered before imaging procedures is parenteral diazepam. Diazepam is the generic name for Valium. The radiographer must be able to identify certain drugs by their trade name and their generic name.

It is seldom possible for a health care practitioner to keep up with all new drugs that are marketed. Those who administer drugs must be able to obtain information concerning the drug from reliable sources before administering a drug they are not familiar with. Some reliable references are *The American Hospital Formulary Service (AHFS) Drug Information*, and the *Physician's Desk Reference*. These references are updated yearly. The radiographer must learn where a reliable drug reference is available in the workplace and consult it as necessary.

DRUG CLASSIFICATION

Although almost everyone understands that there are classifications of drugs, not everyone understands what that classification means. Drugs are classified in various ways depending on the expert that is doing the classification and the reason for the classification. However, drugs are classified by their similarities, such as their medical value or the risk of dependence and misuse. Three methods of classification (used by the United States Department of Veterans Affairs) include chemical structure of the drug; cellular mechanism and organ of the drug's effects; and the therapeutic intent of the drug. Pharmacology classification is known as schedules and is listed in Table 12-1.

Chemical Groups

Drugs affect the body's central nervous system. They affect emotions and behavior. Chemical classification of drugs is grouped depending on the specific chemicals found in the drug. The three main classifications are as follows:

- Depressants: These slow the function of the central nervous system. There is a feeling of relaxation and loss of inhibition. Coordination and concentration are affected and a person's ability to respond to

TABLE 12-1	Drug Schedules		
Schedule	**Characteristics**	**Dispensing Restrictions**	**Examples**
I	High abuse potential; not recognized for medical use; may lead to severe dependence	Limited or no therapeutic use	Heroin, lysergic acid diethylamide, cocaine, and others
II	High abuse potential; accepted for medical use; may lead to severe dependence	Handwritten prescription by a licensed person; no refills; container must have warning label.	Opioids, methadone, morphine, and others; Demerol, OxyContin, morphine
III	Less abuse potential; accepted for medical use; may lead to dependence	Written or oral prescription required; container must have warning label.	Codeine, hydrocodeine with aspirin or Tylenol, nonamphetamine stimulants; Vicodin
IV	Lower abuse potential; may lead to limited dependence	Written or oral prescription that expires in 6 mo	Benzodiazepines, non-narcotic analgesics, Valium, Versed, Halcion
V	Low level of dependence	May or may not require prescription	Antidiarrheals, cough medicines with codeine

situations is slower. Examples include alcohol, opiates, and tranquilizers.

- Stimulants: These speed up the function of the central nervous system. There is an increase in heart rate, blood pressure, and body temperature. The appetite is reduced and there may be insomnia. Examples of stimulants include caffeine, nicotine, and amphetamines.
- Hallucinogens: These distort a sense of what is real. There may be euphoria or panic and paranoia. Effects include gastric upset and nausea. Examples of hallucinogens are ketamine, and lysergic acid diethylamide (LSD).

GENERAL PHARMACOLOGIC PRINCIPLES

Pharmacologic effects of a drug include the mechanism and site of action as well as the effects of that drug. A drug does not have the capacity to change cellular structure but acts to either increase or decrease the rate and range of a normal or an abnormal physiologic process going on within the cells of the body. Drugs are absorbed, distributed, metabolized, and then excreted from the body. As this process takes place, the drug reaches a point at which it has its *intended effect*. This is called the *onset of action*. As it continues to be absorbed, the drug reaches its peak concentration level. This is the time during which the drug attains its maximum therapeutic response. This means that the drug is able to produce its most desired curative or remedial effect. The time during which the drug is in the body in an amount large enough to be therapeutic is called its *duration of action*. As the drug is excreted from the body, the concentration level subsides to a point at which there is little or no intended effect.

Pharmacokinetics

The processes that control absorption, distribution, **metabolism**, and excretion of drugs by the body are called **pharmacokinetics**. People process drugs differently depending on their age, nutritional status, ethnicity, existing physical condition, immune status, state of mind, gender, weight, environmental factors, and time of day.

A drug must be absorbed and taken through the bloodstream to its intended site in order to act. The amount of drug that actually reaches the systemic circulation becomes *bioavailable* or reaches a state of **bioavailability**. Drug absorption varies from person to person and depends on the absorptive surface available. An intended drug surface that is damaged or absent alters the length of time it takes a drug to reach its intended site.

Drugs move to their site of absorption and then must penetrate the cell membrane at that site. This is accomplished by varying methods. One method is *passive diffusion (passive transport)*, which requires no cellular energy. The drug simply moves across a cell membrane from an area of higher concentration to one of lower concentration. This is known as moving down the gradient. When the concentration equalizes on both sides of the cell membrane, the transport is complete. *Lipid solubility* is the most important determinant in deciding whether a drug will cross cell membranes, although water solubility is also important. Most drugs cross cell membranes by passive diffusion.

Active transport is another method of drug absorption. Active transport is necessary to move some drugs and electrolytes, such as sodium and potassium, from outside to inside a cell. This method requires energy from the cell and a carrier molecule, such as an enzyme or protein that forms complexes with drug molecules on the membrane surface, to carry them through the membrane and then leave them by disassociation. This requires energy because the drugs are moving from an area of higher concentration to one of lower concentration, or moving down the gradient. Pinocytosis is a type of active transport in which a cell engulfs a drug particle, forms a protective coat around it, and transports it across the cell membrane.

Drugs taken orally are usually absorbed in the small intestine, which has a large surface for absorption. If a portion of the small intestine has been removed or is scarred, the ability to absorb a drug is reduced.

The quantity of blood flow to absorption surfaces affects the rate at which a drug is absorbed. For instance, a drug is absorbed much more rapidly when it is administered intramuscularly in the deltoid muscle than in the gluteal muscle because the blood flow is greater in the deltoid. A person who is in severe pain or in a state of acute stress may have decreased ability to absorb a drug.

First-Pass Effect

When a drug is taken orally and swallowed into the stomach, it goes from the small intestine to the mesenteric vascular system and then to the portal vein and from there into the liver before it is transported into the systemic circulation. Because of this travel through the gastric and hepatic circulation, a portion of the drug is metabolized en route and becomes inactive. This partial metabolism of a drug before it reaches the systemic circulation is called a **first-pass effect**. In the case of many drugs taken orally, this effect requires that a larger dose of a drug be administered so that a portion of the drug remains to perform its intended effect. Drugs that can be administered by the sublingual, vaginal, or parenteral route avoid the first-pass effect by going directly into the systemic circulation; however, these routes of administration may be contraindicated for other reasons.

Some drugs, after absorption, are moved from the bloodstream into the liver and then through the biliary tract, where they are excreted in the bile or return to the small intestine and back into the bloodstream. This action, called *enterohepatic recycling*, allows the drug to persist in the body for long periods.

 WARNING!

The dosages of most drugs given orally are generally much larger than those given by parenteral routes because they are susceptible to the first-pass effect!

Distribution

After a drug is absorbed into the body, it is distributed to its intended target site. The rate and extent of distribution depends on adequate blood circulation, protein binding, and the drug's **affinity** for **lipoid** or **aqueous** tissues. Drugs move quickly to body organs that have a rich supply of blood, such as the heart, liver, and kidneys. They reach muscles and fatty tissues more slowly.

As a drug travels through the circulatory system, it may come into contact with plasma proteins and bind to them or remain free. If bound to plasma protein, the drug becomes inactive. Only free drugs are able to act on cells. As the free drug acts, there is a decrease in plasma drug levels, which allows a portion of the bound drug to be released and become active. The slow release of the drug allows blood levels of a drug to remain somewhat constant. The health status of the person receiving the drug and the drug itself affects drug distribution.

Metabolism

The process by which the body alters the chemical structure of a drug or other foreign substance is called metabolism or **biotransformation**. These terms are interchangeable. Generally, this process reduces lipid solubility to render the drug ready for excretion.

Most drugs are metabolized in the liver by means of a complex chemical action involving enzymes. These enzymes act on a wide variety of compounds. In certain drugs, tissues from the plasma, kidneys, lungs, and intestinal mucosa may be involved.

Age, health status, time of day, emotional status, the presence of other drugs in the body, genetic variations, and disease states may alter the rate of drug metabolism. An altered metabolic state may allow a drug to accumulate in the body and produce an **adverse reaction**. Conversely, rapid metabolism of a drug may interfere with the intended effect. Drugs administered orally are significantly metabolized by the first-pass effect through the liver, which also alters their metabolism.

Excretion

Excretion of drugs from the body takes place chiefly in the kidneys. Some drugs are excreted virtually unchanged through the kidneys, whereas others are extensively metabolized with only a small amount of the original drug remaining.

Other sites of drug excretion are through the biliary tract and into the feces or through the enterohepatic cycle and later into the kidneys. Gases and volatile liquids used for anesthesia are excreted by the lungs. Sweat and saliva are of minimal importance in drug excretion.

Half-life

The time it takes for a 50% decrease in a drug's presence in the body is called its **half-life**. It is important for a prescribing health care worker to understand a drug's half-life in order to attain a steady-state concentration in the body. To attain this steady state, the same amount of a drug must be taken in, as is eliminated in, each 24-hour period. Drugs with a short half-life need to be administered more frequently than is a drug with a prolonged half-life in order to be at maximum therapeutic level at all times.

A drug's removal from the body is called its **clearance rate**. The clearance rate of a drug is an important consideration because a drug with a slow clearance rate that is given too often may accumulate in the body and reach a toxic level. Contrast media, the drugs most used by radiographers and other imaging professionals, have a very fast distribution through the body. Because they are not metabolized as other drugs are, the contrast is excreted through the kidneys in about 24 hours.

Pharmacodynamics

Pharmacodynamics is the study of the method or mechanism of drug action on living tissues or the response of tissues to chemical agents at various sites in the body. Drugs may alter the physiologic effects in the body in the following ways:

1. By altering blood pressure
2. By altering heart rate
3. By altering urinary output
4. By altering the function of the central or peripheral nervous system
5. By altering changes in all other body systems

Drugs do not produce new functions on tissues or organs of the body. Usually, a primary site of drug action is targeted by a drug that is administered systemically; nevertheless, all body tissues are affected in some way by every drug administered. The beginning and ending point of drug action is generally considered the pharmacodynamic effect. This describes the outcome effects after the drug reaches the site of action.

The particular area for which a drug is intended and that receives the maximum effect of a drug is called the *drug receptor*. The function of a cell is altered but not completely changed by a drug. A drug receptor is a **macromolecular** component of body tissue.

Drug receptors have an *affinity* for a particular drug. This means that there is an attraction between the drug and the receptor. Affinity is the factor that determines the concentration of drug necessary to accomplish its intended effect. If there is a strong affinity at the receptor site, the concentration of drug necessary to accomplish its effect is low. This is referred to as the *efficacy* of the drug. The molecular structure of each drug determines the affinity for a receptor. A very small change in a drug molecule can leave the drug's affinity for a receptor unchanged but drastically change the pharmacologic action of a drug.

Pharmacogenomics

The branch of pharmacology that studies the effect of genetic factors as they are related to drug reactions is known as pharmacogenomics, sometimes called pharmacogenetics. This studies how people's genes affect the way they respond to drugs and, in this manner, the best drug or dose can be prescribed for that particular person.

An example is the drug amitriptyline and depression. This drug is affected by two genes known as *CYP2D6* and *CYP2C19*. Therefore, the physician might test the patient to see whether these genes are present before prescribing the drug amitriptyline.

DRUGS RELEVANT TO RADIOGRAPHY

Table 12-2 is the list of drug categories that radiographers may, at some point in their career, become involved with. The table discusses the uses and effects of those drugs listed under each category.

TABLE 12-2 | **Drug Categories Relevant to Radiography**

Trade Name	Generic Name	Uses	Adverse Effect
Analgesics and anti-inflammatory drugs: Used to reduce pain, reduce fever, and reduce inflammation in tissues			
Motrin Advil	Ibuprofen analgesic drugs (NSAIDs)	Used to treat moderate pain usually related to muscle or neurologic origins	Gastric distress, renal failure, prolonged bleeding time
Aspirin	Acetylsalicylic acid	Used to treat mild pain or fever, arthritic conditions, and inflammatory condition, to prevent **thrombosis**	Tinnitus, nausea, GI bleeding
Tylenol	Acetaminophen	Used to treat moderate pain without anti-inflammatory effects	Liver toxicity, hemolytic anemia, skin rash
Morphine Demerol Duragesic	Morphine sulfate Meperidine Hydrochloride Fentanyl citrate	All are used to control severe pain; all may create dependence; all are kept in locked storage.	Nausea, restlessness, respiratory depression, shock, death
Codeine Percocet Darvon	Codeine sulfate Oxycodone Hydrochloride propoxyphene napsylate	All are used alone and in various combinations with milder analgesics to control less severe pain.	Sedation, clouded sensorium, dizziness, nausea, constipation, dependence
Anesthetics: Drugs that prevent patients from feeling pain during procedures. There are three types—general, regional, and local.			
Diprivan	Propofol	Induces sleep	Nausea, vomiting, dry mouth, muscle aches
Lidocaine	Lignocaine	Used as a local anesthetic to numb a body part	Local effects occurring at site of injection
Nitrous oxide		Can be used for general anesthesia or procedural sedation, also to treat severe pain	Respiratory depression, hypoxia, nausea, and vomiting

TABLE 12-2	Drug Categories Relevant to Radiography (*continued*)		
Trade Name	**Generic Name**	**Uses**	**Adverse Effect**
Antianxiety drugs: Benzodiazepines are used for treatment of anxiety and, in some cases, to treat behavior disorders. Antidepressant drugs: Medications used to treat major depressive disorder, some anxiety disorders, some chronic pain conditions, and to help manage some addictions.			
Xanax Ativan Valium	Alprazolam Lorazepam Diazepam	All are used to reduce anxiety; at higher doses, produce hypnosis, relax muscles, and may reduce seizure activity.	Bradycardia, drowsiness, severe withdrawal reaction with prolonged used; dependence
Celexa Lexapro Zoloft	Citalopram Escitalopram Sertraline	All work to balance chemicals in the brain that affect mood and emotions.	Headache, nausea, vomiting, diarrhea, insomnia
Antiarrhythmics: Used to correct arrhythmias of the heart due to electrical abnormalities in formation or conduction that may be life-threatening			
Quinaglute	Quinidine	Used to maintain normal cardiac rhythm	Hypotension, heart block, liver toxicity
Xylocaine	Lidocaine hydrochloride	Used to treat serious ventricular arrhythmias, also used as a local anesthetic	Cardiac arrest, respiratory depression, convulsions
Cordarone	Amiodarone hydrochloride	Used to treat life-threatening ventricular fibrillations	Pulmonary toxicity, ataxia, hypothyroidism
Antibacterial drugs: Used to specifically treat infections caused by bacteria such as *Staphylococcus*, *Streptococcus*, and *Escherichia coli*			
Augmentin	Clavulanate potassium	Treats pneumonia, ear infections, bronchitis, UTI	Nausea, vomiting, diarrhea, vaginal itching
Levaquin	Levofloxacin	Treats active TB, complicated skin infections	Dizziness, nausea, fast heart rate
Penicillin	Penicillium fungi	Ear, throat, and skin infections	Diarrhea, fever, bruising
Cipro	Ciprofloxacin	Treats pneumonia and other URI	Headache, dizziness, nausea
Anticholinergics: Drugs that block the action of a neurotransmitter that causes involuntary muscle movement associated with certain diseases such as Parkinson			
Atropen	Atropine	To treat conditions such as bradycardia, and reduce salivation and bronchial secretions	Fast heart rate, glaucoma, dry mouth, dizziness, nausea
Ditropan XL	Oxybutynin	Treats overactive bladder	Swelling of the eyes, lips, genitals, drowsiness, confusion, agitation, dementia
Anticoagulants: Used to prevent thrombus formations before surgical and imaging procedures. They are used to prevent extension of thrombi after myocardial infarction.			
Heparin	Heparin sodium	Inhibits formation of fibrin clots; used to maintain potency of venous catheters	Hemorrhage, thrombocytopenia, allergic reactions
Coumadin	Warfarin sodium	Prevention of emboli in chronic atrial fibrillation, DVT, heart valve damage	Hemorrhage, hematuria, hepatitis
Menadione	Vitamin K_3	Assists in normal clotting of blood	Skin rash, muscle stiffness, dizziness, chest pain

(continued)

| TABLE 12-2 | Drug Categories Relevant to Radiography (*continued*) |

Trade Name	Generic Name	Uses	Adverse Effect
Anticonvulsant drugs: All are used to prevent and treat seizures such as epilepsy.			
Tegretol Zarontin Dilantin	Carbamazepine Ethosuximide Phenytoin	Controls seizures, pain, and bipolar disorder	Dermatologic reactions, aplastic anemia, cramps, drowsiness
Antidiabetics: Drugs developed to stabilize and control blood glucose levels and to help manage diabetes			
Glucophage	Metformin	Used for type 2 diabetes to control high blood sugar	Nausea, vomiting, stomach upset
Precose	Acarbose	Used to treat type 2 diabetes in combination with insulin	Diarrhea, gas, bloating
Antiemetics: Used to treat motion sickness, nausea, and vomiting. All are used for similar purposes but belong to various drug categories and have various adverse effects.			
Compazine Transderm-Scop Dramamine Vistaril	Prochlorperazine Scopolamine Dimenhydrinate Hydroxyzine	Nausea and vomiting Patch for N/V Motion sickness Anxiety, itching	Because each of these have various adverse effects, the radiographer is responsible for becoming familiar with them.
Antihistamines: Used to treat anaphylactic shock, upper respiratory disorders, acute urticaria, edema, hypersensitivity reactions, motion sickness, and nausea. Some are used OTC as sleep medications.			
Benadryl	Diphenhydramine	Used to prevent anaphylaxis	Drowsiness, dizziness, dry mouth
Chlor-Trimeton	Chlorpheniramine	Used to treat symptoms of colds and allergies	
Phenergan	Promethazine	Used for sedative effects and for motion sickness	
Antihypertensive drugs: Calcium channel blockers that reduce calcium flow to the heart and relax smooth muscle tone and reduce muscle spasm			
Cardizem	Diltiazem	Used to treat **angina** and hypertension	Peripheral edema, bradycardia
Calan	Verapamil hydrochloride	Used to treat angina, cardiac arrhythmias, hypertension	Peripheral edema, bradycardia
Antiviral drugs: Have relatively limited use, but general uses are treatment of herpes, AIDS-related infections, cytomegalovirus, RSV			
Zovirax Symmetrel Sustiva	Acyclovir Amantadine Efavirenz	To treat herpes and HIV	Headache, nausea, diarrhea, many other adverse effects
Amphocin	Amphotericin B	To treat systemic fungal infections	Headache, fever
Lotrimin	Clotrimazole	To treat topical fungal infections	Skin irritation, burning
Bronchodilators: Used to make breathing easier by relaxing the muscles in the lungs and widening the bronchi			
Adrenalin	Epinephrine	All are used to treat long-term conditions where the airways may become narrow and inflamed.	All may cause trembling (particularly in the hands), headaches, dry mouth, and cough.
Atrovent	Ipratropium		

TABLE 12-2	Drug Categories Relevant to Radiography (*continued*)		
Trade Name	**Generic Name**	**Uses**	**Adverse Effect**
Proventil	Albuterol		
Spiriva	Tiotropium		
Cathartic and laxatives: Increases the passage and motility of feces			
Dulcolax	Bisacodyl	All are used to help in the passage of fecal material.	All may cause bloating, cramps, nausea, and dehydrations.
Senokot	Senna	Used for short-term constipation	Cramps, diarrhea, stomach discomfort
MiraLax	Polyethylene glycol 3350	Used for short-term constipation	Cramps, diarrhea, stomach discomfort, vomiting
Coagulants: Drugs that help the blood to form clots. It is the opposite of anticoagulation.			
Amicar	Aminocaproic acid	An antifibrinolytic agent used to induce clotting after surgery	Headache, stomach pain, loss of appetite, nausea, vomiting, diarrhea
Menadione	Vitamin K_3	A vitamin K that assists in the normal clotting of blood	Skin rash, muscle stiffness, difficulty in breathing, dizziness
Corticosteroids: Used as replacement therapy in diseases of the adrenal glands, for relief of inflammatory symptoms, for severe allergic reactions, and for relief of stress caused by trauma or other stress reaction resulting in physical insults to the body			
Cortef	Hydrocortisone	Short acting	Hyperglycemia, moon face, peptic ulcers, behavioral disturbances, edema, infection
Cortone	Cortisone	Short acting	Insomnia, dry and thinning skin, slow wound healing, headache
Medrol	Methylprednisolone	Intermediate acting	Nausea, vomiting, heartburn, headache, dizziness
Decadron	Dexamethasone	Long acting	Headache, dizziness, insomnia, weight gain
Antiseptic and disinfectant agents: Used in hospitals and health care settings for skin and equipment cleansing by inactivating microorganisms			
Hexachlorophene	Hexachlorophene	Used as a surgical scrub and bacteriostatic skin cleanser	There may be effects on the respiratory system, skin, and eyes when the chemicals are not used as prescribed.
Cortane-B	Chloroxylenol	Antiseptic and disinfectant used for skin disinfection and surgical instruments	
Diuretics: Help rid the body of sodium and water by helping the kidneys release the sodium into the urine, which helps remove water from the blood.			
Lasix	Furosemide	Increases the amount of urine by drawing extra water out of the blood	Dizziness, lightheadedness, headache, blurred vision
Aldactone	Spironolactone	Used to treat high blood pressure and heart failure as well as edema	Dizziness, lightheadedness, headache, drowsiness, nausea
Bumex	Bumetanide	Used to reduce edema	Dizziness

(*continued*)

TABLE 12-2	Drug Categories Relevant to Radiography (*continued*)		
Trade Name	**Generic Name**	**Uses**	**Adverse Effect**
Hormones: Can be used to treat cancers or to replace hormones that are lost because of disease or age			
Prempro	Medroxyprogesterone	Helps reduce the symptoms of menopause	Stomach pain, nausea, vomiting, bloating, breast tenderness
Prefest	Estradiol/norgestimate	Also relieves menopause symptoms but with high amounts of estrogen	Stomach pain, nausea, vomiting, bloating, breast tenderness
Femhrt	Norethindrone acetate	Helps reduce the risk of cancer of the uterus while reducing the symptoms of menopause	Stomach pain, nausea, vomiting, changes in weight or appetite, breast tenderness
Sedatives and hypotonic drugs: Commonly called tranquilizers. They have a relaxing and calming effect by acting on the CNS.			
Xanax	Alprazolam	Used to treat anxiety and panic disorders	Drowsiness, dizziness, headache, memory impairment, depression
Ambien	Zolpidem	Used to treat insomnia	Drowsiness, tiredness, headache, difficulty keeping balance
Vasodilators: Affect the muscles in the walls of the arteries to prevent them from narrowing. Open the blood vessels. **Vasoconstrictors:** The opposite of vasodilators			
Corlopam	Fenoldopam mesylate	Used to treat severe hypertension	Chest pain, heart palpitations, fluid retention, headache
Adrenalin	Epinephrine	Can be used to restore cardiac rhythm in cardiac arrest. Also used as OTC agent for asthma	Dizziness, sweating, vomiting, irregular heartbeat, difficulty breathing

CNS, central nervous system; DVT, deep vein thrombosis; NSAIDs, nonsteroidal anti-inflammatory drugs; N/V, nausea and/or vomiting; OTC, over the counter; RSV, respiratory syncytial virus; TB, tuberculosis; URI, upper respiratory infection; UTI, urinary tract infection.

CONTRAST MEDIA

Millions of imaging procedures worldwide involve the use of some form of contrast media to aid in the visualization of a body part or system. The radiographer must have a fundamental understanding of contrast media makeup, pharmacokinetics, and possible reactions. Contrast media are categorized as drugs because they can be absorbed into the systemic circulation and may produce an allergy-like or physiologic response on the body. The radiographer must use extreme caution when preparing contrast media for injection or ingestion.

Types of Contrast Media

Contrast media are required to visualize areas of the body when the organ or system of interest is too similar to the surrounding area. There are three types of contrast media—negative, positive, and radionuclides. Negative contrast media make the organ appear darker on the image. This is known as being **radiolucent**. When an anatomic area is filled or outlined by a positive contrast agent, the organ appears to be **radiopaque**, meaning white or light on the image. Radionuclides are the third type of contrast; they emit radiation and are used in nuclear medicine.

In a number of applications, such as double-contrast barium studies, air is the preferred medium that is used with the positive medium. Excellent double-contrast esophageal images can be obtained when the patient swallows air together with the barium preparation. This is accomplished by having the patient drink barium through a large-bore straw that has holes in the sides that draw in air.

There are commercial preparations that have carbon dioxide added to the barium suspension. The patient is asked to drink the canned preparation as soon as it is opened so that the carbon dioxide is released in the esophagus and stomach. This is similar to drinking a carbonated beverage. Effervescent granules are used to induce air into the stomach during an upper GI examination. The patient places the granules in the mouth and uses a small amount of barium to wash it down. The esophagus can be viewed immediately and the stomach fills with gas shortly after. The patient is instructed not to "burp" because this will release the gas.

Carbon dioxide has been used for double-contrast studies of the lower GI area because it is absorbed faster than air and it is believed that its use results in greater patient comfort. The use of either air or carbon dioxide allows the barium (or other positive contrast) to "outline" the anatomy, rather than coat it, which may hide small abnormalities such as small polyps or other areas on the lining of the organ. Negative contrast media used in these ways have decreased because computed tomography (CT) and magnetic resonance imaging (MRI) have replaced procedures that were once performed with these gaseous materials. However, the most common radiographic examination done is the chest study. In this case, the patient takes in a deep breath to fill the lungs with air, thus allowing the lungs to become radiolucent and to be "seen through."

To sum up the characteristics of negative contrast: (1) It has a low atomic weight—*therefore, it will* (2) decrease the organ density—*because it* (3) absorbs less radiation photons—*which causes a* (4) greater image density; (5) it is radiolucent, meaning it can be seen through; and (6) it is rapidly absorbed by the body.

Radiopaque contrast media (positive) are what the radiographer works with most frequently. There are two categories of positive media—insoluble (barium) and soluble (all others). Barium does not dissolve in water to any significant degree; it is merely suspended in solution. Mixing is necessary so that the barium crystals remain dispersed in water. If the container is allowed to stand, the barium crystals settle to the bottom.

Barium is termed as "thick" and "thin" types. This refers to the viscosity of barium and does not infer any difference in radiodensity. "Thick" barium is a paste that is used for esophageal swallows, whereas the "thin" barium is the liquid form used for stomach and bowel studies.

Soluble media contain iodine in some form. Iodine is used because it is readily available, has a nonmetallic atomic number, and is easily exchangeable with other ions. Water-soluble contrast media are **hypertonic**, causing water and electrolytes to be drawn into the bowel, causing dehydration. The high **tonicity** also causes dilution and reduces the degree of contrast.

The atomic numbers of barium and iodine are high and absorb photon energy that creates a white space where the contrast-filled organ would be on the image. This is very different from the black area that negative

contrast creates. Positive contrast media: (1) Have a high atomic weight—*therefore they* (2) increase the organ density—*because it* (3) absorbs more radiation—*which causes* (4) decreased image density; (5) they are radiopaque (meaning they cannot be seen through); (6) they are readily excreted unchanged through the liver or kidneys (only water-soluble contrast); and (7) they are relatively nontoxic.

Beam Attenuation Characteristics

Intravascular radiopaque contrast media are used primarily to add density to vasculature structures of an organ. This allows normal and abnormal anatomies to be studied by the radiologist. Positive agents are effective photon absorbers in the body because they are derivatives of tri-iodinated benzoic acid.

Barium is the most common type of contrast used in imaging the GI system. Barium is a metal and does not dissolve; therefore, it is suspended in solution. The metallic component of barium makes it an ideal substance for use as a contrast medium. Gastrografin is another type of contrast used for GI imaging.

All positive contrast media, except barium, used in diagnostic imaging contain iodine, and are known as iodinated contrast media (ICM). The high atomic numbers of iodine, barium, and bromine give them the ability to decrease radiographic density on the image receptor. Iodine, with an atomic number of 53, is able to absorb the x-ray photons, thus allowing the area of interest to be seen on the radiographic image as a white area (Fig. 12-1). Barium has the atomic number of the

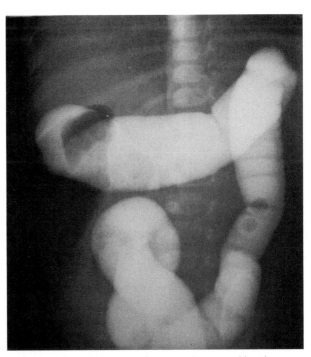

FIGURE 12-1 White area of interest is created by the use of barium. This area is said to be radiopaque.

metal barium (56) and is able to accomplish the same absorption of x-ray photons and the same radiopaque image. The higher the atomic number of the contrast media, the more it absorbs the photons of the radiographic beam that creates a white area on the image.

ICM are used in the examination of the GI tract, kidneys, gallbladder, pancreas, heart, brain, uterus, spinal column, arteries, veins, and joints. Contrast media are used to increase the visibility of body cavities, organs, and the vascular system in diagnostic imaging, fluoroscopy, and other imaging modalities such as CT and MRI. The CT technologist works with contrast more often than does a technologist working elsewhere in the department because more contrast-related procedures are now done in the CT department than in the past. Gadolinium-based contrast media (GBCM) are radiodense and can be used for opacification in CT and digital subtraction angiography instead of iodinated radiographic contrast. Gadolinium has an atomic number of 64. GBCM are considered to have no nephrotoxicity at approved doses for MRI. Special imaging procedures are discussed in Chapter 14.

Pharmacologic Profile

Differences in radiopaque contrast media can cause significant changes in radiodensity of tissue substance, which is related to the amount of iodine in the contrast. Two common iodinated substances are iothalamate and diatrizoate. Each of these contains methylglucamine (meglumine) salts or sodium salts, or a combination of the two. Meglumine compounds are less toxic but are more viscous than are sodium compounds. All positive contrast media are made up of a cation (a positive charge) and an anion (a negative charge). The cation is either the sodium or the meglumine compound. The anion is basically the same in all positive media, with the exception of one side chain, and determines the rest of the makeup of the contrast.

Ionic and Nonionic Contrast Media

The chemical structures of nonionic and ionic contrast media differ significantly. A common error is made in thinking that nonionic means there is no iodine, which is untrue. There is iodine in both ionic and nonionic contrast.

The early contrast media were salts of iodinated benzoic acid derivatives. Because they are salts, they consist of a positively charged cation and a negatively charged anion. These salts are strong acids and are completely dissociated (ionized) in solution. For every three iodine atoms in solution for contrast, two particles for osmolality exist (one anion and one cation). These are known as high-osmolar contrast media (HOCM). The ratio between the number of iodine atoms present and the number of particles in solution are the osmolality and ionicity of contrast media. Both of these have a bearing on the toxicity of the media.

The cation was eliminated from the ionic media because cations contain no iodine and give no diagnostic information. However, it was responsible for as much as 50% of the osmotic effect, which increases the risk of adverse reactions. The cations were replaced with hydroxyl groups, which did not add to the osmolality.

Figures 12-2 and 12-3 show positive contrast media that are ionic and nonionic.

The development of radiopaque, iodinated intravascular contrast media of lower osmolality (low-osmolality contrast media [LOCM]), both ionic and nonionic, has made better and safer contrast media available. These contrasts have an osmolality that is closer to human plasma and thus are less likely to cause an adverse reaction.

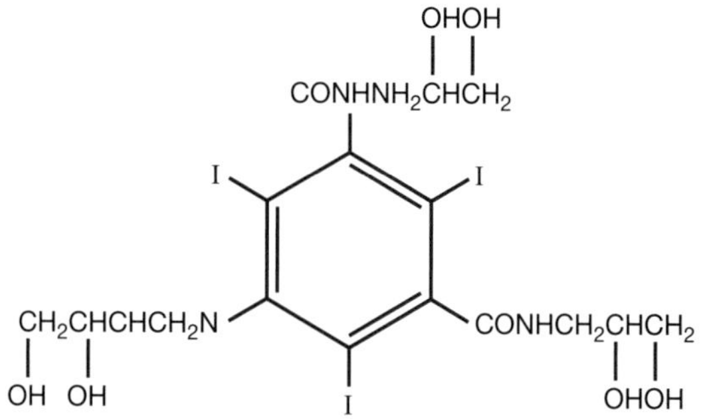

FIGURE 12-3 Iohexol contains six hydroxyl groups, making this a nonionic contrast media. (Reprinted with permission from Linn-Watson T. *Radiographic Pathology*. 2nd ed. Wolters Kluwer; 2014.)

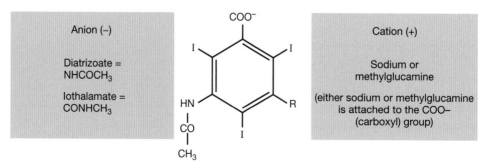

FIGURE 12-2 Diatrizoate and iothalamate differ in the composition of their side chain. (Reprinted with permission from Linn-Watson T. *Radiographic Pathology*. 2nd ed. Wolters Kluwer; 2014.)

A great deal of research into the chemistry and molecular structure, toxicity, and solubility of contrast materials has resulted in the development of iodinated compounds that can be safely used in intravascular diagnostic radiology. The express purpose of these media is to provide contrast enhancement and improved diagnostic images.

Osmolality of a contrast is a significant factor to consider when adverse reactions may cause severe complications. Conventional ionic media are significantly hyperosmotic to body fluids such as blood because they dissociate into separate ions in solution. This can cause adverse effects, such as cardiac problems, vein cramping and pain, and abnormal fluid retention. Contrast media that have hypo-osmolality (less osmolality) than the body fluid result in fewer and less severe **side effects**. Thus, nonionic contrast media are advantageous in this respect, and there is no appreciable difference in image quality when compared with the ionic media.

Table 12-3 compares the iodine concentration and the osmolality of the various types of contrast media.

TABLE 12-3 Iodine Concentration and Osmolality for HOCM and LOCM

Product	Chemical Structure	Salt Concentration (%)	Iodine Concentration (%)	Osmolality
Nonionic Intravascular Contrast Agents				
Omnipaque 140	Iohexol	0	14	322
Omnipaque 180	Iohexol 38.8%	0	18	408
Omnipaque 240	Iohexol 51.8%	0	24	520
Omnipaque 300	Iohexol 64.7%	0	30	672
Omnipaque 350	Iohexol 75.5%	0	35	844
Ultravist 150	Iopromide	15	150	328
Ultravist 240	Iopromide	24	240	483
Ultravist 300	Iopromide	30	300	607
Ultravist 370	Iopromide	37	370	774
Optiray 160	Ioversol 34%	16	160	355
Optiray 240	Ioversol 51%	24	240	502
Optiray 300	Ioversol 64%	30	300	651
Optiray 320	Ioversol 68%	32	320	702
Optiray 350	Ioversol 74%	35	350	792
Isovue 200	Iopamidol 40.8%	20	200	413
Isovue 250	Iopamidol 51%	25	250	524
Isovue 300	Iopamidol 61.2%	30	300	616
Isovue 370	Iopamidol 75.5%	37	370	796
Visipaque 270	Iodixanol 55%	27	270	290
Visipaque 320	Iodixanol	32	320	290
Ionic Intravascular Contrast Agents				
Conray	Iothalamate/meglumine	60	28.2	1,400
Conray 30	Iothalamate/meglumine	30	14.1	600
Conray 43	Iothalamate/meglumine	43	20.2	1,000
Conray 400	Iothalamate/sodium	66.9	40	2,300
Reno-DIP	Diatrizoate/meglumine	30	14.1	1,450
RenoCal-76	Diatrizoate/combo	66 Meg, 10 Sodium	37	1,690
Hypaque 76	Diatrizoate/combo	Meg 66, 19.6 Sodium	37	>2,016

(continued)

TABLE 12-3	Iodine Concentration and Osmolality for HOCM and LOCM (continued)				
Product	**Chemical Structure**	**Salt Concentration (%)**	**Iodine Concentration (%)**	**Osmolality**
Hexabrix 32	Ioxaglate/combo	Meg 39.3, 19.6 Sodium	19.6	600
Ionic GI Agents				
Gastrografin	Diatrizoate/combo	Meglumine	37	1,940
Ionic Uroradiologic Agents				
Hypaque-Cysto	Diatrizoate/meglumine	30	14.1	1,515
Cysto-Conray	Iothalamate/meglumine	17.2	8.1	Instilled for **retrograde** cystography
Conray	Iothalamate/meglumine	43	20.2	1,000

GI, gastrointestinal; HOCM, high-osmolar contrast media; LOCM, low-osmolar contrast media.

Absorption, Distribution, Metabolism, and Elimination

The pharmacologic properties of absorption, distribution, metabolism, and elimination were discussed in the previous paragraphs. Contrast media behave in the same manner as do other drugs.

Any type of contrast cannot provide the differences in contrast needed for imaging unless it arrives at its intended target. Of course, with barium, the patient either drinks the preparation or has it inserted through a tube, either nasogastric (NG), nasoenteric (NE), or rectally. Iodinated contrasts are most often introduced into the body through the systemic circulation. Increased circulation provides better absorption. The concentration of the drug (how much iodine it contains) also affects the imaging factors. As explained under beam attenuation, the more iodine, the more x-ray photons are stopped from hitting the image receptor, which, in turn provides a better image.

It is the blood stream that distributes the contrast to the area for which it was intended. Metabolism occurs in the liver, which then eliminates it through bile or by sending it to the kidneys and out through the urine. However, some radiographic contrast can cause renal damage, which is why it is so important for the radiographer to perform an allergic history before any contrast administration.

Interactions, Indications, and Contraindications

Drugs that have similar mechanisms of action can either enhance the activity of each other or can inhibit the activity. Detrimental effects may occur if the drugs given in the imaging department combine with the drugs a patient is taking. An example would be giving ibuprofen to a patient who is taking warfarin because this may increase the patient's risk of stomach bleeding.

Because most contrast media are used in the performance of CT examinations, and because the use of contrast extends the time of the examination itself, the ordering physician reviews the need and **indications** for the use of the contrast. A major indication is suspected lesions seen on noncontrast brain scans.

Before giving a patient contrast media, a complete allergic history must be performed (Display 12-1). Each health facility has its own form that must be filled out before performing any contrast-related studies. Through the use of the patient history, the radiographer should be able to determine whether there are any possible **contraindications** to the use of the contrast.

The technologist must review the form after a patient has completed it to ensure that the patient has understood the questionnaire and has answered it as completely as possible.

Possible contraindications when using IV contrast media that present an increased risk for an adverse reaction include the following:

- Previous reactions to contrast
- Asthma
- Allergies
- Heart disease
- Renal disease

A previous or preexisting nephrogenic systemic fibrosis in a patient is an absolute contraindication when using gadolinium contrast. Gadolinium is used in MRI to image the brain and spinal cord, inflammatory joint disease, bowel disease, or neoplastic conditions of organs such as the liver or kidney. However, if a patient states that they have a history of diabetes, hypertension, history of vascular disease, history of smoking, they are older than age 60, have a known history of kidney disease or a family history or renal disease, or a body mass index

DISPLAY 12-1

Patient Precontrast Questionnaire for Radiology

NAME: _____ Date of Birth: _____

Your Doctor's Name: _____ Today's Date: _____

1. Reason for Examination _____

2. DO YOU HAVE ANY SYMPTOMS AND FOR HOW LONG? _____

_____

_____

3. Please answer these questions by circling either YES or NO
   1. Have you had a prior reaction to contrast?   YES   NO
   2. Do you have multiple myeloma?   YES   NO
   3. Do you have asthma?   YES   NO
   4. Do you have heart disease?   YES   NO
   5. Do you have kidney disease?   YES   NO
   6. Do you have any history of cancer?   YES   NO
   7. Do you have diabetes? If yes, how long: _____   YES   NO
   8. Are you taking Glucophage, Glucovance, Metaglip, Avandamet, Fortamet, Riomet, metformin, Actoplus Met, or interleukin? (circle)   YES   NO
   9. Have you had a mastectomy or lymph node dissection?   YES   NO
      Which side? _____
   10. FEMALES ONLY:
   Is there any chance of pregnancy? YES   NO

   ALLERGIES:

   _____

   _____

   _____

   PRESENT MEDICATIONS:

   _____

   _____

   Reviewed by: _____

   MEDICAL HISTORY:

   _____

   _____

   PREVIOUS SURGICAL HISTORY:

   _____

   _____

   FOR ALL RADIOLOGICAL STAFF TO COMPLETE.
   Have prior examinations been reviewed?

   _____ Laboratory Data   eGER = _____   Creatinine = _____   Date Drawn = _____
   _____ Patient Assessment:

(continued)

DISPLAY 12-1

Patient Precontrast Questionnaire for Radiology (*continued*)

Alert: YES   NO   *Procedure explained:* YES   NO   *Pt. Acknowledges understanding:* YES   NO

CONTRAST INJECTION:

Contrast: _____, Volume _____ mL, Location # _____ g in

_____, Power injection   or   Hand injection

ADDITIONAL NOTES: (If none, cross out):

_____

DISCHARGE INSTRUCTIONS:

1. Drink several extra glasses of fluid today.   YES   NO

2. Diabetic instructions given   YES   N/A

RN/Physician Signature: _____

Technologist: _____

Date: _____   Time: _____

(BMI) over 30, an estimated glomerular filtration rate (eGFR) should be completed before the MRI.

Appropriateness of an Examination

Every clinician must make the decision as to which diagnostic test to order for their patient. Considerations about the type of contrast media that would be used in the examination, along with the risk and contraindications, must be taken. The American College of Radiology (ACR) publishes an appropriateness criteria manual to help physicians and others make the best decision when ordering procedures based on the condition of the patient. The manual is divided into the various areas of the body, allowing physicians to review the specific area, such as lower extremity venous diseases, vertebral compression fractures, and biliary obstruction.

Conditions that must be reviewed before giving the patient any contrast include the patient's condition, age, and weight; lab values such as blood urea nitrogen (BUN), eGFR, and creatinine; and allergic history. For example, a patient that is suspected of having a perforated bowel or a ruptured appendix would not have barium used as a contrast medium. If barium were to get into the peritoneal cavity, it could cause barium granuloma or peritonitis because the barium would dissociate from the fluid and not be absorbed by the body. Instead, a water-soluble contrast with a high enough iodine content that it cannot be diluted would be preferable. Aqueous contrasts are also used when there is a possibility of impactions.

The age and weight of the patient play a role in the choice of the contrast for the examination. Because of the

decreased metabolism in elderly patients, the radiologist may decide to decrease the amount of contrast used in CT examinations. Body weight has been suggested as the best factor for estimating the contrast dose needed for consistent enhancement in abdominal CT. However, if the patient is obese, a larger dose, based on the weight, may be too much because of contrast distribution in adipose tissue. This leads to other indications that need to be used for dose calculations that are beyond the scope of this chapter.

Variables the physician considers when selecting a contrast medium are as follows:

1. Its ability to mix with body fluids
2. The viscosity
3. The ionic strength
4. Its persistence in the body
5. The osmolality
6. The iodine content
7. The potential for toxicity

Most contrast media are water based, and the body will absorb water-based contrasts in time. A limited number of procedures require an oil-based contrast agent. These may be excreted from the body in a natural manner or may be removed at the end of the procedure.

Preparation

Patient preparations for studies that require contrast media will vary with the type of procedure that is ordered. For lower GI examinations (more commonly known as barium enemas), the patient must remain

NPO for approximately 6 hours before the examination time. In addition, patients must have some form of large-bowel cleansing. Imaging departments usually have directions that are given to patients on what to eat and when, when to take the cleansing preparations, and a phone number to call if there are any questions. Many departments even provide a special kit that is given to each patient that includes a solution or pills for cleansing the large bowel.

When a patient is undergoing an upper GI series that may include the esophagus, stomach, or the small bowel, the patient has no special preparation other than to remain NPO for a certain number of hours before the examination. Other examinations that utilize contrast media usually don't require a special type of preparation before the contrast is given.

While the patient is in the imaging department and ready for the examination, the technologist is duty bound to inform the patient of the administration of contrast and any possible effects that may occur. Informing patients of expected side effects will help prepare them for what is about to happen and to remain calm. The patient must also be informed of any possible adverse reactions and instructed to let the radiographer know immediately if any of those occur.

The radiographer also has to be prepared when a patient is receiving contrast media. To achieve an understanding of the patient's condition, an appropriate and adequate history must be obtained by questioning the patient. Allowing the patient to fill out the allergic history form is not adequate. The radiographer must question the patient regarding any answers that stand out as a possible risk. Screening should include any historical elements that will affect the decision to continue with the administration of contrast. Has the patient had a prior allergic-like reaction to the contrast that is to be used? If so, there is a high likelihood that the patient will experience another reaction. A history of asthma increases the possibility of developing bronchospasm after the administration of contrast.

Preparation of the patient for a contrast examination is multifaceted. Far more than just doing a study prep, it is a complete allergic history as well. Failure to assess the patient for possible allergies can lead to dire consequences. The case study presented in the following paragraphs shows how negligence on the part of the radiographer can lead to fatal consequences.

CASE STUDY

A radiographer is preparing a patient for an **intrathecal** injection before a CT myelogram. She goes to the cupboard in the radiography room where all the contrast media are stored. She selects a particular vial, gathers the needles and syringe, and informs the radiologist that she is ready for him to come in for the injection. The radiologist draws up the contrast and injects it into the patient's spinal canal. The patient has his CT myelogram as planned and is sent home.

When the technologist is cleaning the room after the injection, she finds that the vial will not fit into the sharps container. She then reads the label and discovers that she has used the wrong contrast and that it is *not* for intrathecal injection. She immediately alerts the physician and the supervisor, and the patient is called back. By this time, the patient is already experiencing leg numbness and is having extreme difficulty walking.

The patient is hospitalized and an attempt is made to withdraw the contrast from the spinal canal. However, with the passage of time, the contrast has already been absorbed into the spinal fluid. The patient is kept hospitalized for several days to make sure that the effects are temporary.

The patient does file a lawsuit against the hospital, the radiologist, the technologist, and the radiology administrator. Through discovery, it is found that the hospital radiology department did not follow The Joint Commission recommendations for storage of contrast media. The radiologic technologist did not read the label before handing it to the physician. Nor did she show the physician the label before he drew up the contrast medium. The physician did not question the radiographer because, having worked with her for many years and having never had an issue with her work, he "trusted her judgment."

This unfortunate incident can be looked at as simply an accident; however, it is one that could and *should* have been prevented. There were many errors that were committed, but they all could have been discovered and prevented if the technologist had simply read the label when she removed it from the shelf.

Reactions to Contrast Media

The number of mild and moderate reactions related to the administration of contrast has decreased with the use of LOCM. However, a number of severe and life-threatening reactions still occur without any predictability. Because of this, the technologist must be trained and stay current regarding patient care after contrast is administered. The American Society of Radiologic Technologists (ASRT) requires radiography programs to teach pharmacology, but it is up to the student to remain alert and competent after graduation in recognizing the signs and symptoms of a reaction and the intervention required.

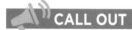 **CALL OUT**

It cannot be stressed enough that the radiographer must know the signs and symptoms of adverse reactions and the medical interventions required to save the patient's life!

Contrast media are not always accepted into the body without any physical or functional changes because of the molecular structure of the compound used. Reactions to contrast media occur most often when the medium is administered IV or **intra-arterially**. When the body reacts to contrast in a manner that is of little or no consequence, the patient is experiencing a side effect. Side effects are common and can be expected to happen in many patients. Expected side effects must be explained to the patient, before the procedure begins, to alleviate anxiety. These include a feeling of warmth and flushing and a metallic taste in the mouth. These effects are usually due to the speed with which the contrast is injected and will pass within a few minutes. Although these side effects are normal and not a true contrast reaction leading to a life-threatening situation, they may cause the patient to vomit, which will delay the start of the procedure and thus the quality of the examination because of contrast elimination.

The body's reactions that are more toxic are considered adverse reactions. Adverse reactions are also known as idiosyncratic reactions. Depending on the osmolality of the contrast, there may or may not be a reaction. The ACR publishes a manual on contrast media that is revised every few years. This manual is an excellent resource for all radiographers who inject contrast media. It fully explains the various types of contrast and their uses, what the possible reactions are, and what interventions should be used to counteract the reactions.

Reactions are divided into sections and then into categories. The two sections of contrast reactions are allergic-like or physiologic. Allergic-like is used rather than allergic reactions because there may be different immunology even though there is a similar clinical presentation. Physiologic reactions are not allergic-like; instead, they are the body's automatic reaction to the contrast. An example would be the "fight or flight" response where the heart rate increases, the pupils of the eyes dilate, and respiration increases. The ACR further divides the reactions into mild, moderate, or severe.

Mild reactions to the contrast are usually self-limiting and may require nothing more than a reassurance from the technologist. These types of reactions seldom progress to the next level and so are not life-threatening. Dermal reactions are usually the least significant of adverse effects associated with contrast media and may not require treatment. However, antihistamines may be warranted if the dermal reactions such as urticarial (hives) persist. If this is the case, the radiographer should observe the patient for approximately 20 minutes to assure that no further reactions occur.

Moderate reactions are more pronounced than minor ones; however, they are not immediately life-threatening. They may require medical attention because they may have the potential to increase in severity. Symptoms include nausea, possible vomiting, urticaria, mild bronchospasm, tachycardia, and mild hypotension. These symptoms may be treated using diphenhydramine for the hives, an inhaler for the bronchospasm, and elevating the legs for hypotension.

The final category of contrast media reaction is severe. They rarely occur but it is essential for all technologists who administer contrast media to understand how unpredictable these reactions are and that they require immediate recognition and treatment. Cardiac or respiratory arrest can and does occur with either allergic-like or physiologic reactions. Symptoms start with anxiety and respiratory difficulty related to bronchospasm, laryngospasm, and angioedema of the upper airway. Severe hypotension and pulmonary edema may also occur, particularly if the patient is already suffering from congestive heart failure. This could lead to sudden cardiac arrest.

Cardiac and pulmonary arrest requires cardiopulmonary resuscitation (CPR) and advanced life-support equipment. It is of utmost importance that the technologist be well versed with current CPR training. Whenever there is contrast media in use, the radiographer must have the "crash cart" (Fig. 12-4) on hand because this contains the medications used for contrast reactions as well as the defibrillator in case it is needed.

Table 12-4 gives the types of reactions and the severity of the reactions. It lists the signs and symptoms, as well as the interventions that are necessary to counteract the reactions.

Delayed Reactions to Contrast Media

Although most reactions occur within 5 minutes of the injection of the contrast medium, some reactions can occur much later, even after the patient has left the imaging department. The incidence of delayed adverse reactions ranges from 0.5% to 9%, with those reactions starting from 3 hours to 7 days following the administration of a medium. Delayed reactions are unusual in that there is a high rate of recurrence. Any reaction or side effect to contrast injection must be documented appropriately according to the facility's protocols. The very minimum that must be documented includes the dose and type of

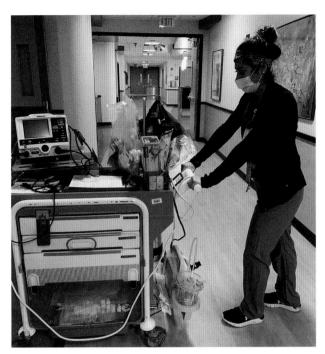

FIGURE 12-4 The crash cart should be located in a fast and easy-to-reach location whenever there is contrast media being injected.

contrast that was injected, any signs and symptoms that the patient exhibited, any treatment and medication that were given to the patient to counteract the reaction, and the patient's response to the treatment.

DRUG SAFETY

All drugs (medications) are potentially harmful. The radiographer must completely understand the implications of any actions when administering drugs or assisting with drug administration. Never administer a drug that has not been specifically ordered by a physician. All health care workers who administer drugs must understand the intended action, contraindications, side effects, and potential adverse effects of any drug they administer.

 WARNING!

The radiographer must remember that contrast media are drugs and the precautions listed in this chapter pertain to these agents as well!

TABLE 12-4	Contrast Reactions and Radiographer's Response and Treatment		
Reaction	**Allergic-Like Symptoms**	**Physiologic Symptoms**	**Response and Treatment**
Side Effect	• Pain at injection site	• Feeling of flushing or warmth • Headache • Nausea and/or vomiting • Metallic taste	• Slow the rate of contrast infusion. • Observe the patient closely, offer reassurance.
Vasovagal Reaction	• Not applicable	• Pallor • Cold sweats • Rapid pulse • Syncope or feeling faint • Bradycardia • Hypotension	• Stop the infusion. • Place the patient in flat or Trendelenburg position. • Notify radiologist or nurse. • Do not leave.
Mild Reaction	• Limited urticaria • Cutaneous edema • Scratchy throat • Nasal congestion • Sneezing	• Limited nausea/ vomiting • Headache/dizziness, anxiety/altered taste • Mild hypertension	• Stop infusion; notify radiology or nurse. • Monitor vital signs. • Prepare for administration of antihistamine.
Moderate Reaction	• Diffuse urticaria • Diffuse erythema • Facial edema • Wheezing/ bronchospasm	• Protracted nausea/ vomiting • Hypertensive urgency • Isolated chest pain	• Stop the infusion but maintain the IV access. • Notify radiologist and nurse. • Take vital signs. • Call for emergency team if symptoms progress rapidly.

(continued)

TABLE 12-4	Contrast Reactions and Radiographer's Response and Treatment (*continued*)		
Reaction	**Allergic-Like Symptoms**	**Physiologic Symptoms**	**Response and Treatment**
			• Prepare to administer oxygen and IV medications, such as Benadryl. • If patient is in respiratory distress, place in a semi-Fowler position. • If patient is vomiting, place them on the side to prevent aspiration. • For patient with hypotension and bradycardia or tachycardia, elevate the lower extremities. • Drugs that must be on hand include epinephrine, hydrocortisone, and diphenhydramine (Benadryl).
Severe Reaction	• Diffuse edema • Dyspnea • Erythema with hypotension • Wheezing/ bronchospasm • Anaphylactic shock	• Vasovagal reaction resistant to tx • Arrhythmia • Convulsions, seizures • Hypertensive emergency	• Call Code Blue. • Notify radiologist and radiology nurse. • Keep the IV site but stop the contrast flow. • Prepare to use automated external defibrillator. • Prepare to help in the administering of oxygen and IV medications such as diphenhydramine (Benadryl).

IV, intravenous; tx, treatment.

The radiographer must adhere to the following rights of drug administration at all times:

1. The right patient (P)
2. The right drug and documentation (D)
3. The right amount or dose (A)
4. The right route (R)
5. The right time (T)

Using the acronym PDART, one can easily remember the six rights. Note that there are two "D"s.

Other precautions that must be taken before any drug is administered are as follows:

1. Read all labels carefully before drawing up or pouring a drug. Check the name, strength, and dosage of the drug.
2. If a drug contains a sediment or appears to be cloudy, do not use until the pharmacist approves the drug.
3. Check the expiration date of the drug on the label. If that date has passed, do not use.
4. Do not use drugs from unmarked or poorly marked containers. Discard them.
5. Measure exact amounts of every drug used. If medication is left over, do not replace it in the container; discard it according to institutional policy.
6. Drugs must be stored in accordance with the manufacturer's specifications. No drug should be stored in an area where temperature and humidity vary greatly or are extreme.
7. If a medication is a liquid to be poured, pour away from the label.
8. Do not combine two drugs in a syringe without verifying their compatibility with the pharmacist. If in doubt, do not combine!
9. Before selecting a medication, check the label of the container three times: before taking it from storage, before pouring it or drawing it up, and after it has been prepared for administration.
10. When drawing up medication for someone else to administer, show that person the label of the drug container. Have the person who will do the administration verbally confirm the name of the drug.
11. When approaching a patient who is to receive a drug, ask the patient for two identifying qualifiers (name and birth date). Do not accept the fact that a patient answers to what is thought to be the correct name. An anxious patient may respond incorrectly. Read the name label on the patient's wrist, if available.
12. After identifying the patient, explain about the drug and how it will be given.

13. A drug history of allergies must be taken before any drug is administered.

14. The radiographer must not administer a drug that was preprepared by another person. All drugs and contrast media must be prepared and administered (or overseen) by the same person.

15. Report and document any drug that the patient refuses to take.

16. Document any drug administered immediately according to department procedure.

17. Do not leave unattended a patient who may be having a drug reaction!

18. A patient who has received a sedative, hypnotic, antianxiety, or narcotic analgesic drug must not be allowed to drive home.

19. A child who has received a medication and is sleeping may not leave the department until fully awake.

20. Patients should be observed for 1 hour before leaving the department alone after receiving any drug.

Patients who receive narcotic analgesics or hypnotics may suffer respiratory depression and shock and must not be left unattended.

Special considerations that must be watched for when administering drugs are further delineated in Table 12-5.

TABLE 12-5 Special Considerations When Administering Drugs

Age Group	Physiologic Changes	Precautions
Pregnant women	Many drugs cross the placental barrier. Drug effects depend on fetal age and can result in harm to the fetus.	Drugs during pregnancy must be avoided or administered only to women who absolutely require treatment. If in doubt, inform patient's physician of possible pregnancy before administering any drug.
Infants	Lack well-developed muscle mass; lack the protective mechanisms of older children and adults. Skin is thin and permeable; stomach lacks mucous barrier; temperature control is poor; they become dehydrated easily and have immature liver and kidneys that cannot manage foreign chemicals.	Only persons educated in drug administration to infants must administer medications to them.
Breastfed infants	May have all drugs in maternal circulation transferred to colostrum and breast milk.	Mothers who are breastfeeding may be advised by the physician to cease breastfeeding for a prescribed time if they are to receive radioisotopes or radiation. All other drug therapies must be evaluated because they may harm the infant. A detailed history must be taken, and no drugs should be administered without establishing that they will not harm the infant.
Pediatric patients	At 1 year of age, liver metabolizes more rapidly than it does in adults; renal function may be more rapid than that in adults. Standard dosage depends on child's weight or body surface. Topical drugs are more easily absorbable through the skin.	Children are not small adults! Physiologic differences vary, and only those experienced in medicating children must administer drugs to them! Topical drugs and solutions, including antiseptics, can cause poisoning in children. Cleanse only with soap and water.
Elderly patients	Blood-brain barrier is more easily penetrated, with increasing rate of dizziness and confusion. Reduced baroreceptor response increases hypotensive effects of some drugs. Liver size, blood flow, and enzyme production decrease, increasing the half-life of some drugs and leading to possible **toxic reactions**. Increased adipose tissue in abdominal area may lead to toxicity from fat-soluble drugs. Decreased renal blood flow and filtration decrease elimination of drugs from the body. Slower gastric emptying time and increase in pH of gastric juices increase risk of gastric irritation.	Drugs affecting the central nervous system and cardiovascular system must be given with extreme caution. Patients must be monitored closely and assisted with ambulation to prevent falls. Do not allow elderly patients who have been given drugs to leave the area unattended.

ROUTES OF ADMINISTRATION

The route the drug and contrast is administrated depends on the drug's absorption, distribution, metabolism, and elimination. Drugs used to treat most illnesses are administered in small dosages at selected intervals, whereas contrast media are often administered in a large dose at one time called a *bolus*. Most drugs used for treating illness that are administered intravascularly are *isotonic*. That is, they have the same concentration of solute as other body fluids; therefore, they exert the same amount of osmotic pressure as the body fluid with which they are combining. Contrast media have osmolality much higher than the body fluid with which they are combining. They are highly viscous, and when administered intravascularly, they prompt a sudden shift in body fluid from the interstitial spaces and cells into the systemic circulation. There are basically five routes by which drugs are administered—**enteral**, tube or catheter, inhalation, **topical**, or parenteral. In the following sections, each of these is described, with particular emphasis on the parenteral route.

Enteral

The enteral routes are broken down into **oral, sublingual, buccal,** and **rectal**.

Drugs taken by mouth and swallowed into the stomach are said to be given *orally*. The medical term for this route of administration is PO. It is often the most efficient and most cost-effective method of drug administration. This route is used if the drug will not be destroyed by gastric secretions and when slower absorption and longer duration of drug activity are desired.

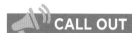

CALL OUT

Do not break or crush enteric-coated tablets because they may act as gastric irritants or become less effective!

A sublingual drug is placed under the tongue and remains there until it is dissolved completely. The patient must not eat or drink until the drug dissolves. It is not to be swallowed or chewed.

A drug administered by the buccal route must be placed against the mucous membranes of the cheek in either the upper or the lower jaw. It must remain there until it dissolves. Drugs given by this route are used for local effect and are drugs such as lozenges.

Drugs may be administered by rectum if a patient is nauseated and unable to retain oral drugs. It is difficult to determine the correct dosage by this route because absorption may be erratic. Lack of fluid in the rectum also makes absorbability questionable. The radiographer has little or no reason to administer drugs by rectum.

Tube or Catheter

Tubes and catheters are methods used to introduce contrast into the stomach, small bowel, large bowel, or urinary bladder. The use of either of these methods requires a retrograde flow of contrast administration and will not show the function of the body part.

Catheters are more common in the urinary bladder. After draining all the urine out of the bladder, contrast is distilled retrogradely and, therefore, does not show the function of the bladder. Similarly, tubes such as NE and NG are merely a way for the contrast or other drugs to be introduced into the organ where the tube is inserted. In the case of the stomach and small bowel, the contrast most likely to be used is Gastrografin or other water-soluble media in the event that there is a blockage in the system. Although rectal is listed in the enteral route, the means by which contrast is introduced is the enema tube with an attached tip inserted into the anus, allowing the contrast (usually barium) to flow retrogradely into the rectum and continue through the sigmoid, descending, and transverse colon.

Inhalation

Drugs that are administered by inhalation include through the mouth as well as through the nose. In both instances, the drugs pass through the trachea and into the lungs. Although this may be the most advantageous method of delivering medication to the lungs, there are some disadvantages because of airway symptoms that will not allow the patient to inhale deeply enough to get a full dose. An intranasal route helps the absorption of the drug by passive diffusion. The respiratory system is a well-vascularized system that facilitates the drug's passage.

Topical

Topical drug administration includes the following:

Drugs administered to the skin for local treatment of lesions or skin conditions

Drugs administered to the eyes, nose, and throat

Drugs administered to the vagina and, in some cases, to the rectum

Drugs applied to the skin for intended systemic effect, called *transdermal application*

It is believed that drugs administered transdermally are absorbed slowly and a constant blood level of the drug is achieved. The radiographer may care for patients with transdermal patches applied at various areas of the body, generally, the upper thoracic area. This route is used most often for relief of chronic pain and for cardiac therapy.

Parenteral

There are several methods of administering drugs by parenteral routes, and they vary depending on the drug to be administered and the route ordered by the physician. The routes include the subcutaneous, intramuscular, intradermal (ID), and IV. Other routes of parenteral administration are the intrathecal, intra-arterial, **intraosseous**, and **intra-articular**. These routes are used only by the physician or specialty nurses.

1. Subcutaneous: Drugs are introduced just below the dermis and epidermis layers of the skin. There are few blood vessels in this area, so absorption is slow. Areas that are most often used for subcutaneous injections include the upper arm, abdomen, the front of the thigh, and the upper area of the buttock behind the hip.

2. Intramuscular: Body muscles, such as the deltoid, rectus femoris, and ventrogluteal or dorsogluteal muscles, are areas where drugs can be injected. The most common site is the dorsogluteal. However, the sciatic nerve and the superior gluteal artery pose a risk.

3. ID: This type of drug administration has the longest absorption rate of all parenteral routes. The injection is into the dermis, which is below the epidermis. The ID route is used for tests for tuberculosis (TB) or allergies. If contrast allergy testing is performed, an ID injection is used.

4. IV: Because the drugs are injected directly into the blood stream, the first-pass effect is bypassed. The effect of the drug is immediate. The most commonly used locations include the median basilic or cephalic veins in the upper extremity. The IV route of drug administration is the only parenteral route by which radiographers are able to administer contrast. It will be further explored in Chapter 13.

5. Intrathecal: By injecting drugs into the subarachnoid space of the spinal cord, the blood-brain barrier is bypassed. Doses can be smaller and there is a smaller chance of side effects than when alternate routes of administration are used. A lumbar puncture is made between L3 and L4 so that the needle is less likely to injure the spinal cord.

6. Intra-arterial: The carotid artery or the vertebral artery is used when an intra-arterial drug administration is necessary. This is used when thrombolytic drugs are needed with higher levels of concentration at the site of a thrombus. Interventional imaging uses the femoral artery to insert a catheter and thread it to the location that is desired to be imaged.

7. Intraosseous: Drugs are introduced directly into the marrow of a bone. Areas where an intraosseous line is placed include the sternum, clavicle, head of the humerus, the distal femur, or proximal tibia. Intraosseous infusions are used when an IV infusion is not possible. It allows the drug to go directly into the vascular system.

8. Intra-articular: Injections are given into the joint space to show musculoskeletal anatomy and pathology. Osteoarthritis in the hip and knee were formerly diagnosed with arthrography that consisted of contrast being injected into the joint. The joint was then manipulated before imaging occurred. Steroids such as Cortisone are injected intra-articularly to manage pain.

Equipment used for parenteral injections is dependent on the route. Any health care worker who plans to administer parenteral medications to children requires special education beyond the scope of this book. All parenteral drug administration requires laboratory instruction and practice before administering drugs to actual patients. The procedures described in the following paragraphs pertain to the average adult patient. The following are some rules that apply to all parenteral drug administrations:

1. All equipment that penetrates the skin, including needles, syringes, and the drug itself, must be sterile.

2. The patient must be correctly identified.

3. The procedure is explained to the patient and the medication (including contrast media) to be administered is identified.

4. If the patient refuses the drug, document the refusal. Do not insist that the patient accept the drug.

5. The skin at the injection site is cleansed with an antiseptic solution until it is as free of microorganisms as possible.

6. The antiseptic chosen will be dictated by the institution. Alcohol-based preparations are commonly used because many people are allergic to povidone-iodine preparations.

7. All persons administering parenteral drugs must wear gloves during the procedure to prevent exposure to blood.

8. There must be a physician's order for all drugs to be administered. This includes contrast media and may include barium mixtures.

9. The five rights of drug administration must be followed.

10. The drug administered must be documented according to the policy of the department.

11. The patient must be observed closely for 1 hour following drug administration for adverse or allergic reactions.

12. A patient who has had a sedative, tranquilizing, or hypnotic drug may *not* drive home alone.

Summary

1. Drug nomenclature is the process of how drugs are named.
   a. The trade name is given by the manufacturer. This may be the name by which most people know the drug.
   b. The chemical name is the formula of the drug and will not change.
   c. The generic name is given after approval.
   d. Diazepam is a generic name and is not well recognized, yet the trade name, Valium, is known. The trade name is better known than the generic name.
2. Drug classification is based on the medical value or the risk of dependence and misuse.
   a. Pharmacology classification includes schedules based on dependence.
      i. A class I drug is not used for medical purposes; class II drugs (opioids) have a high abuse potential; and class V drugs have a low level of dependence and are cough syrups and antidiarrheal medication
   b. Drugs are also classified by chemical groups—depressants, stimulants, and hallucinogens.
3. General pharmacology principles include the mechanism of the drug, the effect of it, and the site of action.
   a. Pharmacokinetics looks at how the drug is absorbed, distributed, metabolized, and then excreted.
      i. Partial metabolism before the drug reaches the systemic circulation is called the first-pass effect. Larger doses are needed because of this.
      ii. Metabolism means that the chemical structure of the drug has been changed.
      iii. Excretion occurs through the kidneys or through the biliary tract and the feces.
   b. Pharmacodynamics is the study of physiologic effects on the body.
   c. Pharmacogenomics is also called pharmacogenetics and studies how genes affect a drug's response on the person.
4. Contrast media are considered drugs because the majority have the same pharmacokinetics as other drugs.
   a. There are three types of contrast. One is radionuclides and is used in nuclear medicine. The other two are negative and positive.
      i. Negative contrast is air (carbon dioxide). It can be used in combination with positive contrast for a "double-contrast" study.
         1. These are known as radiolucent because one can "see through" the medium. Think of the chest image where the patient takes in a large breath, filling the lungs with air. The lungs will appear darker.
      ii. Positive contrasts are called radiopaque contrasts. There are two—barium and water soluble.
         1. Barium is inert and cannot be dissolved in solution. It will separate. It is mixed with water for the use of upper and lower GI studies. A thicker paste-like barium is used for esophagrams.
         2. Soluble contrast contains iodine. It is hypertonic, which means it causes dehydration.
   b. Both ionic and nonionic contrast media contain iodine. Both have a negative anion compound that provides a portion of the makeup of the contrast. The other part is a positive cation, which is either a sodium or meglumine compound that contributes to the osmolality of the contrast.
      i. HOCM created a greater chance of the patient having an adverse effect.
      ii. Contrasts that have an osmolality closer to the human plasma (LOCM) are safer to use and less likely to cause an adverse reaction.
      iii. LOCM are nonionic. HOCM are ionic.
   c. Beam attenuation is affected by the atomic number of the contrast medium. The higher the atomic number, the more x-ray photons are absorbed and less that hit the IR. Thus, the image is "white" or "clear" where the anatomy would be on the image. This gives it a radiopaque look.
      i. The atomic number of barium is 56.
      ii. The atomic number of iodine is 53.
      iii. The atomic number of gadolinium is 64 (gadolinium is used in CT and MRI).
   d. Before injecting contrast media, all patients must be questioned about allergies and fill out a precontrast questionnaire.
      i. Contraindications include previous reactions, asthma, allergies, and heart or renal disease.
      ii. Determine what the patient's medical condition is and find out what medications are being taken.
      iii. Verify the patient's dosage because it relates to age and weight.
      iv. Review the lab values such as BUN, creatinine, and eGFR to avoid renal issues.
      v. Has the patient signed a consent form? Where is the crash cart?
   e. Reactions can occur without warning.
      i. There are vasovagal effects, side effects, and adverse reactions. The ACR has a manual that talks about effects and responses.

    ii. Vasovagal effects are physiologic. They include pallor, rapid pulse, bradycardia, and hypotension.

   iii. Side effects are expected and subside within a short time. Effects include a warm, flushing feeling and an altered taste such as a metallic taste. Reassurance is usually all that is needed and medical intervention is rarely needed in this instance.

   iv. Mild effects include allergic-like symptoms of urticaria, edema, nasal congestion, sneezing, and physiologic effects of nausea and/or vomiting (N/V), hypertension and headache, dizziness, and altered taste.

      1. Medical intervention includes monitoring vital signs, stopping infusion, and getting help if symptoms progress. Do not leave the patient alone and observe closely.

    v. Moderate effects include allergic-like symptoms of urticaria, erythema, bronchospasm, and wheezing. Physiologic effects are N/V and isolated chest pain.

      1. Radiographer must stop the infusion and notify the radiologist. Get ready to help with oxygen and IV medication from the crash cart.

   vi. Severe effects are life-threatening. The patient experiences all of these plus arrhythmia, convulsion, seizures, and anaphylactic shock.

      1. Radiographer must call a code, notify the radiologist, get the crash cart ready with automated external defibrillator (AED), and get ready to help with oxygen and IV medications.

5. Drug safety includes the five rights—patient, drug and documentation, amount, route, and time.

   a. Read the label three times, show it to the person doing the injection, and check the expiration date.

     i. If the label is not readable, do not use it.

   b. Do not mix unless compatibility has been checked.

   c. Throw out drugs that are cloudy or have sediment.

   d. After injection, don't discharge until the patient has been observed for a time for any effects.

6. Drug administration is based on the pharmacodynamics of the contrast. There are basically five routes of administration.

   a. Enteral is either oral, sublingual, buccal, or rectal.

   b. Tube or catheter such NG or NE tubes

   c. Inhalation through the use of aerosols through the mouth or nose

   d. Topical administration is through the skin, eyes, nasal mucous membranes or transdermal patches.

   e. Parenteral routes can only be done by physicians or specialty nurses with the exception of IV. Parenteral routes include the following:

     i. Subcutaneous

     ii. IM

    iii. ID

    iv. Intrathecal

     v. Intra-arterial

    vi. Intraosseous

   vii. Intra-articular

  viii. IV

CHAPTER 12 REVIEW QUESTIONS

1. Drugs that must bear the legend "caution: federal law prohibits dispensing without prescription" include the following:
   a. Hypnotics and narcotics
   b. Alternative drugs
   c. All diet drugs
   d. All analgesics

2. Alternative dietary and herbal supplements are classified as food, not drugs.
   a. True
   b. False

3. The alternative name for Valium is diazepam. Valium is:
   a. The trade name
   b. The generic name
   c. The chemical name

4. Drugs given orally are generally given in larger doses. This is because:
   a. They absorb more slowly.
   b. They absorb more rapidly.
   c. They are unreliable.
   d. Larger doses ensure that some of the drug will remain to perform the intended effect.

5. For a drug to reach its therapeutic effect more quickly, a physician might order:
   a. An initial larger dose and later smaller doses
   b. A smaller initial dose, then a larger dose
   c. A bolus
   d. A maximizing dose

6. Marjorie Merriweather takes oral morphine for chronic pain. After taking the prescribed dosage for 4 weeks, she notices that it no longer seems to be controlling the pain. This reaction is called:
   a. Addiction
   b. Dependency
   c. Tolerance
   d. An adverse reaction

7. Drug absorption varies from person to person. The efficiency of drug absorption is largely dependent on:
   a. The time of day
   b. The sex of the individual
   c. The absorptive surface available
   d. The type of drug

8. Drugs given orally are not affected by the first-pass effect.
   a. True
   b. False

9. Match the following terms pertaining to drugs with the correct definition:

   1. Half-life   a. _____The method of drug action on living tissues
   2. Metabolism   b. _____The effect of a drug that may be life-threatening
   3. Clearance rate   c. _____The process by which the body alters the chemical structure of a drug
   4. Pharmacodynamics   d. _____The time it takes for a 50% decrease of a drug's
   5. Side effect presence in the body   e. _____The removal from the body
   6. Adverse effect   f. _____Unintended but nontoxic effect of a drug

10. Contrast media are categorized as drugs. This is because they are absorbed into the systemic circulation and may produce a physiologic response on the body.
    a. True
    b. False

11. The physiologic effect of a contrast medium on the patients' body that may create an adverse reaction when administered is because of:
    a. Its low viscosity as compared with other drugs
    b. The fact that it is isotonic
    c. Its osmolality particularly when it is higher than blood plasma
    d. Its shift of fluid into the interstitial spaces and cells related to its high viscosity

12. Expected side effects of contrast media administered by intravascular route are: (Circle all that apply)
    a. Feeling of warmth and flushing
    b. Feeling of being short of breath
    c. Metallic taste in mouth
    d. Complaints of itching

13. A patient is receiving an IV contrast medium by bolus. The patient begins to complain of nausea, itching around his eyes, feeling dizzy, and a headache. The radiographer decides the patient is having:
    a. A vasovagal reaction
    b. A mild adverse reaction
    c. A severe adverse reaction
    d. A moderate adverse reaction

Venipuncture

13

KEY TERMS

Bolus: A single, large quantity intended for therapeutic use

Compartment syndrome: When nerves and blood vessels become compressed by the buildup of fluids, decreasing blood flow in the area leading to nerve and tissue damage

Extravasation: The escape of fluid from a vessel into tissue

Infusion: The introduction of a drug slowly through the bloodstream

INTRODUCTION

The professional radiographer who administers drugs is expected to know the safe dosage, the safe route of administration, and the limitations of the drug to be administered. All potential hazards of any drug that is incorrectly or unsafely administered must also be known. If drug administration errors are made because of lack of knowledge, the person who administers the drug is legally liable. Radiologic technology students who are permitted to administer drugs must adhere to the specific ethical and legal guidelines established for drug administration. The student must be supervised by a licensed professional, professional liability coverage must be adequate, and the student must also demonstrate competency before administering drugs without supervision.

The position of the American Society of Radiologic Technologists (ASRT) is that "venipuncture falls within the profession's Scope of Practice and Practice Standards and that it shall be included in the didactic and clinical curriculum with demonstrated competencies of all appropriate disciplines regardless of the state or institution where such curriculum is taught."

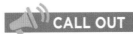
CALL OUT

Any radiographer or radiographic technology student who administers drugs must demonstrate competency before administering drugs without supervision.

CURRENT PRACTICE STANDARDS

According to the ASRT Practice Standards of 2019, the scope of practice for medical imaging professionals allows for administering contrast and medication by parenteral injection through an existing vascular access or through a new one. Other methods of administration include enterally or via an infusion pump or power injector when prescribed by a licensed practitioner.

The ASRT goes on to state that "Federal and state statutes, regulations, accreditation standards and institutional policies could dictate practice·parameters and may supersede these standards." As with all certification and licensing, the student must check the state and employer where employment is sought after graduation. It is incumbent upon the radiographer to apply for the appropriated training and licensing that is required above and beyond the ASRT scope of practice.

With this added responsibility, radiographers can and will be held legally liable in the administration of any drug. Radiographers must be taught the basics of drawing up medications and contrast as well as venipuncture. If the rules of administration, documentation, and observation, as well as knowing the signs and symptoms of reactions (discussed in Chapter 12), are followed religiously, the chances of being found negligent and being named in a lawsuit are greatly reduced.

METHODS

There are various methods of administration that fall under the parenteral route that are part of the scope of practice of a radiographer as stated by the ASRT. Infusion can be either continuous or intermittent. A continuous infusion is also known as a "drip IV" and can take from several hours to days. Contrast media can be hung on an intravenous (IV) pole and slowly administered over the course of 30 minutes to an hour while images are taken at timed intervals. In the case of a mild reaction, a sterile IV solution can be started with medication added to it that reduces the symptoms and to help prevent the reaction from progressing. Intermittent administration is also through an IV infusion but is added as a secondary IV. This is usually done for volume control to limit the amount of medication to children and the elderly.

Another method of drug administration is through direct injection, either by hand or through a power injector. Known as an "IV push," the medication is administered very slowly (1 minute) directly into a vein that has an existing port or an IV line. This type of administration results in an immediate elevation of serum levels and a high concentration to the heart, brain, and kidneys.

Another method is the use of a power injector (Fig. 13-1). These are used routinely in diagnostic and interventional radiology. The use of these injectors ensures there is optimal opacification of the desired anatomy, including the arteries and veins. Computed tomography (CT) and magnetic resonance imaging (MRI) almost routinely use the pressure (power) injector.

Because the injection is made under pressure, standard procedures for operating the injector must be followed in order to minimize any risk of extravasation or air embolism (discussed later in this chapter). Additionally, the use of this type of injection carries risks in pediatric cases. Slower injection rates are required along with smaller doses of contrast.

SITES OF ADMINISTRATION

Sites of drug administration were discussed in Chapter 12; however, a detailed procedure is outlined here for those administrations that can be performed by a radiographer.

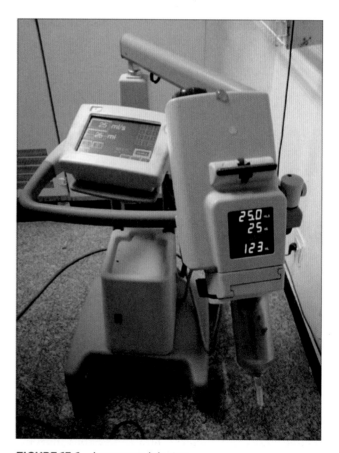

FIGURE 13-1 A pressure injector.

PROCEDURE

Intradermal Injection

1. Select the contrast medium to be tested. Usually, less than 0.5 mL of the medium is used.

2. Select the equipment needed. This includes a tuberculin syringe, a 25G to 27G needle with a 1/2 in length, an alcohol wipe, and a pair of clean gloves.

3. Approach the patient and explain the procedure. Select a site for the test: it is usually administered into the dermis on the inner aspect of the forearm. Areas with excessive hair, scarring, or tattoos must not be used because the results may be difficult to detect.

4. Cleanse the site with an alcohol wipe in a firm, circular motion.

5. Put on gloves.

6. Hold the skin at the area to be injected taut with the nondominant hand.

7. Insert the needle, bevel side up, at a 5° to 15° angle. It should be almost flat against the skin.

8. Inject the drug. A small raised area or wheal should be seen at the injection site (Fig. 13-2).

9. Withdraw the needle but do not massage or cleanse the site. Remove gloves and

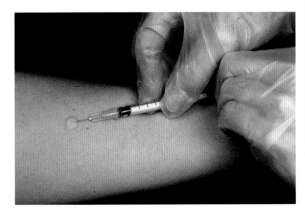

FIGURE 13-2 Performing an intradermal injection.

dispose of the needle according to rules of standard precautions.

10. Instruct the patient concerning the time to read the results of the test. Usually, the time allowed for contrast results is brief. If the patient is allergic to the contrast medium, the area becomes inflamed, and the patient complains of itching at the site. If the patient has a more severe reaction, follow the instructions for allergic reactions. Any reaction must be reported to the radiologist before any contrast medium is administered.

11. Document the procedure and the result of the injection.

Intradermal Administration

Intradermal injections are also called *intracutaneous injections*. For the radiographer's purposes, only the injection used for testing for sensitivity to a contrast medium is discussed. These injections are under the layers of the skin of the inside of the forearm.

Intramuscular Injections

Intramuscular routes for administration of drugs are the dorsal gluteal (anterior, lateral area of the pelvis near the anterior superior iliac spine [ASIS]), the ventrogluteal (lateral aspect of the hip, found by placing the palm on the greater trochanter, the index finger on the ASIS, and making a "V" between the second and third fingers), and the deltoid muscles (the lateral aspect of the shoulder at the mid-deltoid area) (Fig. 13-3A-C). The radiographer must assess the patient before obtaining a site for intramuscular injection. Elderly persons lose muscle mass and may need a shorter needle and a site in which there is an appropriate amount of muscular tissue. The amount of fluid that may be safely administered ranges from 1 to 5 mL. Persons receiving the injection must be relatively large if more than 3 mL of medication is to be injected into the muscle. The radiographer must be educated in a laboratory setting before actually performing this procedure in a clinical setting because incorrect technique may result in harm to the patient. Radiographers in a major facility do not give injections in this manner because it is beyond the scope of practice. However, technologists in rural areas may be schooled in this technique because of multiple roles they have.

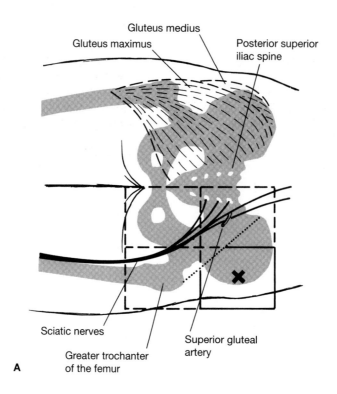

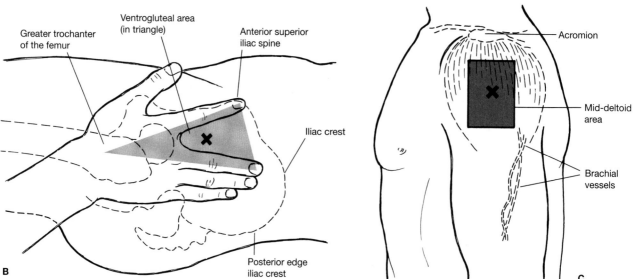

FIGURE 13-3 Sites for intramuscular injection. **(A)** Dorsal gluteal. **(B)** Ventrogluteal. **(C)** Deltoid.

PROCEDURE

Intramuscular Injection

1. Assemble equipment needed. This includes the following: a 3- to 5-mL syringe, an 18G to 22G or 23G needle, a 1-inch-long needle selected for use in the deltoid area or for use on a very thin patient, three alcohol wipes, and a pair of clean gloves.

2. Read the order and identify the drug using the five rights of drug administration. Identify the patient. Assess the patient to determine the site for injection and any

potential allergies to the drug, and explain the procedure to them.

3. Draw up the drug into the syringe. If the medication is an irritating substance such as hydroxyzine, change the needle after it is drawn into the syringe to prevent burning on injection.

4. Position the patient appropriately and cleanse the area with an alcohol wipe. Put on clean gloves and prepare a second alcohol wipe.

5. Place the nondominant hand on the muscle to be injected to support the patient. Quickly insert the needle into the muscle at a 90° angle.

6. With the needle inserted, support the needle with the nondominant thumb and index fingers and draw back on the plunger to aspirate, making certain no blood returns into the syringe. If blood appears in the syringe, withdraw the needle and select an alternative site after changing the needle.

7. If no blood appears, inject the drug into the muscle and quickly withdraw the needle.

8. Wipe the area with the second alcohol wipe. A Band-Aid may be applied if there is a small amount of bleeding following the injection. Remove the gloves.

9. Make the patient comfortable and dispose of the gloves, needle, and syringe correctly.

10. Wash hands and document the procedure.

IV Drug Administration

The area selected for venipuncture requires careful assessment before the procedure is begun. The type of contrast, the length of time for the infusion or bolus, and the age and physical condition of the patient are all to be considered when selecting a venipuncture site.

Veins in the hands and arms should be selected rather than those in the lower extremities unless an emergency precludes this. There is a greater hazard of embolus formation in the lower extremities related to IV infusion. Unless a drug is to be injected by bolus, do not select a vein located over a joint, because any movement dislodges the needle or catheter. If a vein over a joint is selected, the extremity needs to be immobilized. The volar (palm) side of the wrist must not be used because the radial nerve is in that area and the patient may feel extreme pain. Do not select a very small vein for contrast because there is greater danger of leakage into the tissues and pain results. The basilic or cephalic veins are good choices, if available (Fig. 13-4).

Elderly patients must receive special consideration. Their veins are more fragile and have a greater tendency to "roll" as the needle or catheter is inserted. The tissues of the elderly patient are also more fragile, necessitating use of a smaller needle or catheter. The tourniquet is more apt to damage the skin and must be applied with less tension. The elderly patient is also prone to have an adverse reaction to contrast media. This may be the result of medications the patient has taken prior to their admission to the imaging department, a history of diabetes mellitus, or other medical conditions that result in venous thrombosis. Contrast media are more likely to dehydrate the elderly patient; therefore, an IV solution that helps in hydrating the patient is often started prior

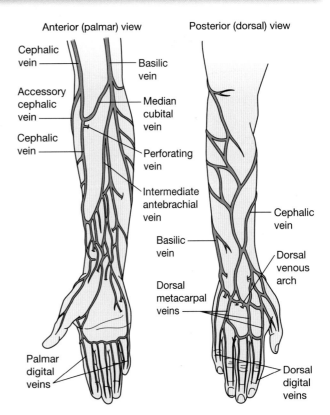

FIGURE 13-4 Basilic and cephalic veins. (From Smeltzer SC, Bare BG, Hinkle JL, et al. *Brunner & Suddarth's Textbook of Medical-Surgical Nursing.* 11th ed. Lippincott Williams & Wilkins; 2008, with permission.)

to the administration of the contrast agent. The elderly patient must be observed closely for any symptom of an adverse reaction as well as **extravasation.**

Pediatric patients are often frightened and have difficulty remaining immobile. Allowing a parent to hold the child's extended arm, if possible, may be the best way to calm the child and maintain immobility during venipuncture. Finding a suitable vein in a small child is often difficult. If the situation permits, a pediatric nurse or pediatric health care specialist should be called upon to perform the venipuncture. Veins on the anterior surface of the forearm are most easily accessible in a child. The size of the butterfly needle or venous catheter must be much smaller than for an adult.

The volume of contrast media is much lower, as is the child's blood volume. The tonicity of the contrast medium must also be considered. Although children do not experience reactions to contrast media as frequently as adults, anaphylactic reactions and other adverse reactions may occur, and the radiographer must be alert for any adverse or allergic symptom. The radiographer must recognize that a child or an infant is unable to communicate feelings; therefore, due diligence is necessary if the patient is a child or an infant. The emergency cart and correct sized equipment must be readily available at any time.

WARNING!

Oxygen administration equipment, pediatric face masks, suction, and all other emergency equipment and drugs must be on hand when a child or an infant is the patient!

There are two main types of IV lines: peripheral and central lines, with the peripheral being the only method by which radiographers may administer contrast media.

The peripheral IV line is a short plastic catheter that is placed into the vein of the hand, forearm, elbow, or foot. For an adult patient, the veins on the dorsal or ventral surface of the forearm should be considered before other areas. The best choices include the cephalic and basilic veins. Avoid using a vein on the same side as breast surgery, a graft, or any site intended for future vascular access on those patients with chronic kidney disease.

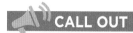
CALL OUT

The peripheral IV route is the only method by which radiographers may administer contrast media parenterally!

A central line is inserted into a vein that communicates directly with the heart's right atrium. A catheter is inserted into a femoral, subclavian, or internal jugular vein. Because these areas have a larger blood flow, a larger quantity of the drug can be used. Radiographers are not permitted to use this method of drug/contrast administration.

VENIPUNCTURE PROCEDURES

Before beginning any procedure that requires venipuncture, the radiographer must think through the process completely. Time wasted getting equipment that wasn't gathered to begin with is frustrating to both the patient and the staff. Documenting errors is far more involved than doing things correctly in the beginning. Understand the administration route and how it is performed completely before beginning. Remember that any invasive procedure requires proper medical aseptic technique for the skin and surgical technique for needles and catheters that are inserted into the patient.

Equipment and Supplies

Needles for parenteral drug administration range in length from 3/8 to 2 in for average use. Longer needles are used for special procedures. Needles may come attached to a syringe of appropriate size or in various sizes packaged separately. Needles are made of stainless steel and consist of the following parts (Fig. 13-5):

- The hub (the part that attaches to the syringe)
- The shaft (the elongated part of the needle)

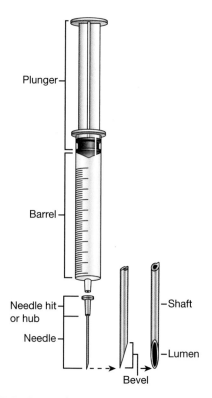

FIGURE 13-5 Parts of syringe and needle. (From Taylor CR, Lillis C, Lynn P, LeMone P. *Fundamentals of Nursing: The Art and Science of Nursing Care.* 8th ed. Lippincott Williams & Wilkins, 2015.)

- The lumen (the hollow tube that runs the length of the shaft)
- The bevel (the sharp angulated tip of the needle)

Selection of the correct size of needle with which to administer a drug is essential. The size of the lumen of the needle can vary from very large to very small. The smaller the lumen, the larger the gauge of the needle (e.g., a 30G needle is much smaller than a 12G needle). The viscosity of the fluid to be injected determines the gauge selected. The area for injection and the condition of the patient determine the length of the needle chosen.

Syringes also vary in size, depending on the amount of fluid to be injected. They generally range in capacity from 0.05 to 50 mL. The parts of the syringe are:

- The tip (the end of the syringe to which the needle is fastened)
- The barrel (the body of the syringe)
- The plunger (the part that fits into the barrel)

Syringes are calibrated in milliliters and minims. One milliliter equals 15 or 16 minims. Syringes are packaged in treated paper or plastic wrappers to maintain sterility, and needles are often attached in the package. The size of the syringe and the size of the needle are printed on the package (Fig. 13-6).

Needlestick injuries are a serious consequence of incorrect handling of injection supplies. The current types of syringes and needles assist in avoidance of this risk. The rules for working with syringes and needles are:

1. Syringes and needles are disposable and are to be discarded after one use.
2. Syringes and needles are to be discarded in puncture-proof containers labeled *sharps container* that are required to be provided in all areas where drugs are administered, even if they contain safety features (Fig. 13-7).

3. A needle that has been used for an injection must not be recapped. If it has a protective mechanism, it must be engaged after use (Fig. 13-8).
4. The used syringe must be held by the barrel and carried immediately to the sharps container (Fig. 13-9).
5. Never place a used syringe and needle back onto a counter to be disposed of at a later time.

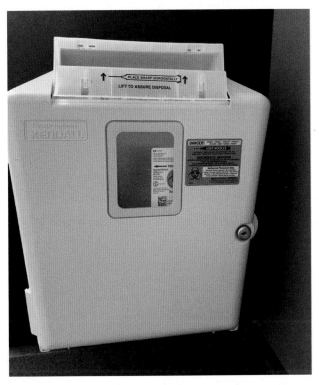

FIGURE 13-7 Sharps containers come in different colors and sizes. Most are red depending on the department in which it is located.

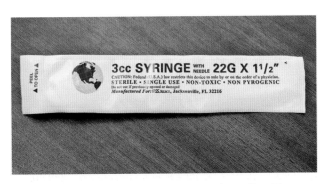

FIGURE 13-6 Packaging for syringe and needles. The contents of this package are sterile until opened.

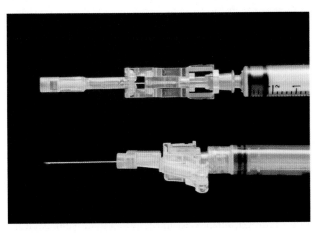

FIGURE 13-8 One type of protective needle device.

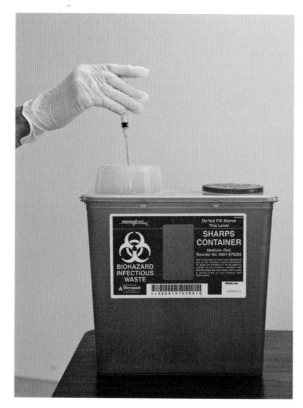

FIGURE 13-9 Discard used needles and syringes in a sharps container.

6. If a needlestick injury should occur, it must be reported as a "critical incident" as soon as possible following the event.

Supplies Needed for IV Drug Administration

1. The following supplies are needed for the administration of an IV drug (contrast medium):

- A butterfly needle (also called a scalp vein needle or a winged needle) or an over-the-needle catheter for a prolonged infusion (either of the correct gauge)
- A tourniquet
- Antimicrobial swabs
- Clean gloves
- The contrast medium drawn up into the correct size syringe or the contrast in a bag or glass bottle for a continuous infusion
- An IV infusion set that includes IV tubing and a drip chamber (Fig. 13-10)
- Clear adhesive dressing or tape for infusion
- An IV pole
- An infusion pump, if required (Fig. 13-11)

Packaging of Parenteral Medications

Drugs intended for parenteral administration are packaged to maintain sterility. If they are intended for IV,

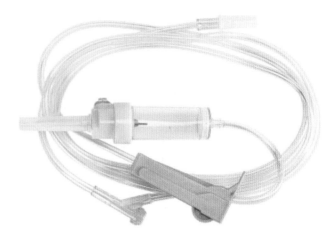

FIGURE 13-10 IV infusion kits such as this will come prepackage in a commercial wrapper.

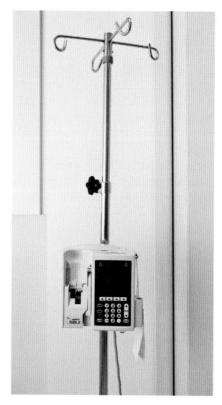

FIGURE 13-11 An intravenous (IV) pump attached to an IV pole.

subcutaneous, or intradermal injection, they are either in an ampule or in a vial. Drugs to be administered IV may be contained in an ampule or a vial if the amount to be administered is small. If a large amount of fluid or drug is to be administered, it is contained in a calibrated glass or plastic container (Fig. 13-12A-D).

An ampule is made of glass and contains a single dose of a drug. The ampule is labeled with the name of the drug, the dosage per milliliter, and the route for administration. A vial is a glass or plastic container with

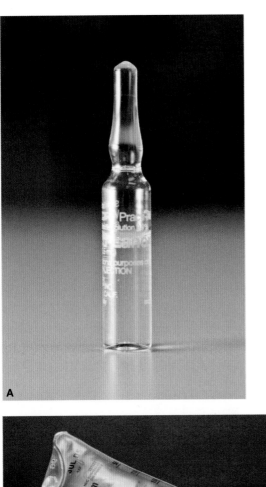

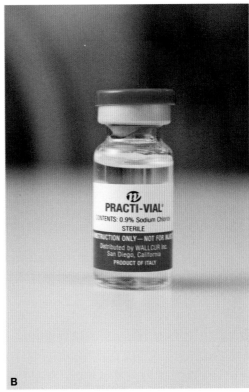

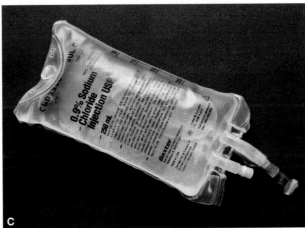

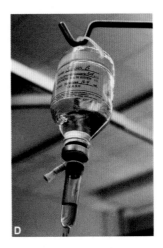

FIGURE 13-12 **(A)** Ampule. **(B)** Vial. **(C)** A collapsible plastic bag used in intravenous (IV) administration of drugs. **(D)** Glass bottle that is used in IV administration of drugs or contrast media.

a rubber stopper circled by a metal band; the band holds the stopper in place. The rubber stopper is protected from contamination by a plastic cap. Some vials are for multidose use. If this is the case, it is considered contaminated after it has been used for 24 hours and must be discarded.

Fluids, contrast media, and medications that are of a large volume (50 to 1,000 mL) are packaged in heavy plastic. Plastic bags containing fluid for IV infusion collapse under atmospheric pressure as the fluid leaves it. The plastic bag has two ports, one for the IV tubing and one to use if other drugs are to be added to the infusion.

Patient Identification and Assessment

As in all other types of diagnostic imaging studies, the patient must be identified by a minimum of two ways, usually stating a full name and also the date of birth. The ordering physician should assess the patient to ensure that the administration of contrast is appropriate. Although guidelines might state that certain actions should be taken when ordering a contrast study, the physician might choose another course of action as necessary based on the condition of the patient or limited resources. Reasons for the

PROCEDURE

Drawing a Drug from an Ampule

1. View the top of the ampule above the neck to see if there is any fluid in the top. If there is, gently tap the cap until the fluid drops down into the ampule (Fig. 13-13).

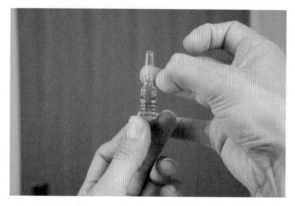

FIGURE 13-13 Be sure to tap the top of the ampule to dislodge any fluid that may be located there. (Reprinted with permission from Craven RF, Hirnle C, Henshaw C., *Fundamentals of Nursing*, 9th Edition. Wolters Kluwer, 2020, p. 503.)

2. The indented area at the neck of the ampule may be opened by simply snapping off the top of the vial.

3. The health care worker must never attempt to snap off the top of an ampule without protecting the hands, because the glass may break unevenly and cause lacerations (Fig. 13-14).

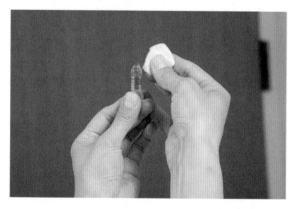

FIGURE 13-14 Protect the hands by placing a gauze pad over the top of the ampule. Break the top so that the broken edge is away from the body. (Reprinted with permission from Craven RF, Hirnle C, Henshaw C., *Fundamentals of Nursing*, 9th Edition. Wolters Kluwer, 2020, p. 503.)

4. If an ampule shatters when broken open, the medication must be discarded because there may be glass shards in the drug.

5. Insert the needle into the ampule and pull back on the plunger to draw the medication into the syringe.

6. If necessary, turn the ampule upside down (Fig. 13-15) to get the last few drops because all medication is needed to make a single dose. The fluid does not come out of the ampule unless the radiographer has injected air into it at the beginning. Injecting air into the ampule is not necessary.

7. If the entire drug in an ampule is not used, it must be discarded because it will not remain sterile after the ampule is opened.

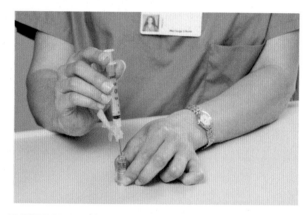

FIGURE 13-15 Place the needle into the ampule. Do not inject air into the ampule. The ampule may be turned upside down if this is not done. Draw the medication into the syringe. (Reprinted with permission from Craven RF, Hirnle C, Henshaw C., *Fundamentals of Nursing*, 9th Edition. Wolters Kluwer, 2020, p. 503.)

PROCEDURE

Drawing a Drug from a Vial

1. Remove the plastic protective cap from the top of the vial.

2. If this is a multidose vial and has been opened previously, check the date and time opened and cleanse the rubber top with an alcohol wipe.

3. Determine the dosage desired from the vial and draw up the equivalent amount of air into the syringe.

4. Insert the needle into the vial and inject the air. Turn the vial upside down so the air rises. This keeps the bevel of the needle in the fluid (Fig. 13-16A and B).

5. Draw the plunger back until the exact amount of drug is obtained (Fig. 13-16C).

6. Remove the syringe from the vial, reread the drug label, and set aside for the physician to see.

7. After the dose has been administered and if there is contrast left in the vial, date and initial it before returning it to the storage area.

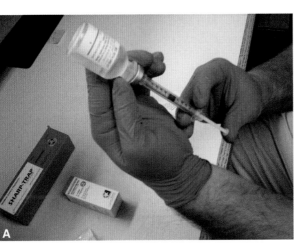
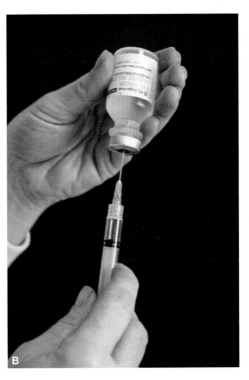

FIGURE 13-16 **(A)** After putting the needle into the vial, inject the amount of air needed to displace the amount of medication desired. **(B)** After injecting the air, pull back on the plunger to draw up the medication.

deviation of published guidelines are documented in the patient's medical record.

Assessment performed by the radiographer prior to contrast administration is the precontrast questionnaire. This alerts the radiographer to possible complications from the contrast. Based on the answers the patient provides, the radiographer can communicate concerns to the radiologist. It is possible that the patient undergoes a test dose prior to the actual study. This small amount of contrast is injected intradermally or subcutaneously to assess any reaction that may occur.

Informed Consent

Informed consent is not the act of signing of a document that states that permission is given to administer drugs and perform the procedure that requires the contrast. Informed consent means that the physician or designee has had a conversation with the patient regarding:

a. The purpose and nature of the procedure
b. How the procedure is performed
c. Possible complications, risks, and benefits
d. Consequences of not having the procedure

The patient has the right to question the physician about these reactions and make an educated decision regarding the procedure. Patients have the right to rescind the consent prior to the start of the exam.

In order for patients to make that educated decision, they must understand what the consent is about. The explanation must be conducted in the language of the patient. A translator must be used if this is applicable. The patient must be of legal age and also mentally competent to understand what is being presented. If this isn't the case, the patient's parent or legal guardian may make the decision if they were involved in the discussion regarding the procedure.

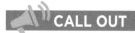

CALL OUT

Consent forms must be signed by both the patient, or representative, and the physician or designee who spoke with the patient.

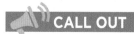

CALL OUT

A copy of the signed informed consent must be made part of the patient's medical record.

Dosage, Calculation, and Dose-Response

The dosage (amount of drug that is given) is dependent on the method of administration and the age of the patient. There are pediatric dose calculators that compute the dose for a child of a given weight. There is a separate calculator that is to be used with adult patients. The health care worker inputs the concentration of the drug, the weight of the patient, and the dose that is to be delivered, and the calculator determines how much one dose will be. In the case of contrast media, vials of contrast contain one dose of contrast that is injected through an IV. Pediatric doses are much less because of the weight of the patient and the immature metabolism of the child.

Dose-response is a cause-and-effect relationship. What happens to a patient when a certain amount of drug is given? Not only the amount of solution but also the concentration of the drug in solution must be taken into account. There is assumed to be little or no effect with very low dosages and toxic effects at very high doses. What is desired is a therapeutic response to occur somewhere between the two extremes of dosages. It must be remembered that just because a high dose is administered the effect is not an automatic higher effect. The outcome could actually decrease the risk to the patient.

When a drug is drawn up in a syringe, the calibrations are done in the metric system. The metric system of measurement has been adopted in most countries as the official standard; in the United States, however, its use is recommended but not required.

The metric system of measurement is used in most medical settings in this country, but the apothecary system of measurement is also used. This means that anyone who administers drugs must understand and be able to use the two systems interchangeably. The radiographer who plans to administer drugs must learn to convert from metric to apothecary measurement, depending on how the physician's order is written.

The metric unit of measure is the liter (L), which contains 1,000 milliliters (mL) or the approximate cubic metric equivalent of 1,000 cubic centimeters (cc). The unit of weight is the gram (g). Kilograms (kg), milligrams (mg), and micrograms (µg) are used in health care. The kilogram is 10,000 g or, in nonmetric terms, 2.2 lb.

Medical symbols and abbreviations are used in health care on a daily basis, and any person who works in this arena is expected to understand them. A list of the most common abbreviations and equivalencies appears in Table 13-1. The radiographer must not make up abbreviations or administer a drug unless there is a complete understanding of correct dosage.

TABLE 13-1	Common Standard Medical Abbreviations		
Abbreviation	**Definition**	**Abbreviation**	**Definition**
PO	By mouth	ac	Before meals
IM	Intramuscular	pc	After meals
IV	Intravenous	hs	At bedtime
STAT	At once	PRN	As necessary
VO	Verbal order	q	Every
SC or SQ	Subcutaneous	qd	Every day
ID	Intradermal	tid	Three times a day
bid	Twice a day	q2h	Every 2 hours
gtt	Drop	mL	Milliliter
cc	Cubic centimeter		

Patient Instructions and Preparation

To help reduce or eliminate the possibility that the patient becomes nauseated and vomits after contrast administration, there are some facilities that require the patient to remain NPO (fasting) approximately 4 hours prior to the procedure. There is a possibility of aspiration when the patient vomits. The use of nonionic low osmolar contrast media (LOCM) reduces the possibility enough that most practices do not require the patient to fast prior to the exam. In fact, fasting itself presents with some concerning possibilities, such as fainting or dizziness. Patients should be instructed to continue taking their prescribed medications, even if they are told to not eat or drink prior to the exam.

General instructions should be printed out and given to the patient prior to the study. For those patients taking an oral contrast like barium sulfate, the patient is instructed to be NPO for a period of time. The contrast comes already mixed, but the patient must be reminded to shake the bottle well before drinking it. Timing is important to make sure the contrast is in the proper location by the time the scan starts. Patients should start drinking 1.5 hours prior to the appointment and drink one-third of the bottle every 15 minutes. The last one-third should be consumed at the appointment.

Other instructions should be given regarding diabetic drugs that the patient may be taking. Also, the patient must be given a phone number to call in case there are questions, or the need to cancel arises.

Some patients are required to have lab tests done to determine renal function. Values of blood urea nitrogen (BUN), estimated glomerular filtration rate (eGFR), and creatinine may cause the ordering physician to decide that a particular contrast is not appropriate. As an example, if eGFR is less than 30 mL/min and the patient is known to have chronic kidney disease, gadolinium-based contrast is withheld because of the increased risk of fibrosis in the kidney.

Standard Precautions

As stated in Chapter 12, contrast media are drugs and the precautions listed pertain to contrast as well. Those precautions are:

✓ The six rights
✓ Read the label three times; check for name, expiration date, cautionary labels, and strength of the drug.
✓ Check for color change, sediment, and cloudiness.
✓ Ensure the patient has filled out an allergic history and that it has been confirmed and is in the patient's record.
✓ If the person who is administering the drug did not draw it up, it is incumbent on them to check the label or not administer the drug at all, especially if that person did not see the drug being drawn up.
✓ All administration of any type of drug must be documented and entered into the patient's record.

Needle safety is very important. Once a needle has been used, it should be disposed of, along with the syringe, immediately in the sharps container. If a needlestick incident should occur, it must be reported as soon as possible and a critical incident report should be filled out.

Performing Venipuncture

Contrast media may be given by bolus or by infusion. A **bolus** is a designated amount of a drug that is administered at one time, usually over a period of several minutes. An **infusion** usually refers to a larger amount of a drug, fluid, or fluid containing a drug or electrolytes that is administered over a longer period ranging from hours to days. Both methods require venipuncture; each requires different equipment.

Prior to approaching the patient to begin the actual invasive procedure of the vein, the infusion must be assembled and made ready for the connection to the needle.

PROCEDURE

Preparing for an IV Drug Administration

The following must be completed prior to insertion of a needle into a vein:

1. Assemble the proper contrast to be administered, an IV infusion kit, gloves, tape, and a scalp vein needle (Fig. 13-17) if appropriate. If the administration is through an existing line, the contrast should be drawn up in a syringe with a clean, unused needle attached.

2. Prepare the containers (collapsible bag or glass bottle) for the IV tubing. Opening a new bottle by removing the metal tab from the bottle leaves the top sterile. Caution: Do NOT remove the metal band surrounding the black rubber stopper! Remove the blue topper from the bag. This area is sterile and should remain so. Be careful not to touch the end (Fig. 13-18).

3. Open the IV tubing and straighten out, removing all kinks. Place the clamp near the drip chamber and close it by rolling the thumb valve down to the bottom of the clamp (Fig. 13-19).

(continued)

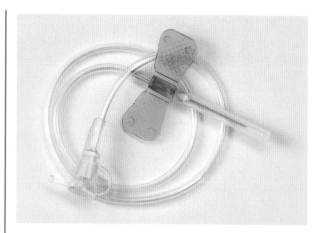

FIGURE 13-17 Intravenous (IV) scalp needle used in IV administrations. (Courtesy of Shutterstock/ANGHI.)

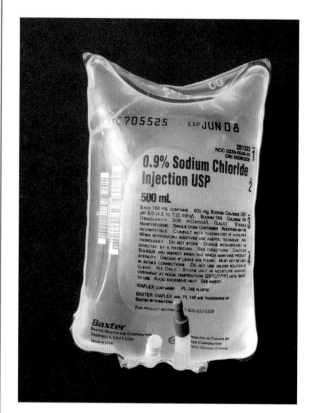

FIGURE 13-18 Collapsible bag showing the blue-capped port in which to put the spike of the intravenous line.

4. Remove the cap on the spike of the drip chamber. This is sterile. Do not touch it. Put the spike into the rubber stopper of the glass bottle or the tab of the bag (Fig. 13-20). If using a bottle, do NOT push the spike into the vented opening. This is to allow air into the bottle. This opening is smaller than the opening to use for the tubing.

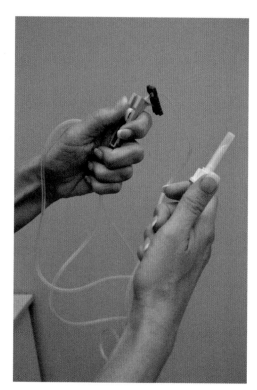

FIGURE 13-19 Close the clamp by rolling it to the bottom.

5. Hang the container on the IV pole. Squeeze the drip chamber until it is half full (Fig. 13-21). Do NOT fill it as the drops from the container must be seen to make sure the fluid is still flowing.

6. Raise the pole until the container is 18 to 24 in above the patient. Open the clamp and allow the fluid to flow through the tubing to displace and remove any air

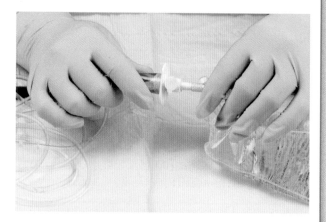

FIGURE 13-20 Place the spike of the drip chamber into the port opening of the container. (Courtesy of Shutterstock/MedstockPhotos.)

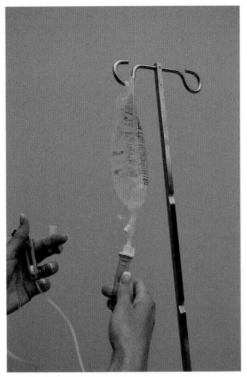

FIGURE 13-21 Insert the top of the intravenous line into the solution container.

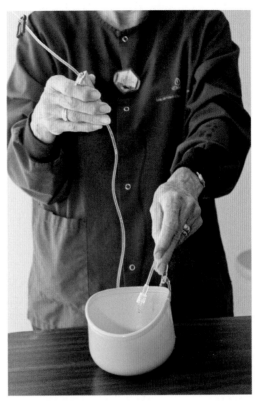

FIGURE 13-22 Prepare the intravenous line for use by bleeding the air from the tubing.

in the tubing. Be sure to clamp the line closed once the air is gone (Fig. 13-22).

7. Drape the tubing over the IV pole and take to the patient.

PROCEDURE

Performing Venipuncture

The following procedure should be followed when performing venipuncture:

1. Approach and identify the patient, and assess for latex or iodine allergies. Explain the procedure and answer any questions there might be.

2. Perform a hand wash.

3. Secure the tourniquet over the site selected in such a manner that it can be removed by pulling on one end (Fig. 13-23A and B).

4. Instruct the patient to make two or three tight fists to force more blood into the veins to make them more visible.

5. Put on clean gloves. Gloves need not be sterile; however, all other equipment used that cleans or penetrates the skin must be sterile.

6. Cleanse the area for the venipuncture with an antiseptic swab or alcohol swab using firm strokes from center of site to outside. Do this at least three times using a separate swab each time. Allow the area to dry.

7. Hold the skin taut above or below the insertion site. Insert the needle or catheter bevel side up into the vein (Fig. 13-24).

8. When the needle enters the vein, blood returns into the flashback chamber immediately. If no blood returns, the venipuncture was not successful. If this is the case, remove the needle and obtain a new needle to start the IV and select a new site. Apply pressure to the failed area with a sterile gauze pad until bleeding stops. If the second effort fails, call a member of the IV team or another team member who will be able to start the IV.

(continued)

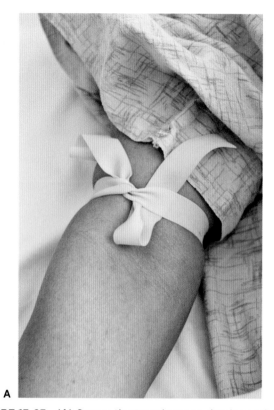 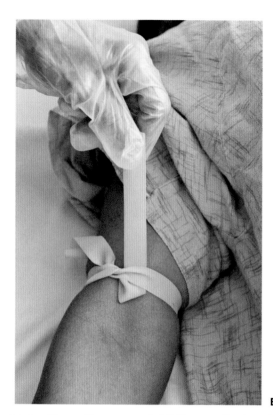

A   B

FIGURE 13-23 **(A)** Secure the tourniquet so that it may be removed by pulling one end. **(B)** Remove the tourniquet by pulling one end.

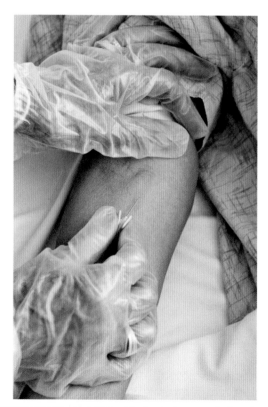

FIGURE 13-24 Hold the skin taut above or below the insertion site.

9. If blood returns, release the tourniquet, instruct the patient to relax, thread the needle 1/8 to 1/4 in further into the vein, and connect the syringe containing the contrast medium if a bolus is ordered. If an infusion is started, remove the needle from the catheter, thread the catheter into the vein, and connect the IV tubing (Fig. 13-25). Secure the catheter with narrow nonallergenic tape and/or a transparent dressing.

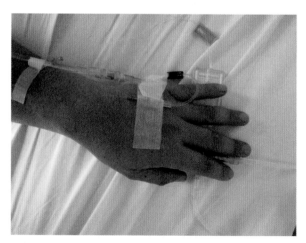

FIGURE 13-25 Connect the intravenous tubing to the catheter of the needle and secure with tape. (Courtesy of Shutterstock/Kittinand Intham.)

10. A bolus is administered at the rate ordered. An infusion is begun at the rate ordered by the physician.

11. Document the procedure, including the time the IV was started and the contrast medium injected. The radiographer must sign all documentation.

12. The needle should be left in place to leave an open line until the procedure is complete. This provides quick and easy availability to inject medication to counteract an adverse reaction to the previously injected contrast.

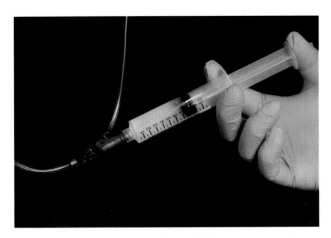

FIGURE 13-26 Use a port on an existing intravenous line to inject contrast using a syringe.

If the contrast is to be administered through an existing port, the contrast should be drawn up into a syringe. Find a "piggyback" port located on the already established IV line. Clean it with an alcohol wipe. Next, using a new needle, insert it into the rubber port. While pinching off the IV line above the port (to prevent that medication from flowing into the contrast and diluting it), inject the contrast from the syringe into the IV line (Fig. 13-26). Once the contrast has been injected, release the IV line and remove the syringe and needle. Immediately place these into the sharps container. Observe the patient as in any other contrast administration.

Site Observations

Once the venipuncture procedure is complete and the infusion is in place, stay with the patient if possible, leaving only to take images as required. Check the site for redness or swelling. Look at the tubing to make sure there are no kinks or bends that would inhibit the flow of drug. Continue to converse with the patient to assess their ability to respond coherently and to determine if there is a change in the pitch and tone of the voice.

CARE OF THE PATIENT WITH AN IV INFUSION IN PLACE

If the IV infusion site is the antecubital vein, the patient's arm must be secured so as to immobilize the elbow

joint. The arm may be secured using an elastic bandage applied to avoid circulatory impairment. Assess the site frequently to ensure that there is no discomfort or impaired circulation.

The infusion site must be assessed every 30 minutes to be certain that the contrast medium is not infiltrating into the surrounding tissues. Ask the patient about any pain or discomfort, and inspect the surrounding tissues for swelling, coldness, or redness. If there is any such condition, discontinue the infusion and ask the physician for direction. If the solution is infusing too slowly, reposition the arm and assess the flow. The IV standard must be positioned 18 to 24 in above the injection site. A large amount of fluid infusing too quickly may result in fluid intoxication or pulmonary edema, both of which are life-threatening. The symptoms of this may be headache, syncope, flushing of the face, complaints of feeling tightness of the chest, shock, and cardiac arrest.

 WARNING!

The radiographer must never place pressure on the needle when administering a bolus of drug or contrast. The fluid must be able to flow into the vein with ease!

Emergency Medical Treatments

Once a patient has been injected with or ingested large amounts of contrast media, the radiographer must be attentive to the patient's reactions. Whether a pressure injector or hand injection has been used, the radiographer must continue to communicate with the patient in a two-way conversation. Being attentive to any change in tone or pitch of the patient's voice is one of the first indications of laryngeal swelling. Never leave the patient alone (except to take images). If any onset of contrast reaction is observed, help should be summoned.

Appropriate Codes

If the patient is experiencing a severe reaction, a Code Blue must be called. The radiographer must know how to do this as time cannot be wasted looking up phone numbers or what type of code must be called. Most health care facilities have a specific phone number that is called that the operator answers immediately. The caller should announce "Code Blue" along with the location of the emergency. Also, state if the patient is a child or neonate to alert the emergency team that the patient is not an adult. An example of a call would be "Code Blue; pediatric; CT 3." The operator will announce on the overhead speaker the call three times. When the code has ended, the radiographer needs to alert the same operator so that an "all clear" announcement can be made.

Emergency Cart

The crash cart (Fig. 13-27) is a set of drawers and trays that are on wheels so that it can be moved from one area to another quickly. The contents of the cart may vary from different areas of the hospital, but for those located in the imaging department, the contents are needed to treat a person in or near a cardiac arrest or respiratory arrest because of a contrast medium reaction. In addition, a defibrillator, suction devices, and bag valve masks are on the cart. The common emergency medications that are found in the cart are listed in Table 13-2. In addition, drugs for intubation such as succinylcholine and for peripheral and central venous access are found on the cart.

Accessory Equipment

In addition to the medications listed in Table 13-2, an IV pole, an oxygen tank holder, sharps container, and an

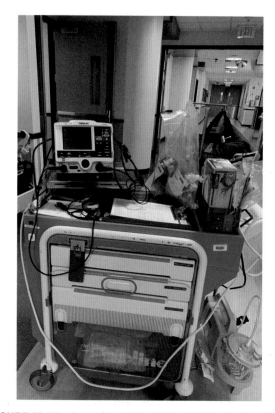

FIGURE 13-27 A crash cart that is located in the imaging department.

automated external defibrillator (AED) are found on the outside of the cart. A back board may also be located on the back of the cart. Although the equipment located inside the cart varies from one imaging department to another, most have the following:

Alcohol wipes and iodine cleansing swabs

Airway equipment (laryngoscope, endotracheal tubes, tracheal tubes, oxygen flow meter, nasal cannulas)

Blood pressure equipment (stethoscope, pressure cuff)

Scissors and hemostats

Syringes, needles, and tourniquets

Sterile gloves, gauze, bandages, tape, and adhesive pads

Various tubes (nasogastric [NG], suction, Levine)

Radiographer's Response

During the course of the emergency medical treatment, the radiographer must be on hand to assist as needed. In almost all cases, the Code Blue team handles the emergency; however, the radiographer must be able to relay to the physicians what happened, when it happened, what was done to react to the patient's condition, and what the vital signs were before the team arrived. The radiographer's responsibility is to document everything that took place prior to calling the Code Blue. Documentation is critical. As stated elsewhere in this book, if it isn't documented, it didn't happen. The time that each event happened must be logged on the facility's unusual occurrence report. Once the report is completed, it must be signed and entered into the patient's medical record. In the event that there is litigation stemming from an adverse reaction and emergency intervention, documentation is necessary to help determine if the proper steps were taken for patient care.

COMPLICATIONS

Drugs administered IV act very quickly. Any complaint of itching or feeling of congestion or fullness in the chest or throat is a cause for ceasing drug administration. The radiographer must not wait for further evidence of complications. Stop the infusion or bolus and notify the physician.

Infiltration

When an IV infiltrates, the fluid that should have been carried through the veins seeps into the tissues. Some drugs are extremely irritating to tissues if allowed to infiltrate. The result may be pain, swelling, and **compartment syndrome**. Symptoms usually begin within 8 hours or up to 48 hours. The patient may experience throbbing, tingling or numbness, swelling, or discoloration. In severe cases,

TABLE 13-2	Common Emergency Medications		
Drug	**Route**	**Concentration**	**Volume**
Epinephrine	IM, IV, SC, ET, IO	1.0 mg/mL	1 mL ampule
		1.0 mg/mL	1 mL vial
		1.0 mg/mL	30 mL vial
		0.1 mg/mL	10 mL syringe
		0.01 mg/mL	5 mL syringe
Dopamine	IV	0.8 mg/mL	250 and 500 mL bag
		1.6 mg/mL	250 and 500 mL bag
		40 mg/mL	5, 10, and 20 mL vial
		80 mg/mL	5 and 20 mL vial
		80 mg/mL	10 mL syringe
		160 mg/mL	5 mL vial
Atropine	IV, ET, IO	0.05 mg/mL	5 mL syringe
		0.10 mg/mL	10 mL syringe
		0.30 mg/mL	1 and 30 mL vial
		0.40 mg/mL	1, 20, and 30 mL vial
		0.50 mg/mL	5 mL syringe
		0.80 mg/mL	0.5 mL syringe
		1.0 mg/mL	10 mL syringe
Lidocaine (direct IV administration)	IV, ET, IO	10 mg/mL	5 mL syringe
		10 mg/mL	20, 30, and 50 mL syringe
		20 mg/mL	5 mL syringe
Lidocaine (IV mixture)	IV	40 mg/mL	25, 50 mL vials
		40 mg/mL	25 and 50 mL syringe
		100 mg/mL	10 mL vial
		200 mg/mL	10 mL vial
Lidocaine (premixed IV infusion)	IV	2 mg/mL	500 and 1,000 mL bag
		4 mg/mL	250 and 500 mL bag
		8 mg/mL	250 and 500 mL bag
Sodium bicarbonate	IV, IO	0.5 mEq/mL	5 and 10 mL syringe
		0.9 mEq/mL	50 mL syringe
		1.0 mEq/mL	10 and 50 mL syringe
Vasopressin	IV, IM		20 units/mL
Amiodarone	IV		150 mg/3 mL vial

ET, endotracheal; IM, intramuscular; IO, intraosseous; IV, intravenous; SC, subcutaneous.

the patient may need surgery on the area of infiltration to relieve the pressure, which restores blood flow. If it is left untreated, the limb may need to be amputated.

Extravasation

Extravasation is fluid that leaks into the tissue around the injection site. This differs from infiltration in that tissues are damaged, where infiltration of the fluid does not damage the tissue. Where there is extravasation, it must be treated as a medical emergency, and immediate action is required. It is more common and severe in pediatric patients. Elderly patients are at increased risk for extravasation because the patient may unknowingly dislodge the needle because of a confused state of mind; the elderly patient may have reduced pain sensation and not tell the technologist of a problem at the site, and because the skin is fragile and veins roll quite easily.

Extravasation is associated with needle placement in the dorsum of the hand, foot, ankle, and near joints. Butterfly needles cause extravasation more readily than a cannulated needle, so these should be avoided if possible.

Signs of extravasation are as follows:

1. Patient complains of moderate-to-severe pain, burning, or stinging at the injection site.
2. Redness and/or swelling and possible leakage of fluid (contrast) at the site
3. The infusion does not flow freely, and resistance is encountered when an attempt to adjust the flow rate is made.

Responses to extravasation include:

1. Explain to the patient what is suspected and what is about to be done.
2. Stop the infusion but leave the needle in place.
3. Slowly aspirate any remaining contrast from the needle.
4. Remove the needle.
5. Place a cold (or warm) pack on the site and elevate the part.

Phlebitis

Phlebitis means inflammation caused by an irritation in a vein, such as an IV catheter. The vein becomes swollen because of the IV. This type of phlebitis is not usually serious but it can lead to other infections within the bloodstream. Symptoms include redness, warmth, tenderness, and swelling of the surface of the skin around the injection site. Treatment involves applying a warm compress to the affected area after removing the IV. Elevating the arm helps. It should resolve within a few days to a week.

Air Embolism

An air embolism developing from peripheral IV lines is rare; however, symptoms of one need to be discussed so that the radiographer can identify what is occurring and take the necessary steps to rectify the situation. An air embolism occurs when one or more air bubbles enter the vein and block it. These bubbles can travel to the brain, heart, or lungs. Minor air embolisms may show no symptoms or very mild ones. If the patient is experiencing difficulty breathing, chest pain, hypotension, or cyanosis, get help immediately as these are signs of a severe air embolism, which may lead to respiratory failure or a heart attack.

Drug Incompatibility

Drug incompatibility occurs when two or more drugs are combined in the same syringe, tubing, or bottle. It creates physical and chemical changes that are noticeable, such as precipitation, and changes in color or consistency of the drug. Precipitation is likely when oppositely charged drug salts are mixed in strong concentrations. Incompatibility of drugs is hazardous and any person administering a drug that is mixed with another must be absolutely certain that the two are compatible and not cause complications.

Low Fluid Level

When the fluid level within the IV container falls below the level of the spike, there should be enough fluid left in the drip chamber to keep any air out of the tubing. There should be no air entering from the bottle or collapsible bag, nor should there be blood backing up from the insertion site unless something interferes with the IV. Air cannot get into the body if the container runs dry.

DISCONTINUATION

An infusion is not discontinued without a physician's order to do so except in situations that call for immediate action. Patients who are receiving IV drugs do not wish to have an IV restarted if it is not necessary, because the procedure is uncomfortable. The radiographer must be certain that the IV infusion is to be discontinued and the catheter withdrawn at the termination of a procedure before proceeding.

To discontinue an IV, gather the following equipment: dry sterile 2 × 2 in gauze sponges, clean disposable gloves, and a roll of tape.

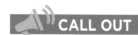
CALL OUT

The radiographer must not discontinue an IV without orders from the physician!

PROCEDURE

Discontinuing an IV

1. Identify the patient; wash hands.

2. Stop the solution that may be continuing to be instilled.

3. Disconnect the IV line from the needle, making certain that the hub or the needle or catheter is clearly visible and still in the patient (Fig. 13-28).

4. Prepare a sufficient strip of tape to cover a small pressure dressing.

5. Loosen the tape that holds the needle or catheter in place (Fig. 13-29). Do NOT untape the actual insertion site.

6. Open the sterile gauze sponge pack using aseptic technique.

7. Put on clean gloves.

8. Gently withdraw the needle or catheter from the vein completely (Fig. 13-30).

9. Apply pressure to the site with the dry, sterile sponge until bleeding stops—about 2 minutes.

10. When the bleeding stops, place a sterile gauze sponge folded in half over the site of insertion, and tape it in place using some pressure over the sponge. Inform the patient that this dressing may be removed in 1 or 2 hours.

11. Dispose of the materials correctly. Remove gloves and wash hands.

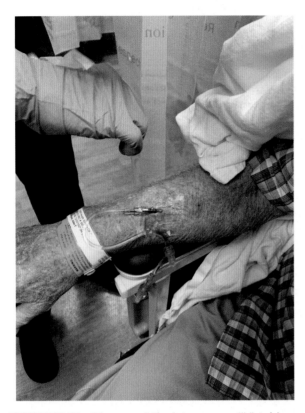

FIGURE 13-28 Disconnect the intravenous (IV) tubing from the catheter of the needle prior to removing the IV needle.

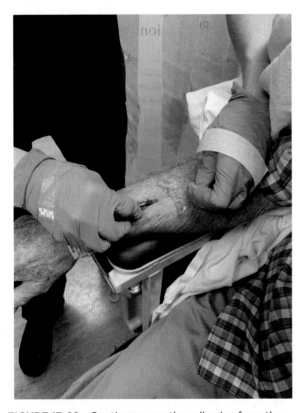

FIGURE 13-29 Gently remove the adhesive from the site, being careful not to dislodge the needle.

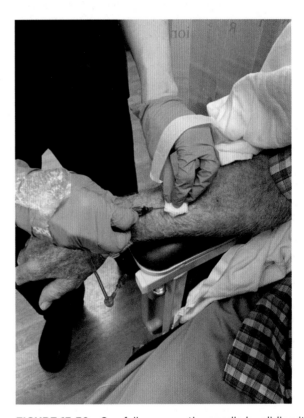

FIGURE 13-30 Carefully remove the needle by sliding it down the arm and placing a gauze pad over the needle site.

DOCUMENTATION OF ADMINISTRATION

Licensed physicians, dentists, podiatrists, and optometrists can prescribe, dispense, and administer drugs. Under specific circumstances that vary from state to state, nurse practitioners, physician assistants, and pharmacists may order and dispense drugs.

No health care worker may prescribe or administer drugs that are not ordered by a person licensed to do so. In health care settings, an order must be dated, written, and signed by the physician. If the patient is in a diagnostic imaging department, the order for the procedure is considered to be the order for the contrast injection.

The written request for an examination using IV contrast media should include the medical necessity for the examination, the type of contrast to be used, and the manner in which the procedure is performed. Medical necessity for the procedure is demonstrated by including the signs and symptoms of the patient's problem, a relevant history, the current diagnoses, and a specific reason for the procedure requested. This request must come from the patient's physician.

When a radiographer, acting under the supervision of a radiologist, administers a contrast medium to a patient, it must be recorded in the patient's medical record. The time of day, the name of the contrast, the dose, and the route of administration must be included in the documentation. The radiographer, or whoever administers the medication, must also sign the medical record for identification purposes. The supervising physician then countersigns the entry. The documentation of administration of contrast media vary according to institutional protocol. In most cases, the use of contrast media is stated in the radiologist's report following the procedure.

If a patient is to be discharged with a prescription, it will be written on the physician's personal order form. The order includes the following:

> The patient's full name, the date, and the time the order is written
>
> The date and time(s) that the drug is to be taken
>
> The generic or the trade name of the drug
>
> The dosage and the route of administration
>
> The physician's signature

An example of a physician's order for a hospitalized patient might be as follows:

> 7 AM July 19, 2022
>
> Give Tramadol, 5 mg by mouth (PO) at 8 AM
>
> J. Glucose, MD

Another type of order that is encountered is the stat order. This means that a physician gives an order for medication to be administered immediately. This order must also be written and signed by the physician. The most common "stat" order the radiographer receives is for a radiographic image to be taken, such as in a "stat" mobile chest radiograph.

In the radiographic imaging department, the radiographer frequently assists with medication administration rather than actually giving the drug. If this is the case, after receiving a verbal order from a physician to procure a drug to administer, the radiographer does the following:

1. Obtain the drug from the locked drug storage area or the pharmacy location.
2. Verify that it is the correct drug by checking the label before taking it from the area.
3. Obtain the correct supplies for the particular route of administration and prepare the drug; that is, draw it into a syringe or pour it into a glass for oral administration as appropriate and read the label a second time.
4. Put the medication, the package from which it was taken, and other items that are needed for administration in an area that is available to the radiologist or other physician.
5. Hold the package (bottle and vial) at the physician's eye level and state the name and dosage of the drug that has been prepared as the physician prepares to administer the drug. Be sure that the physician reads and acknowledges the drug.
6. Assist the physician to administer the drug to the patient.
7. Document the drug in the correct area.

Every institution has a slightly different manner of documentation. It is the radiographer's responsibility to learn the correct method. Many institutions use the Medication Administration Record (MAR) format of documentation. MAR must be recorded immediately after the administration. It cannot be completed prior to the administration. It must contain the following information:

1. Patient's name
2. Name, strength, and quantity of the drug
3. How the drug is to be administered
4. Date and time the drug is to be administered
5. Name of the person administering the drug
6. Any changes made to the original order
7. Any reaction that occurred (if this is the case, an unusual occurrence report must also be filled out)

MEDICATION ERRORS, RESPONSE, AND DOCUMENTATION

All professional health care workers are responsible for their actions. It is the legal and ethical obligation of all radiographers to be knowledgeable about any drug that they administer. If a drug is incorrectly administered or an order misinterpreted, the radiographer is legally liable. All federal regulations pertaining to controlled substances must be fully understood. The Controlled Substances Act of the federal government restricts personnel who are legally permitted to administer narcotic and hypnotic drugs or any drug that may cause dependence. It also restricts access to these drugs, which should always be kept in a locked area. Documentation and accounting for these drugs are also carefully controlled.

Medication errors are an area of frequent litigation in diagnostic imaging. The radiographer who is administering or assisting with administration of drugs is frequently implicated in this type of litigation. If an error in medication administration is made or if the patient has an adverse reaction to a contrast medium, the radiographer involved must assess the patient's condition and notify the prescribing physician immediately.

The error or adverse reaction must be included in the patient's chart. An incident report (sometimes called an unusual occurrence report) is also required by the facility. A "misadventure" form or a "misadministration" form is also required. A "misadventure" is one in which the wrong dose or wrong contrast media brought about the same outcome as that expected by the correct drug or correct dosage.

Every detail of the incident must be included in the report, which becomes the property of the department and is not a part of the patient's medical record. Items to include in the report are:

1. Name of the patient, the procedure, and who made the error
2. Time the error was made and what happened
3. Who was notified and when
4. The patient's reaction/condition
5. How the error was remedied

An example of documentation of the wrong contrast administered follows:

Nov. 12, 2021:
Patient: Ida Menge   Procedure CT lumbar spine
Error made by TARyan
08:20 hours Iopamidol 30 mL administered IV. Administered in error instead of Omnipaque.
08:30 hours Dr. Glucophage (radiologist) notified of the error.
08:40 hours Dr. Glucophage assessed patient's condition.
08:45 hours BP 124/70; P 72; R 16. Patient reports no complaints.

The patient must be observed for an appropriate amount of time, and periodic reports on their condition are documented until the patient is discharged from the department. If a drug is administered to the wrong patient, the same procedure is followed. Accurate documentation is the best defense if litigation follows.

CASE STUDY

Mrs. L., a 94-year-old female, is in assisted living and is beginning to have dizzy spells as well as showing signs of dementia. She had a CT of the head with contrast in April. She put on the allergy form that she had asthma. The CT tech read the form but did not question Mrs. L. further. Shortly after the contrast injection was completed, Mrs. L. began to cough and complain of being short of breath. The technologist completed the study, which took only a few moments, and pulled Mrs. L. out of the equipment, lowered the table, and helped her sit up. Within a few minutes, Mrs. L. stated she was feeling much better and was ready to go home. The technologist released her.

In October of the same year, another CT scan of the head was ordered after a rather serious fall where Mrs. L. hit her head on the edge of a sink. She was not sure if she lost consciousness or not. Once again, she was given a precontrast questionnaire to fill out. However, she did not state that she had any type of reaction from her previous contrast, nor did she mark that she had asthma like she did on the form in April. There was a different technologist performing the scan and he did not question Mrs. L. at all regarding her history or her previous study.

Once again, the contrast administration was completed and everything seemed to be progressing as planned with the study. However, Mrs. L. began stating that she couldn't breathe and that she needed to sit up. The technologist stopped the scan, pulled her out of the equipment, and noticed that "a foamy substance" was coming from her mouth. He did not take any vitals, but started "sternal rubs" as he couldn't determine if Mrs. L. was breathing or not. He pressed the "Code Blue" button and immediately returned to Mrs. L.

It was at this point that the technologist tried to find a pulse and found it weak and thready. When the team arrived, they determined that Mrs. L. needed to be transported immediately to the hospital. It took 11 minutes for the ambulance to arrive. During that time, she went into cardiac arrest and was revived by the emergency team. During the transport to the hospital, Mrs. L. expired. The death certificate indicated anaphylactic reaction to contrast as the cause of death.

There were several serious issues that were discovered during the discovery phase of this legal case. One of them involved the precontrast questionnaire that stated if the patient checked even one question as "YES," the radiologist was to be informed prior to the contrast administration. The form also stated that any patient over the age of 65 must have a BUN, creatinine, and an eGFR completed prior to the administration of contrast. None of these were performed.

ISSUES TO CONSIDER

1. Considering the study in April:
   a. Should the coughing and shortness of breath be considered a reaction to the contrast?
   b. Should the technologist have alerted the radiologist that the patient had asthma, even though it was not the normal practice to do so?
   c. What documentation should have been completed and where should it have been filed?
2. Regarding the study in October:
   a. What should the technologist have done when he received the questionnaire from the patient?
   b. Did the technologist provide proper care to Mrs. L. immediately following her complaints?
   c. Considering the outcome of this study, what documentation must be completed for the CT department?
3. Considering the age of the patient and the clinical history, what should both technologists have done after receiving the precontrast questionnaire and prior to injecting any contrast? Why would one want to question the patient further?

SUMMARY

1. The ASRT scope of practice states that imaging professionals are allowed to administer contrast and medication by parenteral injection.
   a. Radiographers can be held liable and so they must be competent in administration, document all administrations and reactions, and understand the symptoms of any reaction that may occur.
2. Methods of parenteral injection for the radiographer include a drip IV, or continuous infusion, and direct injection.
   a. Direct injection can be done through a pressure (power) injector or is done by hand.
   b. Pressure injectors are used most often in CT. They carry a risk of extravasation or air embolism.
3. Radiographers can also administer drugs via intradermal injection, which is used to test the contrast in cases of allergic history.

4. Needle angles for injections are as follows:
   a. Intradermal   5° to 15°
   b. IV   15° to 35°
   c. Intramuscular   90°
5. Needles have a bevel at the tip, which is the point that should be used to puncture the skin and into the vein. This means that the sharp tip goes in first.
   a. Needles are sized by gauge and length. The gauge is the size of the lumen of the needle. The smaller the gauge, the larger the number.
   b. Syringes are sized in milliliters. There are 0.5-mL syringes (very small) to 50-mL (very large) syringes.
   c. Both needles and syringes must be disposed of into a sharps container.
   d. If a needlestick injury occurs with a dirty needle, report it immediately and fill out an incident report.

6. Vials and ampules contain medication that the radiographer will need to know how to draw into a syringe.

7. Patients must be identified by at least two identifiers just like any other time in doing a study. In addition, a contrast allergic history must be completed.

   a. Before any type of contrast study is performed, the patient must sign an informed consent form and it must be on file with the patient's medical records.

   b. Patients must be given written instructions to follow in regard to medications and if they can eat prior to the exam. Time frame for completion of any lab tests that must be done is important to be understood by the patient.

8. Radiographers should be familiar with the different types of abbreviations that are used in health care.

9. The radiographer must be competent in the performance of venipuncture,

   a. The patient must be watched for reactions for about 30 minutes.

   b. If an emergency should occur, the radiographer must know how to call a "Code Blue" and the location of the radiologist and the crash cart.

10. Complications of venipuncture may not occur very often, but when they do, they can happen very quickly.

    a. Extravasation and infiltration are the most common complications. The difference is that in infiltration, there is no damage to the tissue, whereas in extravasation, there is damage.

    b. Other complications are air emboli, phlebitis, drug incompatibility, and the fluid level falling below the level of the bevel of the spike on the IV line.

11. Discontinuation of an IV must be ordered by a physician. Disconnect the IV tubing from the needle prior to withdrawing the needle from the vein.

12. Documentation of the administration must include the patient's name, date, time, amount, route, and any reactions. The radiographer and physician must sign the documentation. All documentation must be filed in the patient's medical record.

    a. When medication errors occur, there must be documentation that includes not only what was discussed earlier but also an unusual occurrence report or incident report. This must also be scanned into the patient's medical record.

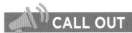 **CALL OUT**

Each of the procedures listed in this chapter is demonstrated on "The Point." Viewing these short vignettes is extremely helpful in learning the exact method for these important skills necessary for the radiographer, particularly one that is planning to go into CT.

CHAPTER 13 REVIEW QUESTIONS

1. The radiographer who administers a drug incorrectly is not held liable for the error.
   a. True
   b. False

2. If the radiographer is required to administer an unfamiliar drug, information must be sought before administering the drug. Where would such information be found?
   a. The encyclopedia
   b. The radiographer's textbook
   c. *The Physician's Desk Reference*
   d. From colleagues

3. Intradermal administration of a contrast would be used as a test for contrast adverse reaction.
   a. True
   b. False

4. How should a used ampule be disposed of?
   a. Wrap it in a paper towel and throw in the trash.
   b. Put it in the sharps container.
   c. Throw it in the biohazard waste.
   d. Tape it into a plastic bag, then throw into the trash.

5. Match the following medical abbreviations with the correct term:
   a. PO _____ 1. Milliliter
   b. IV _____ 2. At once
   c. STAT _____ 3. Every day
   d. PRN _____ 4. Intravenous
   e. Qd _____ 5. By mouth
   f. mL _____ 6. As necessary

6. Which of the following may be a cause of a complication at the contrast injection site?
   a. Anaphylaxis
   b. Extravasation
   c. Asthma
   d. Elevated BUN

7. Mrs. Ida Menge (age 94) returns to the department after being allowed to use the restroom. The radiographer observes that her skin is very dry and fragile, and she states that she has not had anything to eat or drink for 12 hours. The radiographer is to inject a bolus of contrast media and proceed with the study. He takes scout images, completes the allergic history form, and prepares the media for injection. He approaches the patient and assesses her arms for an injection site. The patient's veins do not look promising; however, the cephalic vein on her right arm appears to be the most likely to be successful.

After gathering the material and proceeding with the injection, the vein rolls, and the venipuncture is not successful. The radiographer understands that he has only one more opportunity to begin the procedure without calling another staff member to assist him with the venipuncture. How should he proceed?

a. The radiographer should pull back the needle and attempt to reinsert it into the vein.

b. The radiographer should release the tourniquet, remove the needle, and apply pressure to the site. He should then attempt to reinsert a second needle into a vein in the vicinity of the cephalic vein.

c. The radiographer should gently massage the arm, apply a warm compress to the site, instruct the patient to drop her arm over the side of the table briefly, and then attempt the venipuncture.

d. The radiographer should withdraw the needle and instruct the patient to go home and return when she is better hydrated.

8. After attending to Mrs. Menge, the radiographer is sent to discontinue an intravenous infusion for Mr. Domingo. The radiographer approaches the patient and observes that his arm is cold and edematous at the infusion site. How should the radiographer proceed?

a. He should identify the patient and turn off the infusion pump. He should then obtain a sterile gauze and remove the catheter from the vein. Finally, he should inform the patient that the swelling will subside "in a few minutes" and leave the area.

b. He should identify the patient, observe the site, and call the radiologist.

c. He should identify the patient, observe the site, discontinue the infusion, and place a sterile gauze over the infusion site. He should apply pressure to the infusion site with the gauze and notify the radiologist of the problem.

d. He should identify the patient, assemble needed supplies, perform hand hygiene, and observe the site. When he notes the problem, he should stop the infusion, notify the radiologist, remove the catheter from the vein, elevate the arm, and apply a warm compress to the area of infiltration.

9. List the items that must be included in the incident report if a drug is administered in error.

10. Which of the following is a possible complication that can occur from venipuncture?

a. Air embolism
b. Phlebitis
c. Infiltration
d. All of the above
e. None of the above

11. List the three times that the label of a contrast media should be read.

12. Needles and syringes must be disposed of in:

a. Lead containers
b. Sharps containers
c. Plastic bags
d. The trash can

An Introduction to Advanced Imaging Modalities

14

OBJECTIVES

After studying this chapter, the student will be able to:

1. Explain the process of dual-energy x-ray absorptiometry.

2. Describe computed tomography and explain related patient care.

3. Describe interventional radiography and explain related patient care.

4. Explain the procedure of mammography.

5. Describe magnetic resonance imaging and explain related patient care.

6. Explain the procedure of nuclear medicine.

7. Define positron emission tomography.

8. Describe radiation therapy and explain related patient care.

9. Describe the procedure of sonography.

10. Define the procedures of arthrography and myelography.

11. Identify advanced levels of certification and educational requirements.

KEY TERMS

Certification: The American Registry of Radiologic Technologists' (ARRT) certification indicates having passed an examination that has met the recognized educational and ethical eligibility requirements

Claustrophobic: Suffering from claustrophobia, which is the fear of being in a confined place

Dehydration: Deprivation of water

Diagnostic mammogram: An x-ray examination of the breast of a person who has a breast symptom or who has had a positive breast screening

Dorsiflex: To move the toes and forefoot upward

Hypoglycemic: Pertaining to an abnormally small concentration of glucose in the circulating blood

Hypotension: An abnormal condition in which the blood pressure is not adequate for normal perfusion and oxygenation of the tissues

Isotope: Two or more forms of an element having the same atomic number but different atomic weights

Postprimary certification: The ARRT requires an initial certification and registration in specific disciplines that support postprimary categories

Radioisotope: Radioactive atoms having the same number of protons, which refer to radiopharmaceuticals

Radiopharmaceutical: Radioactive compound used in nuclear medicine

Restenosis: Recurrence of stenosis after corrective surgery on the heart valve; narrowing of a structure

Screening mammogram: An x-ray of the breast on a person who does not have symptoms; also known as a baseline mammogram

Sonographer: Diagnostic medical sonographer uses equipment that produces high-frequency sound waves to produce virtual or real-time images

Transducer: A handheld device used in sonography, which sends and receives sound waves

INTRODUCTION

Patients undergoing advanced imaging procedures require special consideration. Many of these patients have been informed that they may have life-threatening illnesses and the procedure they are about to undergo will either confirm or rule out this threat. Many of the advanced imaging procedures are not without pain and risk, and most patients find them anxiety provoking. Even something as innocuous as the diagnostic setting can cause the patient distress.

The atmosphere into which the patient is received is often intimidating for the patient. The environment includes an imaging room, an operating room, or a room where specialized equipment, the patient, and the health care team can be accommodated for the procedures. The health care team may either be masked and gowned or is hidden behind protective screens, which may require that they address the patient by microphone. This, combined with the prospect of a shortened life span, often elicits patients' feelings of helplessness, vulnerability, and fear.

Patients receiving radiation or proton therapy may be in various stages of the grieving process. They know that they have a potentially terminal illness and that the prescribed treatment is being administered in an attempt to improve the quality and length of their lives or provide them some relief from pain. Working in these diagnostic and treatment areas, one must have exceptional technical skills and superior communication and patient teaching skills. In these areas of patient care, the physician, the registered nurse, the technologist, the **sonographer** or the therapist, and other health care specialists work together as an interdependent team. Each depends on the other for safe and successful diagnostic and treatment outcomes. All patient care skills presented in the previous chapters of this text need to be applied in these areas.

The intent of this chapter is to provide an introductory overview of various diagnostic imaging procedures and related disciplines, which may be a potential area(s) of specialization. Most of the imaging involve additional training and/or education. Detailed technical discussion of these procedures is beyond the scope of this text and is mentioned only when relevant to patient care instruction.

BONE DENSITOMETRY

Bone densitometry is also known as dual-energy x-ray absorptiometry (DEXA, or DXA) scan, or a bone density scan. Bone densitometry uses low-dose radiation levels to image certain areas of bone to measure bone mineral loss. It is a quick, accurate, and painless test used to measure bone density with established standards. The examination is performed by the technologist on an outpatient basis. Images are usually performed in one or more of the following areas: the lower spine, hip, or forearm. Images done on the heel or wrist are not as accurate, and therefore, not as helpful, as those taken of the spine and hip. The procedure is conducted

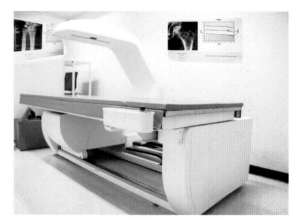

FIGURE 14-1 Bone densitometer table. (Courtesy of Shutterstock/April stock.)

with the patient lying on a padded table (Fig. 14-1). DXA scans most often diagnose osteoporosis and other conditions that cause bone loss and a patient's susceptibility for fractures. The radiologist interprets the images and provides a report to the referring physicians. Figure 14-2 shows a hip scan showing bone density loss in the neck area.

DEXA is strongly recommended for the following types of patients:

- Postmenopausal women not on estrogen
- Having a history of hip fracture or smoking
- Men with rheumatoid arthritis, chronic kidney or liver disease
- Taking medications that are known to cause bone loss such as prednisone
- Having hyperthyroidism

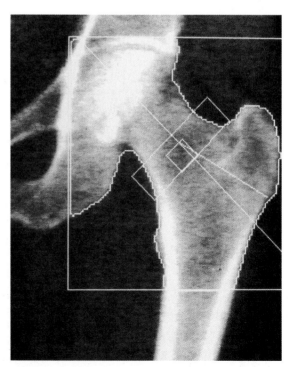

FIGURE 14-2 Dual-energy x-ray absorptiometry scan of a hip with chart to define bone loss. (Courtesy of Shutterstock/Sarah.)

Bone densitometry is of limited use in patients with spinal deformity such as scoliosis, or those with spinal surgeries. CT scans are more useful in these cases.

Patient Care and Education Before a DXA Scan

Patients should be questioned about their last menstrual period to rule out any chance of pregnancy. Additionally, it should be determined if the patient has had any examination involving barium or an injection of contrast for a computed tomography (CT) scan, as the contrast may interfere with the detection of bone mineralization. No special diet or fasting is required, with the exception of withholding calcium supplements for at least 24 hours prior to the exam. The patient removes all metal objects, including body piercing, before lying on the table. Inform the patient that the examination takes about 10 to 15 minutes. During the procedure, the patient will be asked to hold still and hold their breath for a few seconds to avoid blurring the images. After the images have been taken, the patient is free to leave with no specific directions.

COMPUTED TOMOGRAPHY

CT scan is a diagnostic imaging procedure that can be used to scan body tissues and organs combining x-ray and computer technology. CT produces multiple cross-sectional images (Fig. 14-3) of body organs, which can be reconstructed into accurate three-dimensional images. Because CT has higher radiation doses compared with general radiographic imaging procedures, an emphasis must be placed on minimizing radiation for the patient and the technologist. Radiation protection practices must include protocols that reduce radiation for all patients and in particular pediatric patients. CT is a highly effective method of diagnosing disease processes of bones and intracranial, soft-tissue structures of the chest, abdomen, pelvis, and organic pathology. Head, neck, thorax, spine, musculoskeletal, abdomen, pelvis, cardiovascular, CT-guided drainage, aspirations, and biopsies

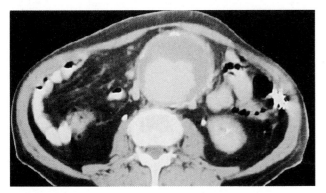

FIGURE 14-3 Abdominal computed tomography.

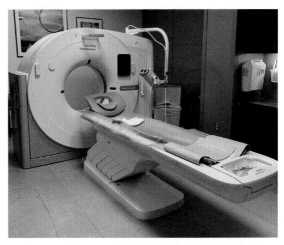

FIGURE 14-4 Computed tomography scanner and gantry.

are a few of the procedures performed with CT imaging. CT procedures are performed on inpatients, outpatients, the critically ill, and pediatric and trauma patients.

The CT equipment is a large machine with a narrow table that slides into a donut-shaped tunnel. Inside the tunnel, known as the gantry, are the x-ray tube and detectors located across from each other (Fig. 14-4). The beam and detector rotate around the patient, imaging multiple slices of the body in one rotation. A workstation is in a separate room behind a large window where the technologist operates the scanner and can monitor the patient's condition both visually and verbally through a speaker and microphone.

Contrast media may be introduced by injection to increase tissue density for body and brain scans. Barium solutions may be used to increase organ density of the gastrointestinal (GI) organs.

Patient Care and Education Before CT

The patient may be receiving contrast media; therefore, all precautions and questioning that precede administration of that drug are included in pre-CT patient care. The technologist must spend time explaining the procedure to the patient in order to alleviate anxiety. Tell the patient that it is important to lie still to ensure clear images. Allow the patient to inspect the equipment and to express any feelings of claustrophobia or fear of the procedure. The technologist should inform the patient that communication through a microphone in the CT room is possible at any time, and that there will be someone to observe, hear, and communicate with the patient at all times.

The technologist must establish a feeling of trust in the patient. It can be frightening for patients to feel that they are in a room alone when receiving an intravenous (IV) injection and going into the equipment that has a small opening. The extremely anxious patient who is in pain and unable to lie quietly may need an analgesic or a sedative medication if this can be prescribed. However, the new generation machines are extremely fast in obtaining images, which is beneficial for children, the elderly, and the critically ill who may find it difficult to stay still.

Inform the patient there may be feelings of nausea, warmth, flushing, and a metallic taste after the contrast is administered. Instruct the patient to immediately speak up if there is any pain. Explain the amount of time that the study will take. The patient must sign an informed consent before receiving a CT scan. The patient's medical history and history of allergies must also be taken before this procedure is begun if contrast is administered. In addition, if the patient has known allergies to contrast media, specific protocols must be in place to address allergies.

Benefits Versus Risks

CT scans have become such a common and routine exam performed that patients rarely ask why a CT is ordered over another type of procedure. However, the radiographer must be prepared to answer any questions that come up regarding the benefits or risks that are involved in CT.

CT is painless and, except for an IV injection for contrast administration, it is noninvasive. Unlike magnetic resonance imaging (MRI), any metal objects in the patient's body will not prevent the scan from being performed. CT is fast and cost-effective. In a medical emergency, CT can demonstrate internal injuries and bleeding. Surgery might be prevented through a diagnosis made by CT scanning.

The risk in having a CT scan comes from the use of an injected contrast medium. As discussed in Chapters 12 and 13, the allergic reactions that can happen are rare, but must be prepared for in the event they do happen. Patients may have a fear of the amount of radiation that is being used to take the images. Patients must be assured that the amount of radiation is low, and that their physician has determined the benefit outweighs any risk of the CT scan.

CT of the Abdomen and Pelvis

Patients who are to have CT of the bowel and abdominal organs are allowed only clear liquids for at least 2 hours and, in some cases, nothing to eat or drink 4 to 6 hours prior to the examination. They may receive a barium contrast agent to drink before the scan. The contrast media may be injected intravenously, which improves the quality of the abdomen and pelvic CT.

The radiographer must spend time explaining the procedure to the patient before beginning this examination, as previously discussed. For the bowel and abdominal CT scan, inform the patient to listen carefully for instructions to breathe, hold the breath, and release the breath. Tell the patient to expect many of these instructions. Patients that are kept informed are more cooperative and relaxed while the examination is in progress.

Patient Care After CT

Patients who have received any type of sedative or antianxiety medication may not self-drive. Patients who have come from their homes and plan to return home should be accompanied by a person who can drive them or assist them to get there safely.

When contrast is injected and the procedure is complete, the IV line is discontinued as ordered by the physician, as described in Chapter 13. The patient is then allowed to sit up with assistance. The patient should sit quietly on the table for several minutes before being assisted back to the dressing room, wheelchair, or gurney. If the patient is hospitalized, they may be transported to their hospital room. If going home, assist the patient to the dressing room, if needed, to get dressed. It should be routine to observe the patient for at least 1 hour for adverse reaction to drugs and for general instability before discharging the patient from the department. This may not be possible; therefore, the patient must be instructed to watch for any type of adverse reaction such as hives, cough and/or wheezing, or difficulty breathing. The patient who has received contrast media should be told to increase fluid intake to at least 3,000 mL and avoid caffeine for the next 24 hours to aid in excretion of the agent from the body and to prevent **dehydration**.

Any adverse reactions that occurred during the CT and any medications that the patient received must be recorded on the patient's electronic medical record. Record the time the procedure began and ended, the patient's tolerance of the procedure, and the instructions that the patient received for postprocedure care.

INTERVENTIONAL PROCEDURES

When a radiographer decides to become an interventional radiographer, the primary responsibilities are to set up and operate the equipment needed for interventional procedures. Working alongside the physician and nurses, the technologist assists in both cardiac and vascular interventional studies. Education includes digital subtraction angiography anatomy, indications, contraindications, complications, equipment (Fig. 14-5), patient care, and pharmacology. Each body system is broken down to

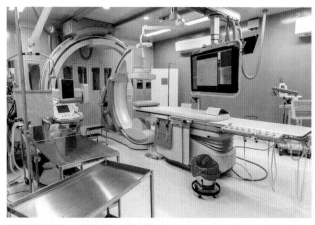

FIGURE 14-5 Biplane interventional equipment. (Courtesy of Shutterstock/Illonajalll.)

include dialysis management and neurologic, thoracic, and abdominal procedures.

Cardiac interventional procedures (Fig. 14-6) are performed by radiologists or cardiologists to diagnose coronary artery patency and, if indicated, treat atherosclerosis of the coronary arteries by nonsurgical means. These procedures include but are not limited to coronary angiography, aortography, pulmonary angiography, shunt detection, thrombolysis, embolization, ablation, biopsies, and coronary angioplasty/stent placement. Cardiac interventional procedures are performed in a cardiac catheterization laboratory with digital fluoroscopy imaging capabilities.

The role of a member of this highly technical team is to participate in the education of the patient, assessment, and general care. One member of the team, either a radiographer or a nurse, performs a surgical scrub, dons gown and gloves, and prepares the sterile instruments. Another member of the team performs a sterile skin prep and drapes the patient for the procedure. All members of the team must be alert to any symptoms of respiratory or cardiac distress, be able to monitor vital signs accurately, assist with drug and contrast media administration, apply surgical aseptic technique, and communicate with the patient in a therapeutic manner. Each member of the team must have special education in the problems and potential complications that may result from the procedure. The patient and the medical team must wear radiation protection apparel (shielding) to protect themselves from unnecessary exposure to radiation during these lengthy procedures, which involve the use of fluoroscopy and digital imaging.

The most common sites for insertion of the arterial catheter are the right and left brachial and femoral arteries. The area surrounding the site of catheter insertion is surgically prepared, usually with an iodophor antiseptic as described in Chapter 11. This area is injected with a local anesthetic, and the artery is accessed with a large-bore needle containing a stylet to prevent return blood flow. When the artery has been accessed, the stylet is removed. A guidewire is then inserted through the needle into the artery, and the needle is removed. A catheter is passed over the guidewire into the artery with fluoroscopic guidance. The guidewire is removed, and the catheter is left in place and manipulated to visualize all vessels desired to diagnose potential areas of cardiac pathology. This process is known as the Seldinger technique.

A low-osmolar contrast medium is injected through the catheter, and the cardiac vessels are observed to assess cardiac output; locate and assess the severity of occlusive coronary artery disease; and diagnose congenital heart abnormalities, aneurysms, or other cardiac abnormalities. Treatment of diseased arteries may be performed at the time of the cardiac catheterization. If the coronary arteries are occluded and would benefit from percutaneous transluminal coronary angioplasty, or if the patient has an evolving myocardial infarct, a balloon-tipped catheter is introduced through a guidewire. After the site of occlusion is reached, the balloon is inflated to compress the plaque that is causing the occlusion.

If there is reason to believe that vessel **restenosis** will occur, a stent may be used to maintain patency of the vessel. A stent is an object that provides support and structure to a vessel. It is introduced in the same way that the balloon is introduced and is left in place when the catheter is removed. Some of the potential complications from these procedures are cardiac arrhythmias, embolic stroke, allergic reactions to the contrast media, and infection or hemorrhage at the catheter insertion site.

Vascular Interventional Radiography

Vascular interventional procedures use the same technology and the same surgical aseptic technique as cardiac interventional procedures to observe major blood vessels throughout the body. The kidneys (Fig. 14-7), adrenal glands, brain, and abdominal aorta are the most common organs to be assessed by this method. The aorta is the typical route to access the vessels of the lower extremities for diagnosis of circulatory impairment of the lower extremities. Potential complications from vascular interventional procedures are much the same as with coronary angiography. If the kidneys are the focus of the procedure, renal failure is an added potential problem. If the adrenal glands are the focus, fatal hypertensive crisis may occur if the patient has the disease pheochromocytoma. Medication to prevent this is administered several days before the procedure.

Patient Care Before and During Interventional Procedures

Interventional nurses have the primary role to perform most patient care duties and responsibilities before, during,

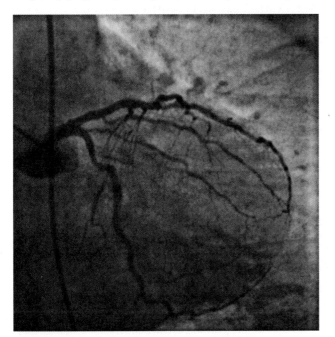

FIGURE 14-6 Cardiac catheterization image.

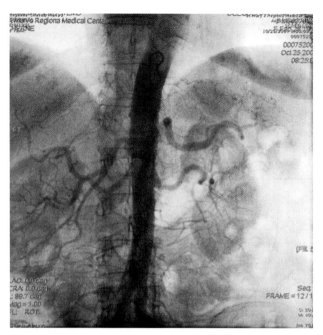

FIGURE 14-7 Arteriogram image.

and after these procedures; however, it is important that the technologist is also knowledgeable to participate in patient care. The technologist must evaluate the requisition and patient and carry out patient teaching and assessment immediately before the procedure. The technologist must monitor the patient during the procedure and provide follow-up patient care. The process varies somewhat depending on the body organ to be assessed, but the process is largely similar:

1. An informed consent is signed after the patient receives instruction from the physician about all that is involved in the procedure, including all potential adverse effects.
2. As with all x-ray procedures, the technologist must ask female patients if there is a chance of pregnancy.
3. Inform the patient before the procedure of the possible immediate need for coronary surgery if complications arise or outcomes from the catheterization indicate the need.
4. For angiography of the heart, the patient must abstain from food and fluids for 4 to 8 hours before the procedure; however, for angiography in areas other than the heart, the patient is often asked to be well hydrated before the examination.
5. Instruct the patient to empty the bladder; to remove dentures, jewelry, and clothing; and to put on a patient gown.
6. When the patient enters the catheterization laboratory, an explanation of the procedure should be done at this time.
7. Allow the patient to express any anxieties or concerns about what is to occur.

8. Assess the patient for allergies to iodine or any medications to be administered.
9. The peripheral pulses are often identified and marked with a pen, so that they may be quickly assessed during and after the procedure.
10. If ordered, medication is administered to alleviate anxiety.
11. The patient is transferred to the procedure table and placed in a supine position.
12. The area of catheter insertion is shaved and scrubbed with an antiseptic solution.
13. A peripheral IV line is started for access and to facilitate administration of drugs as needed. The leads for monitoring the heart rate are placed and connected to the oscilloscope.
14. If the patient is a child, allow a toy to be brought in to calm any anxiety.
15. Inform the patient about instructions to cough or take deep breaths during the procedure to ease feelings of nausea or light-headedness. Coughing may also correct arrhythmias.
16. A local anesthetic may be administered before arterial puncture.
17. The artery is accessed, the guidewire is inserted, and the catheter is placed over the wire.
18. The patient is informed that the contrast is about to be injected and is told that a burning or flushed feeling may be felt and to not be concerned.
19. If the angiography is of the adrenal glands, blood pressure must be monitored continually to assess for evidence of a malignant hypertensive crisis.
20. Images are taken in a timed sequence to demonstrate the arterial and venous blood flow to the organ being studied.
21. Nitroglycerin to dilate blood vessels and other drugs may be administered during the procedure.

Patient Care and Education After Interventional Procedures

Patient care after cardiac interventional and vascular interventional radiography procedures is relatively uniform and must be carried out meticulously to prevent circulatory deficit, thrombus formation, or hemorrhage. In most instances, the patient is transported to the recovery area or to an intensive coronary care area to be monitored after interventional procedures. The technologist must understand the monitoring and care required after these examinations. The patient may be extremely fatigued, and any movement required after the procedure must be done with adequate assistance so there is little demand on the patient. Monitor the patient's pulse rate on the side of the invasive procedure every 15 minutes for 1 hour and then every hour until an 8- to 12-hour period is complete, and no complication has been detected. The blood pressure is monitored on the side opposite the invasive procedure at the same time intervals. The pulses distal to the site of catheter insertion must also be monitored at frequent, regular intervals for 24 hours after the procedure. After femoral catheterization, the patient should be instructed to move the toes and **dorsiflex** the feet frequently. Also, instruct the patient to keep the legs straight and still. Assess the extremities for coldness, cyanosis, pallor, numbness, size of one extremity compared with the other extremity, and tingling. Instruct the patient to inform the nurse if they have any of the latter symptoms. If a circulatory deficit occurs, surgical intervention may be necessary to correct the problem. The patient should also inform the nurse of any feeling of wetness at the site of the catheter insertion; this may indicate hemorrhaging.

If a femoral artery was used for the catheter insertion, inform the patient that they must remain in bed rest for 10 to 12 hours after the procedure to prevent hemorrhage. A weight or sandbag is often placed over the site of catheter insertion to apply pressure. The patient should also be told to apply pressure at the insertion site when coughing or sneezing. Do not raise the patient's head more than 20° during the immediate postcatheterization period.

If the brachial site was used for catheter insertion, the arm on the side of insertion is kept straight with an arm board for several hours, but the patient may be up as soon as the vital signs are stable. Regardless of the site of insertion, the patient must be monitored for 24 hours for external bleeding or for bleeding into the tissues surrounding the catheter insertion site.

Instruct the patient who has received contrast media to increase fluid intake to prevent dehydration and **hypotension**. This may be contraindicated in some patients with congestive heart failure. Patients are often given IV fluid replacement therapy during these procedures, but they should be made aware of the need for increased fluid intake.

Record the time that the procedure began and ended, any drugs or contrast agents administered, and the patient's tolerance of the procedure on their electronic medical record. Also, record the instructions given to the patient after the procedure.

MAMMOGRAPHY

Mammography is a radiographic procedure that uses low-dose radiation with a specialized x-ray machine to image the breast. Mammography is performed on a routine basis for early diagnosis of breast cancer and on an acute care basis if a lesion, lump, or nodule found in the breast is suspected of being cancerous. The American Cancer Society (ACS) recommends that women aged 40 years and older have a **screening mammogram** every year and a yearly physical examination of the breasts. A screening mammogram typically includes two projections of each breast, whereas a **diagnostic mammogram** includes additional projections of the area of interest. A mammogram procedure ranges in time from 15 to 30 minutes.

Mammographic procedures are regulated by the Mammography Quality Standards Act (MQSA) of the federal government, which includes **certification** of the facility, equipment, and personnel. Certification is issued by the U.S. Food and Drug Administration (FDA) with a certificate. This certificate signifies having met the federal quality standards. A decade ago, the FDA approved 3D mammography, also known as breast tomosynthesis, as a preferred method over standard mammography. The American Society of Breast Surgeons released a position statement recommending a 3D diagnostic mammogram be performed yearly. It has been shown that 3D digital screening detected a higher percentage of cancers with fewer false positives than standard 2D digital mammography. Figure 14-8 shows how 3D imaging of the breast provides a much clearer image of an area under suspicion than the standard 2D mammogram did.

The 3D mammographic image is similar to CT in that it takes multiple slices of the breast at various angles, which can then be reconstructed to view the breast tissue one

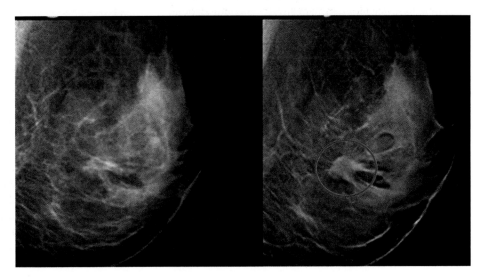

FIGURE 14-8 The image on the left is made with a standard mammography unit. The image on the right is the same breast but imaged with a three-dimensional unit.

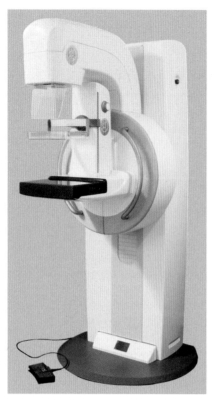

FIGURE 14-9 A three-dimensional mammography unit. (Courtesy of ShutterStock/Radiological imaging.)

slide at a time. This can be likened to turning the pages of a book, with a slightly different picture on each page.

3D mammography is used for breast cancer screening when the patient shows no symptoms or signs of breast cancer. It is also used to determine the cause of thickening or a suspicious lump. In the case of cancer screening, both 3D and 2D (standard) mammography are used. This eliminates the need for follow-up imaging when an abnormality is found. The 3D tube moves from one side to the other above the patient's head to collect images. Standard mammography tubes do not move (Fig. 14-9).

A medical history is taken before an initial mammogram and updated yearly. If a patient has breast implants, the mammographer must be informed prior to the procedure because special techniques will be used to move the implants during the mammogram.

No contrast media are used for routine mammography. The radiographer should instruct the patient to wear an item of clothing that can be easily removed to the waist. Deodorant or powders in the axillary region should not be used before the examination because they may cause the appearance of pathology because of the content of the deodorant. The patient's breasts are exposed and positioned between an image receptor and a compression device. Radiographic images are taken from a minimum of two projections (Fig. 14-10A and B). During the procedure, the breasts are compressed tightly to remove skin folds and air pockets. It is usually known by women presenting for mammogram that the procedure can be uncomfortable. They may, therefore, be anxious when they arrive for the procedure. If the patient is having the mammogram because of suspected pathology, the mammographer must ask the patient to identify the area that is suspect so that additional care is taken to obtain optimum images of that area. Make every effort to preserve patient privacy and minimize anxiety.

With digital imaging, the images are evaluated by the mammographer for positioning and image quality

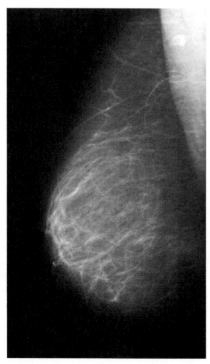

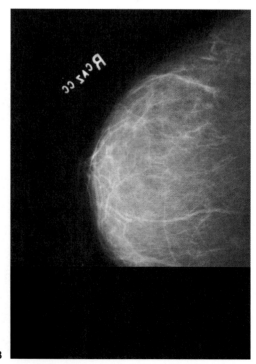

FIGURE 14-10 (A) Mammogram: medial lateral oblique projection. **(B)** Mammogram: cranial caudal projection.

right away. The radiologist interprets the mammogram; a report is provided to the patient's physician. The patient is notified in writing about the results of their mammograms within 30 days. The patient must be notified as a result of federal law found in MQSA.

MAGNETIC RESONANCE IMAGING

MRI is another sophisticated noninvasive procedure used for diagnosing neoplasms as well as vascular, soft tissue, orthopedic areas, central nervous system (CNS), and breast pathologic conditions (Fig. 14-11).

MRI is performed by placing the entire body, or a body part, on a table and into an opening (Fig. 14-12) where a strong magnetic field with radiofrequency properties produces images of body organs and tissues to rule out infections, neoplasms, and acquired and/or congenital anomalies. MRI procedures of the brain (for strokes or head injuries), spine (cervical, thoracic, and lumbar), thorax (to include the breast), abdomen, pelvis, and the musculoskeletal area are commonly conducted. In addition to these procedures, there are many special MRI procedures that exist, for example, MR angiography and MR cardiac studies.

MRI images are easily accessed by physicians to assist them in the diagnosis of diseases in adult and pediatric patients. An MRI has many diagnostic advantages; among them is the absence of radiation that may harm body cells. Although radiation is not a concern for MRI procedures, there are other safety considerations. These considerations require screening patients and other personnel who may have access to the MRI area. In addition, the MRI technologists and other personnel must have an understanding and follow specific guidelines to determine safe and unsafe areas, devices, and objects

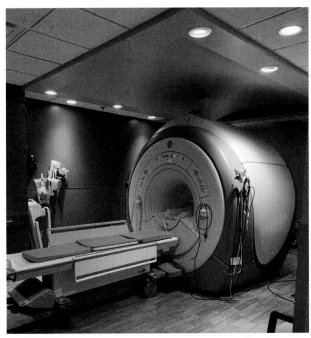

FIGURE 14-12 Magnetic resonance imaging equipment.

in the MRI environment. Another significant advantage of MRI is that the bone can be eliminated to visualize specific organs. New procedures and techniques are continually being developed in MRI.

Patient Care and Education for MRI

Patient education is the key to successful imaging when MRI is the diagnostic procedure selected. Inform the patient the procedure may take from 25 to 60 minutes to complete. **Claustrophobic** fears are common and emerge when the patient is faced with possibly spending 15 minutes to over 1 hour in a cylinder, in a large room, alone. In some instances, a claustrophobic patient may require sedation or some antianxiety medication prior to the procedure to facilitate the MRI procedure. For persons with severe claustrophobia, open MRI is available. In open MRI, the patient is not completely enclosed in a chamber, which decreases the feeling of being enclosed in a small space.

Patients may have two or three examinations ordered at once depending on the patient's level of tolerance for the procedure. Accurate information and instruction help to alleviate these fears. Inform the adult patient of the need to lie in a supine position without moving during the scanning. Also, the patient must be told of the repetitive knocking sounds during the entire examination. The patient may wish to wear earplugs for ear protection.

Explain to the patient that monitoring is ongoing, and the technologist is just on the other side of a glass window. The patient will be constantly observed, and communication with the patient is frequent during the procedure. Show the patient that there is a microphone through which to communicate with the staff. The

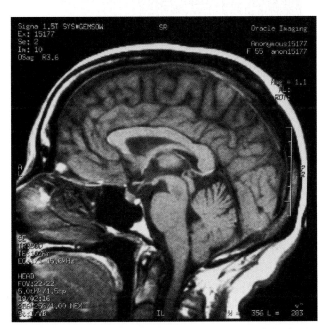

FIGURE 14-11 A magnetic resonance imaging of the brain.

technologist can help decrease the patient's anxiety by speaking to the patient frequently and letting the patient know how much time is left before the examination is completed. The patient should be allowed to examine the MRI equipment and ask any questions that they may have before beginning the procedure. If the patient is a child, a parent may be allowed to sit beside the cylinder and talk to the child during the MRI, but department policies must be followed. Infants should be fed shortly before being placed in the cylinder.

A medical history, as previously described, must be taken before the MRI. History of allergies must be included. If the patient is to receive a contrast medium, the institution may require the patient to sign an informed consent. Many MRI studies do not require the use of contrast; however, a rare earth element, gadolinium, may be required. Known as gadolinium-based contrast media (agents), GBCM(A), they provide contrast enhancement to areas of the spine or brain. It is useful in determining scar tissue from normal tissue after surgery of the spine.

Although reactions such as a rash, sweating, itching, and hives are not common, there are two areas of concern when GBCM are used. They may irritate the veins at the injection site and cause inflammation. More importantly, in patients with compromised renal function, these contrasts have been known to cause nephrogenic systemic fibrosis/nephrogenic fibrosing dermopathy (NSF/NFD). Symptoms may not occur until after the patient has left the imaging department, making it difficult to assess the actual number of these reactions. Patients experience thickening skin, difficulty bending the joints, and difficulty breathing because of fibrosis of the diaphragm and pulmonary vessels. Nephrogenic fibrosis can be fatal. Therefore, it is vital that the radiographer perform a complete allergic history on the patient; get the results of the blood urea nitrogen (BUN), creatinine, and glomerular filtration rate (GFR); and consult with the radiologist prior to injection of GBCA if warranted.

WARNING!

ALWAYS get an allergic history and kidney function tests before injecting GBCA!

There is an extensive MRI safety questionnaire form that patients and all individuals in the MRI area must fill out. Instruct all patients to remove all metal jewelry, dental bridges, clothing with metal closures, belts, metal-containing prostheses, hair clips, and shoes before entering the scanner room. Purses and wallets containing credit cards must be left outside in a secure place because MR deactivates credit cards. The radiographer is responsible for placing the items safely away and for informing patients where their belongings are being kept.

Patients who receive antianxiety or sedative drugs before MRI and those who have a history of asthma and

receive contrast media should be monitored during the procedure. There are pulse oximeters made for use in the MRI chamber.

MRI is contraindicated for people who have metallic implants, such as internal pacemakers, implanted heart valves, metal orthopedic implants, cochlear implants, or surgical clips. It may be contraindicated for pregnant women because the effects of MRI on pregnancy are unknown at present. Patients on life support equipment or infusion pumps or who are critically ill may not receive MRI because the monitoring equipment cannot be used in the scanner room. Other items that prevent MRI are an implanted insulin pump, bone growth stimulator, internal hearing aid, cochlear implant, neurostimulator, metal eye prostheses, vena cava clot filter, an intrauterine device or diaphragm in place, some surgeries, claustrophobia, regular need for oxygen administration, and any metal device.

Patient Care After MRI

There are no special patient instructions or teaching responsibilities after MRI unless the patient has received medication or a contrast agent. If the patient has received drugs or contrast media, the instructions are the same as for other invasive imaging procedures.

Children are sometimes sedated for this examination. If this is the case, the patient is monitored throughout the examination and, until fully recovered from the drug, by a nurse proficient in this field. Sedating children requires special evaluation that is not discussed in this text.

NUCLEAR MEDICINE IMAGING

Nuclear medicine is a diagnostic tool that, with the use of a radioactive pharmaceutical (also called an **isotope** or a tracer), creates images of the lungs, kidneys, heart, bones, thyroid, and GI and urinary systems. The pharmaceutical (Fig. 14-13) emits radiation from the patient's body that is detected by a scintillation or gamma camera. Nuclear medicine imaging is frequently the diagnostic imaging technique of choice to detect or rule out malignant lesions. In addition to diagnosing diseases, nuclear medicine procedures have therapeutic uses. Specific nuclear medicine procedures are performed in the nuclear medicine department to address infection, metabolism, function, and tumors. Many procedures are conducted in adjunct with other imaging modalities to support the diagnosis and treatment of the disease processes.

Patient Care Before Nuclear Medicine Scans

Before the nuclear medicine examination, the patient must be informed about the small amount of **radioisotope** and exposure to a minimal amount of radiation. Patients who

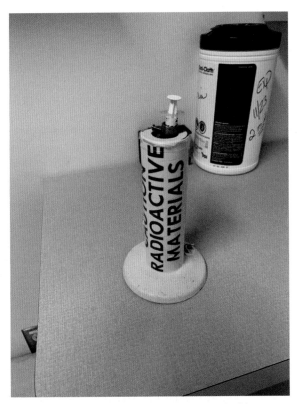

FIGURE 14-13 The radioactive pharmaceutical is contained in a lead container known as a "pig."

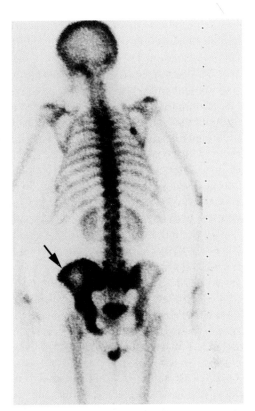

FIGURE 14-14 This nuclear medicine bone scan shows an uptake of isotope (hot spot) in the ribs where a patient had an old fracture. The arrow points to a cold spot in the pelvis where no isotope accumulated, indicating an area where there was no blood flow.

are pregnant or who have renal or hepatic disease should be carefully screened before being scheduled for this diagnostic procedure. The patient should be informed that the isotope will be excreted within 24 hours, and there are no residual radiation effects. After explanation of the study, the patient must sign a consent form, which is then filed into the medical record. Depending on the organ to be diagnosed, the patient may receive an IV injection of the isotope. The patient may also be given a radioactive tracer compound by inhalation or oral route. Depending on the nuclear medicine procedure, the examination may begin immediately after the administration of the **radiopharmaceutical** or a delay can vary from an hour to several days after the administration of the isotope. Only one radionuclide procedure should be scheduled in a day because one may interfere with another. The isotope accumulates in areas of pathology called "hot spots." An area of decreased uptake of the radionuclide may indicate circulatory impairment and is called a "cold spot" (Fig. 14-14).

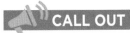

CALL OUT

The patient must not receive more than one nuclear medicine procedure in a day. Other contrast media may interfere with the examination!

Types of Nuclear Studies

Nuclear imaging is used to diagnose or treat conditions of the blood, thyroid, heart, gallbladder, lungs, skeletal system, and kidneys and to determine the stage of cancer.

- Blood flow can be tracked through the body by injecting a small amount of radioactive tracer, which is tagged on the red blood cells (RBCs). These scans are most often done to find the site of bleeding in the colon or other parts of the GI tract.
- Thyroid scans require the patient to take a pill that contains radioactive iodine, which is collected in the thyroid. A scanner detects the amount of radiation emitted from the thyroid and sends it to a computer that displays the images. Nodules may show increased or decreased uptake of the iodine.
- Gallbladder scans are known as hepatobiliary iminodiacetic acid (HIDA) scans; and the scan checks to make sure bile is moving through the body in a normal way. It can determine if there is leakage of bile anywhere; find gallstones, cholecystitis, dilated bile ducts; and determines if the liver is functioning properly.
- Pulmonary ventilation/perfusion scans test the ventilation (breathing) and perfusion (circulation) in all areas of the lungs. These are two separate

scans that involve inhalation of a radioactive gas and an injection of radioactive albumin into the vein. These scans are done when it is suspected that a pulmonary embolus is present, that there may be abnormal circulation within the lungs (shunting), or to test function in patients that have pulmonary diseases such as chronic obstructive pulmonary disease (COPD).

- Bone scans can be performed on the whole body or just on a specific area. The whole-body scan takes about 4 hours over a 2-day visit. In the first visit, the radioactive isotope is injected into a vein and the body is scanned on the next day. Bone scans are used primarily to detect the spread of metastatic cancer. Because cancer cells spread and multiply rapidly, they show as hot spots on the scan. Bone scans are also done to show osteomyelitis or osteitis versus cancer (such as Ewing sarcoma).

- Renal scans show how the kidneys are functioning. This is done by seeing how blood flows into and out of the kidneys; how urine flows through the kidneys, ureters, and bladder; and how much each kidney is cleaning the blood. A tracer is injected into a vein that is followed with the gamma camera to track radioactivity. These scans can take from 45 minutes to 3 hours.

- Cancer may absorb more or less of a tracer than normal tissue, allowing the gamma camera to pick up the pattern of radioactivity. Nuclear medicine is often used with other imaging tests to give a complete picture of what is happening with the patient's body.

Patient Care After Nuclear Medicine Scans

After nuclear medicine imaging, if an IV agent has been administered, assess the area for redness and swelling before discharging the patient. The patient must be cautioned to rise slowly to prevent postural hypotension. Do not allow the patient to leave the area until the images are reviewed for clarity. Instruct the patient to resume usual dietary and medication pattern unless contraindicated by the physician.

Positron Emission Tomography

Positron emission tomography, known as PET, often combines the qualities of nuclear medicine imaging with CT or MRI to study blood flow and volume, metabolism to diagnose tumors, and staging cancers. This has greatly increased the diagnostic ability of nuclear medicine imaging with the use of special cameras and computer program systems (Fig. 14-15A through C).

When PET is combined with CT, the examination is called PET-CT. The body organ studies using PET have

had great success to the CNS, cardiovascular, respiratory, endocrine, GI, genitourinary (GU), skeletal, and the hematopoietic systems. PET is able to assist in the diagnosis of numerous diseases, including Alzheimer disease, brain tumors, cardiac disease, and physiologic changes in psychiatric diseases (Fig. 14-16). It is one of the most innovative techniques currently used. Unfortunately, it is a very expensive procedure that requires sophisticated specialized equipment, specialized computer software, and a team of scientists and health care specialists to carry out the diagnostic procedures. More facilities are opting to install PET-CT scanners (Fig. 14-17) because of the high cost of the equipment and technology. The patient inhales or is injected with a radioisotope. The isotopes emit subatomic particles called *positrons* (positively charged electrons). A nuclear medicine technologist injects the radioisotope; after 45 minutes to an hour, the PET scan takes place. The usual time frame for the procedure including postinjection time is 2 to 3 hours.

Patient Care for PET

The patient must have a clear explanation of the PET procedure. The patient must understand that there will be radiation exposure that is minimal and that a radioactive material, either by injection or by inhalation, will be administered depending on the organ to be studied. The procedure takes 30 to 90 minutes. An informed consent form is required by most institutions.

There may be a food or fluid restriction 1 hour before the examination. The patient should not take caffeine, nicotine, or alcohol for 24 hours. The patient should also not receive sedative or tranquilizing drugs. All these interfere with the examination. Diabetic patients may receive insulin 3 to 4 hours before the procedure. Patients who are pregnant or breastfeeding may be restricted from this examination. Immediately before the examination, the patient is instructed to empty the bladder.

After the examination, the patient should be assisted to rise or leave the examining table because of possible dizziness caused by orthostatic hypotension. Instruct the patient to increase fluid intake for 24 hours and to urinate frequently to eliminate the isotope from the body.

The patient receiving PET is often elderly and may have symptoms of dementia. If this is the case, the technologist must recognize that the patient is unable to follow directions and may need to be closely guided through every aspect of the procedure. The strangeness of the environment may be frightening to a person with symptoms of dementia. Because excessive anxiety may affect the results of the examination, a family member or a familiar caretaker may need to remain with the patient to decrease their anxiety.

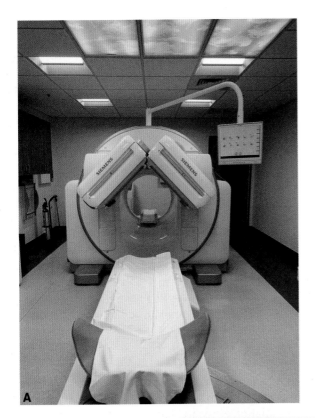
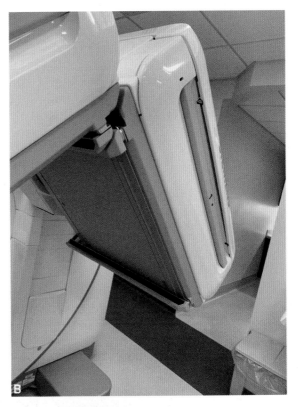
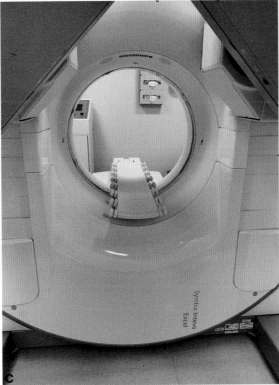

FIGURE 14-15 **(A)** Nuclear medicine camera with a computed tomography (CT) component. **(B)** Nuclear medicine cameras. **(C)** CT gantry that allows the table to be pushed through after a nuclear medicine study.

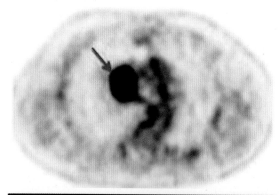

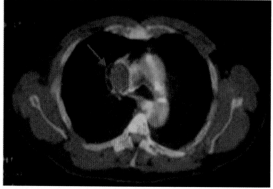

FIGURE 14-16 PET/CT scan of a male smoker. The arrow is pointing to a large cancer mass pushing on the right bronchus.

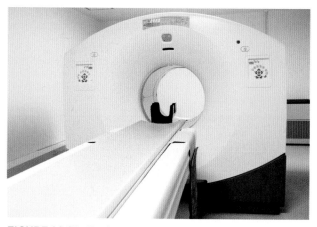

FIGURE 14-17 Positron emission tomography scanner equipment. (Courtesy of Shutterstock/Alexander Gatsenko.)

RADIATION THERAPIES

At least half of the patients with a diagnosis of cancer receive external radiation therapy during the course of the disease. This form of treatment is used to cure the disease, to control malignant tumors that cannot be removed, to prevent spread of the tumor, and to decrease pain when the cancer metastasizes to the bones, brain, or soft tissues. Radiation therapists who work in the area of radiation therapy receive specialized education.

The size, location, and degree of sensitivity of the tumor to radiation are the deciding factors when the plan of therapy is devised. The sensitivity of the cells surrounding the tumor is also a factor in the plan. The intent of therapeutic radiation is not to kill all tumor cells immediately. All cells react differently, and some may repair the radiation-induced damage and begin to reproduce again. For this reason, radiation for treatment of cancer is administered in a series of divided doses for an established period. In this manner, tumor cells that survive the initial radiation are eventually destroyed.

When a patient's physician prescribes external radiation therapy, the patient is sent to the medical oncologist for an initial consultation prior to the first radiation treatment. The consultation involves simulation to precisely prepare for the patient's first treatment. During this simulation, the patient is evaluated with the use of CT to confirm the accuracy of anatomy for the development of a specific treatment plan. Patients receive pinhole size tattoos to pinpoint the area of radiation for each of their treatments. The tattoo marking ensures that the same area of tissue receives the radiation therapy with each treatment. The plan of treatment usually extends daily for several weeks.

At the time that the treatment plan is made, show the patient the treatment room. The patient should be allowed to ask any questions concerning the treatment. Inform the patient that they can communicate by microphone with the radiation team and vice versa. If the patient is in pain, pain medication may need to be administered 30 minutes before each treatment. Also, explain to the patient that the radiation treatments themselves are painless and that there is no danger of the patient carrying radiation out of the treatment area.

Proton Therapy

Proton therapy is a form of external beam radiation treatment. Proton therapy, also known as proton beam therapy, delivers a beam of positively charged particles, known as protons, directly to the tumor. The benefit of proton therapy over conventional radiation therapy is that the proton works at the end of its desired pathway with very little effect on tissues that surround the area. In other words, the "scatter effect" that is such a problem in external radiation therapy is markedly decreased. This allows the dose to the tumor to be increased with no harmful effects to surrounding tissues.

Because the beam can be "targeted" for precise locations, proton therapy is now used to treat cancers of the head and neck, lung, prostate, brain, breast, GI system, liver, pancreatic, ocular and other eye cancers, sarcomas, lymphomas, and pediatric cancers. As an example, the heart and lungs are in close proximity to the breast. Regular radiation therapy irradiates the heart and lungs during the treatment of breast cancer, which in turn increases the risk of long-term side effects. However, because a proton beam can be limited to providing radiation only to the breast tissue, it is a superior method of treating the cancer.

The National Association for Proton Therapy, NAPT, was founded in 1990 to help educate patients and physicians about the benefits of proton therapy. According to the NAPT, there are currently 40 regional proton therapy centers in the United States and over 200,000 patients treated worldwide. As more therapy centers are opened, the equipment becomes more streamlined; however, the cyclotron, which produces the stream of protons, must still be located in a "vault" of high-density concrete far underground. Patients never see this massive piece of equipment, which weighs 15 tons or more.

Patient Preparation for Proton Therapy

The patient preparation for proton therapy is preceded by a diagnostic workup that includes a 3D CT scan to determine the area of treatment. A mold of the patient's body (Fig. 14-18) is made for tumors below the neck, and if the head and neck are the areas of treatment, a form-fitted mask is made to fit the treatment area. During each session, patients lie in the mold made only for them, thus ensuring meticulous patient positioning so that the calculated dose of protons is delivered to the area each time.

Inform the patient that although no one else is in the treatment room, the therapist will be in contact by microphone. If claustrophobia or pain is a problem for the patient, a mild antianxiety or analgesic drug may be prescribed 20 to 30 minutes before treatment. The actual treatment may only last a few minutes; however, preparing the patient may cause the entire time spent in the department to be approximately 20 minutes. Many therapy treatments require daily visits, Monday through Friday, for up to 3 months.

When caring for patients having proton therapy, one must understand that these patients, like patients receiving external radiation therapy, may be grieving because they have had a diagnosis of life-threatening illness. Their care requires extra sensitivity from the health care team, as described in the previous section.

SONOGRAPHY

Sonography, or ultrasound, is a method of visualizing the soft-tissue structures of the body for the diagnosis of diseases without the use of radiation or contrast media. It is a noninvasive, painless procedure that requires the skill of a specially educated technologist known as a diagnostic medical sonographer. Ultrasound (Fig. 14-19) uses high-frequency sound waves to search for pathologic changes in body organs. Images are displayed on a monitor in real time in addition to recording images in analog, digital, and Picture Archiving and Communication Systems (Fig. 14-20).

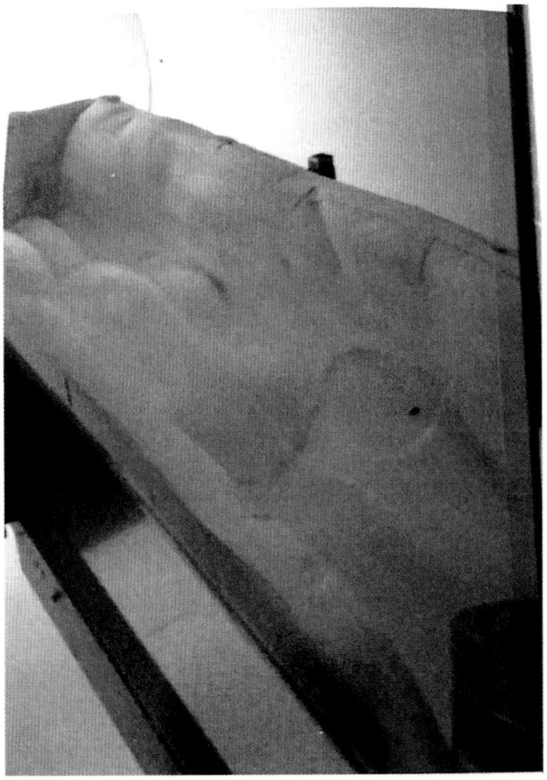

FIGURE 14-18 A mold is made for each patient to provide exact positioning for each treatment. This mold was made for a 6-ft male with prostate cancer.

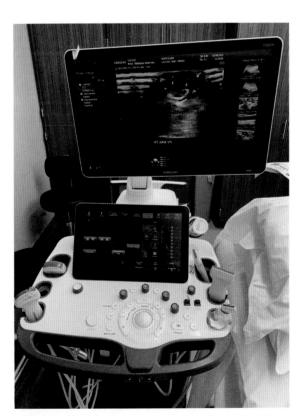

FIGURE 14-19 This ultrasound machine is small and compact so that it can be moved to a patient's bedside, if needed.

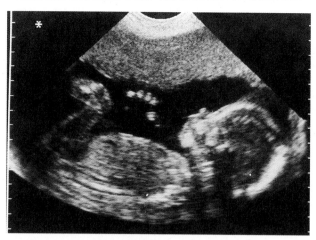

FIGURE 14-20 This ultrasound image shows the side view of a well-developed fetus. The head is down, face up. The thigh and knee can be seen at the left of the image.

This form of imaging is useful in obstetrics for fetal monitoring, in neurology for diagnosing brain disorders, and in urology for diagnosing urinary bladder, scrotal, prostatic, and renal pathologic conditions. It is also used to diagnose vascular, pancreatic, biliary, spleen, GI tract, thyroid, venous, lymph node, eye, and breast pathologic conditions. Echocardiography is a noninvasive method of looking at the chambers of the heart, the performance of the mitral and tricuspid valves, and the thickness of the myocardium and septum (Fig. 14-21).

Patient Care for Sonography

Patient care considerations for sonographic examinations include verification of the patient and examination, an explanation of the procedure, assisting patient with transfer

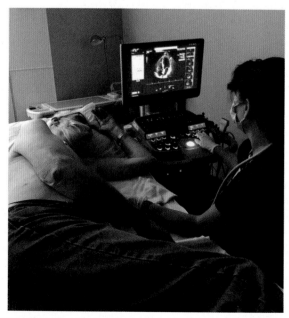

FIGURE 14-21 Echocardiography is an ultrasound study of the heart where the blood flow can be traced through the chambers of the heart.

and movement for positioning, assisting patient with medical equipment, and responding to common emergencies.

If a patient is to have a barium study as well as an ultrasound examination, the ultrasound examination should be scheduled to precede the barium study because residual barium in the GI tract will interfere with effective ultrasound examinations. If a patient has a tendency to have large amounts of gas in the bowel, the gas interferes with visualization. A patient with this problem should be instructed to eat low-residue foods for 24 to 36 hours before the examination and be scheduled at a time when the bowel is relatively gas free.

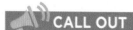
CALL OUT

Ultrasound studies must be performed prior to contrast studies to prevent interference of the sound waves by the contrast!

Active children or patients who are unable to remain quiet because of pain, emotional illness, or anxiety must be scheduled at a time when they can be accompanied by a person who can keep them calm and relaxed. Use of sedative drugs may also be recommended by the physician.

Patients should be informed that this is a painless, noninvasive procedure. A lubricating gel is used as the conductive agent. The sonographer applies the gel. A **transducer** is held by the sonographer and is moved over the surface to be examined, creating images that will show on the monitor.

Some examinations require the patient to fast after midnight. Other ultrasound procedures require the bladder to be filled with fluid. If either of these is required, it must be explained to the patient prior to the study.

Wound dressings, scars, and obesity are all factors to be considered when ultrasound is the imaging technique prescribed. Dressings must be removed, and lubricating gel cannot be applied over an open wound. Scars and obesity prevent good visualization. A clear sterile patch may be worn over wounds if ordered by the physician.

Patient care after sonography is the same as thoughtful patient care after any diagnostic imaging procedure. The lubricating gel must be carefully removed, so that the patients' clothing is not soiled by it. Patients who are in a weakened condition must not be left alone, and any assistance the patient needs must be provided. Patients who have had sedative medication must not be allowed to drive home or return to their hospital room unattended.

MISCELLANEOUS FLUOROSCOPIC-GUIDED PROCEDURES

There are several medical procedures that incorporate image guidance with fluoroscopy, CT, MRI, or ultrasound. When fluoroscopic guidance is used for a procedure, the radiologic technologist is an integral member of the health care team. The technologist is often involved with the imaging portion of the procedures for nerve blocks, lumbar punctures, hip injections, or shoulder injections for MRI. These procedures can be performed in the operating room, the diagnostic imaging x-ray room, pain clinic, and other approved locations. The primary duty of the technologist is to set up and operate the fluoroscopic x-ray equipment. As with any other x-ray procedure, the technologist must ensure safe radiation practices for the patient and all individuals present during the procedure. The technologist may also be involved in obtaining the patient consent and verifying that the correct patient is receiving the correct procedure in the correct area of interest according to department protocols. The technologist may participate in setting up the sterile tray, explaining the procedure to the patient, and assisting with positioning the patient for the examination. At all times, the technologist must maintain sterile fields, especially when manipulating the fluoroscopic equipment during the procedure.

Arthrography

Arthrography is the diagnostic imaging examination of a joint. The indications for this procedure are continual complaints of incapacitating joint pain. The joints of the shoulder, knee, ankle, wrist, or hip can be visualized by this diagnostic imaging procedure (Fig. 14-22). Abnormalities that can be diagnosed are joint capsule abnormalities, synovial cysts, and joint and ligament pathologic conditions. The preferred methods of diagnosing some joint conditions are CT or MRI. Figure 14-23 shows an MRI image of a hip arthrogram.

There is no restriction of food or fluids for arthrography. The patient's history of allergies to local anesthetics,

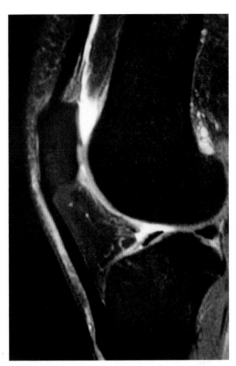

FIGURE 14-23 Magnetic resonance imaging hip arthrography. The arrow indicates a tear in the labrum. (Courtesy of Shutterstock/edwardolive.)

iodine, and contrast agents must be taken. Pregnancy is a contraindication to having this procedure because fluoroscopy is used. Explain the procedure to the patient and adequately answer any questions. A consent form is required to be signed.

The area where the joint will be punctured for instillation of contrast media must be cleansed as for surgical prep. The puncture area is anesthetized with a local anesthetic. The patient and staff wear protective clothing to shield them from radiation. A radiopaque contrast or air contrast or both are used to visualize the joint in question fluoroscopically while it is put through the range of motion and the contrast media fill the joint space. After administration of the contrast, images are taken during this time. If fluid is removed from the joint, it may be collected in a sterile specimen tube and sent to the laboratory for analysis.

After arthrography, if it is a knee or ankle joint, an ace bandage may be applied to the site, and the patient should be instructed in the method of application. The patient should also be told that there may be some swelling or discomfort and, possibly, some crackling noise heard as the contrast is absorbed. The patient may be told to use ice applications for the swelling, and the physician may prescribe pain medication. Advise the patient to see the physician immediately if there is redness, warmth, or drainage at the site of needle insertion.

Myelography

Myelography (myelogram) is a radiographic examination of the spinal cord in which contrast media are injected

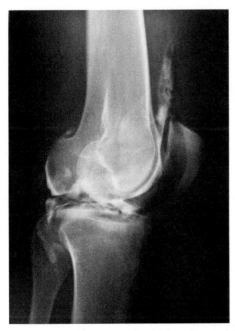

FIGURE 14-22 Knee arthrography with radiographic imaging.

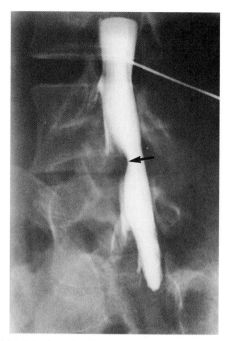

FIGURE 14-24 Standard radiography of a lumbar myelogram. The arrow is pointed to a filling defect in the spinal cord from a ruptured disc.

into the subarachnoid or epidural spaces of the spinal cord. After the injection, x-ray or CT is used to image the spinal canal to detect pathologic conditions such as a herniated intravertebral disk, tumors, malformation, and arthritic bone spurs, under digital fluoroscopic conditions. Figure 14-24 shows a herniated disk with standard radiographs and Figure 14-25 shows a herniated disc using CT imaging.

Patient Care and Education in Myelography

A consent form must be signed by the patient or an appointed person before this procedure is begun. Assess the patient for potential allergic reaction to contrast media. Instruct the patient to increase clear fluid intake and omit solid food for 4 hours before the examination to be well hydrated and to not become nauseated because of food in the stomach. Food and fluid restrictions may vary depending on the contrast agent used. The patient should empty the bladder and bowels before this examination.

Also, instruct the patient to stop taking all drugs 24 hours before the examination. Drugs that may enhance the possibility of seizure activity are particularly important to omit. This includes phenothiazines, tricyclic antidepressants, CNS stimulants, and amphetamines. Patients with a diagnosis of diabetes mellitus must be instructed by their physician on how to prevent a **hypoglycemic** or hyperglycemic reaction during preparation for myelography.

Myelography should not be performed on patients with multiple sclerosis, inflammation of the meninges, Pott disease, infections or bloody subarachnoid fluid, increased intracranial pressure, or a recent myelogram. Radiopaque contrast media are used for this procedure so all precautions taken when these drugs are administered apply. Myelograms may also be contraindicated in patients who are prone to seizures. Seizure-prone patients may receive medication to reduce the possibility of seizures before the examination. Physicians may order medication to reduce the patient's anxiety in preparation for this procedure.

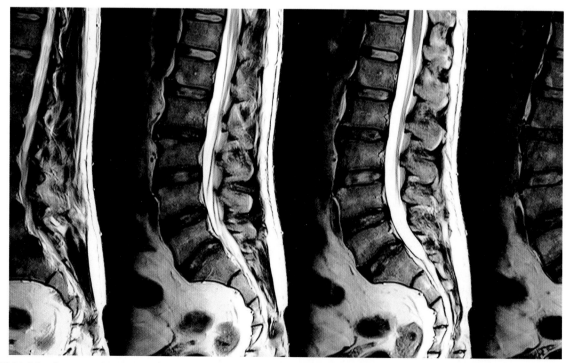

FIGURE 14-25 Computed tomography imaging of a lumbar myelogram. The arrows are pointing to the contrast media in the spinal canal. (Courtesy of Shutterstock/Tomatheart.)

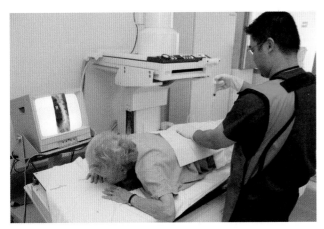

FIGURE 14-26 Patient receiving intrathecal drug administration during myelography.

The area into which the contrast media are to be injected intrathecally is prepped as for other sterile invasive procedures (Fig. 14-26). If standard x-rays are to be done, the radiographer should inform the patient that the table will be tilted during the examination, but that a footrest and shoulder harness prevent a fall. However, this is rarely done now, as CT is less taxing on the patient.

Baseline vital signs should be taken before the myelogram begins and then monitored during the examination. Inform the patient that the examination takes from 30 to 60 minutes to complete.

Report any unusual symptoms or complaints the patient has while the myelogram is in progress to the physician performing the procedure. Specimens of spinal fluid are often collected during this procedure and should be correctly labeled, bagged, and taken or sent to the laboratory immediately.

After a myelogram procedure, the outpatient is monitored for 4 to 8 hours with the head of the bed slightly elevated at a 35° to 45° angle during recovery to avoid a spinal headache.

Also, encourage the patient to increase fluid intake, not to engage in strenuous physical activities, and to avoid bending for a couple of days. The radiographer should inform the patient to notify the physician immediately if there is trouble urinating or a fever, drowsiness, stiff neck, seizures, or paralysis develops. Other complications of myelography are arachnoiditis (inflammation of the delicate spinal cord covering) and meningitis. Any unusual reactions that the patient had to the contrast agent or in general are recorded on the patient's chart. Also, record the time that the procedure began and ended, specimens sent to the laboratory, and the patient's tolerance of the procedure. Instructions given to the patient for post-myelogram care are included in the chart.

POSTPRIMARY CERTIFICATIONS

All of the studies discussed in this chapter require education that is specific to the modality. Students may wish to continue their education after radiography by obtaining training in 12-month programs that may lead to access to a registry type examination or to a certificate. Display Table 14-1 helps the student determine which postprimary pathway may be best to pursue if desired. **Postprimary certification** is required in many areas in order to practice.

DISPLAY TABLE 14-1

Educational Requirements and Certifications

The following modalities offer ARRT certifications:

Modality	Required Education	Primary Certification	Postprimary Certification	Subcategory Certification
DEXA Scans	Certified and registered with ARRT, ARDMS, or NMTCB	ARRT in Radiography or NMT or Radiation Therapy	ARRT (BD) or NMTCB (BD)	
CT	Associate Degree **plus** Certification in Radiography from ARRT	ARRT in Radiography	ARRT (CT)	
Interventional	Certified and registered with ARRT, ARDMS, or NMTCB	ARRT in Radiography	ARRT in Cardiac Interventional Radiography	

(continued)

DISPLAY TABLE 14-1

Educational Requirements and Certifications (*continued*)

Modality	Required Education	Primary Certification	Postprimary Certification	Subcategory Certification
Mammography	Associate Degree **plus** Certification in Radiography from ARRT	ARRT in Radiography	ARRT (M)	
MRI	Associate Degree **plus** MRI program		ARRT or NMTCB or ARDMS	
Nuclear Medicine	Associate Degree **plus** Nuclear Medicine program	NMT from ARRT NMTCB from the Nuclear Certification Board		Nuclear Cardiology Technologist PET/SPECT
Radiation Therapies	Associate or bachelor degree in radiation therapy **OR** in a closely related field with an additional 12-month certificate program in radiation therapy	ARRT in Radiation Therapy (ARRT (T))		Certification is available in Proton Beam Therapy
Sonography	Graduate of a 2-year degree accredited sonography program **OR** Graduate of a 1-year certificate program after training in another health care field	Registered Diagnostic Medical Sonographer (RDMS)	RD Cardiac Sonographer (RDCS) Registered Vascular Technologist (RVT) Registered Musculoskeletal Sonographer (RMSK) Certified Diagnostic Ophthalmic Sonographer (CDOS)	There are multiple point-of-care ultrasound (POCUS) certificates available: Abdominal aortic aneurysm Abdominal trauma Cardiac Gastrointestinal Hepatobiliary/ spleen Lower extremity Deep vein thrombosis Lung Musculoskeletal Obstetrics Renal/ genitourinary

ARDMS, American Registry for Diagnostic Medical Sonography; ARRT, American Registry of Radiologic Technologists; CT, computed tomography; DEXA, dual-energy x-ray absorptiometry; MRI, magnetic resonance imaging; NMT, Nuclear Medicine Technology; NMTCB, Nuclear Medicine Technology Certification Board; PET, positron emission tomography; SPECT, single-photon emission computerized tomography.

Summary

1. Bone densitometry is also known as DXA or simply as a bone density scan.
   a. It is used to see the levels of calcium in the bone.
2. Computed tomography is also known as CT scan. Old terminology is computed axial tomography (CAT).
   a. CT uses higher radiation levels than other modalities.
   b. CT is used to diagnose diseases of the bones, brain, chest, abdomen, pelvis, and the organs.
   c. Patient care in CT involves the use of injected contrast media. Informed consent must be signed and on file.
      i. If the patient has received a sedative and is an outpatient, there must be someone to drive the patient home.
   d. Because of the radiation and contrast injection, physicians weigh the risk of the study to the benefit of the diagnosis before prescribing the patient to undergo the study.
3. Interventional procedures involve catheterization of blood vessels for diagnostic purposes or for therapeutic purposes. Vascular or cardiac procedures are performed by a team of professionals to diagnose coronary artery patency and treat atherosclerosis.
   a. Sites for arterial catheter placement include the brachial or femoral arteries.
   b. The procedure to catheterize the artery is known as the Seldinger technique and is performed under sterile procedures.
   c. Angioplasty is used to inflate a balloon to compress plaque that is causing an occlusion in an artery.
   d. Complications include cardiac arrhythmia, embolic stroke, infection, hemorrhage, or allergic reaction to the contrast.
   e. The vessels of organs, such as the kidneys or brain, can be studied through vascular interventional radiography.
   f. Patient care includes obtaining an informed consent, monitoring the patient for adverse effects of the contrast and/or the procedure, and to explain to the patient the procedure itself.
4. Mammography uses low-dose radiation to image the breast tissue for the early detection of breast cancer.
   a. ACS recommends women aged over 40 having a screening mammogram yearly.
   b. 3D mammography, aka breast tomosynthesis, is recommended; 3D detects a higher percentage of cancer with fewer false positives.
   c. MQSA set the standards for image quality, technologist education, patient reporting, and facility equipment.
5. MRI is performed with the use of a strong magnetic field that causes the nuclei of the body part being imaged to spin on its axis. As they relax and return to a normal position, they give off energy that is picked up by machine.
   a. MRI is used to produce images of the vascular, orthopedic areas, CNS, and soft tissues of the body. It is used to rule out infections, to evaluate head injuries, and respiratory, GI, and GU disorders. MRI can also be used to see the vessels and is known as MR angiography.
   b. Strict safety protocols are in place for all personnel in the area.
   c. Some patients suffer from claustrophobia and may require some sedation, or the use of an open MRI equipment.
   d. Some exams require contrast, which may be a gadolinium-based media. These may irritate the veins at the site of injection and cause inflammation.
6. Nuclear medicine picks up radiation given off from the body after radioactive pharmaceuticals (isotopes or tracers) are injected into a vein.
   a. Nuclear medicine can show function of an organ. It is used to show increased or decreased blood flow, sites of bleeding, and differentiate between cancer and infection, or locate a pulmonary embolus.
   b. Cold spots are decreased uptake of isotope and hot spots are increased uptake of isotope.
   c. Positron emission tomography is used in conjunction with nuclear medicine and CT or MRI.
      i. PET is able to help diagnose diseases such as Alzheimer, brain tumors, cardiac diseases, and psychiatric diseases.
   d. Different types of nuclear medicine scans include thyroid, gallbladder, pulmonary ventilation/perfusion, renal, bone, and heart studies.
7. Radiation therapy is used to treat cancer.
   a. Doses are divided into small doses so that eventually all cells within the tumor are killed.
   b. External radiation deposits radiation into the body on its pathway to the tumor, causing excessive exposure to areas that are not intended to be exposed.
   c. Proton therapy is a form of external beam radiation that uses protons instead of photons. These protons deposit most of the dose to the tumor and are not scattered along the way.
      i. Proton therapy is used to treat cancers of the head, neck, lung, prostate, brain, breast, GI system, liver, pancreas, eye, sarcomas, lymphoma, and pediatric cancers.

8. Sonography is better known as ultrasound. High-frequency sound waves are used to image pathologic changes in the body.

   a. It is used in obstetrics for fetal monitoring, for vascular, GI, GU, eye, and other areas of the body to diagnose pathology.

   b. Patient care and education for sonography concern scheduling. Contrast studies must be performed after sonography. Additionally, patient may need to eat a low-residue diet to reduce abdominal gas or to drink copious amounts of water to fill the bladder.

9. There are several exams that were done with x-ray after the injection of contrast media, but these have been replaced by the use of either CT or MRI.

   a. Arthrography is imaging of joints like the hip, knee, ankle, or shoulder after injection of contrast media. CT or MRI is used to perform the images.

   b. Myelography is imaging of the spinal canal after an intrathecal injection of contrast. CT has replaced x-ray imaging and demonstrates pathology much clearer than standard radiography did.

   c. Both procedures require a signed consent form.

10. Certifications and licensures are available in advanced modalities through either the ARRT or other agencies specific to the modality itself.

CHAPTER 14 REVIEW QUESTIONS

Match the modality with the correct description.

1. Radiopharmaceuticals are used to see areas of disease.
2. Uses high-energy protons to attack cancer cells
3. Uses a contrast medium injected into the joints
4. Sound waves are used to see the heart.
5. Ionizing radiation used to visualize bone and tissue
6. Assesses the density of the lumbar spine
7. Contrast injected intrathecally
8. Powerful magnet used to image tissue and bone
9. Use of sound waves to diagnose different pathology
10. Catheterization of arteries for diagnostic purposes

A. CT
B. Interventional
C. DXA scan
D. Nuclear medicine
E. Sonography
F. Arthrography
G. Myelography
H. Echocardiography
I. Proton therapy
J. MRI

11. Which of the following is performed under fluoroscopic guidance AND either CT or MRI?
    a. Arthrography
    b. Bone density
    c. Sonography
    d. Mammography

12. Which of the following involves a computer to produce 3D images of the body, with no radiation involved?
    a. CT
    b. Mammography
    c. MRI
    d. Nuclear medicine

13. Single-photon emission computerized tomography, HIDA, and ventilation and perfusion scans are all a type of:
    a. CT
    b. Mammography
    c. Interventional
    d. Nuclear medicine

14. Which of the following provides the best method for early detection of breast cancer?
    a. Sonography
    b. 3D mammography
    c. DEXA
    d. PET

15. PET is used in conjunction with either CT or MRI. PET also uses which of the following?
    a. Sound waves
    b. High-energy protons
    c. Contrast medium
    d. Radioisotopes

SUGGESTED READINGS

CHAPTER 1

American Hospital Association. Federal agencies with regulatory or oversight authority impacting hospitals. Published 2018. Accessed February 12, 2022. https://www.aha.org/system/files/2018-01/info-regulatory-burden-federal-agencies.pdf

Assmus A. Early history of x rays. Published 1995. Accessed November 27, 2017. http://www.slac.stanford.edu/pubs/beamline/25/2/25-2-assmus.pdf

Bushong S. *Radiological Sciences.* 10th ed. Elsevier; 2013.

Callaway WJ. *Mosby's Comprehensive Review of Radiography.* 6th ed. Elsevier; 2013.

Nurse Journal. Radiology nurse careers and salary outlook. Accessed February 8, 2021. www.nursejournal.org

Orth D. *Essentials of Radiologic Science.* 2nd ed. Wolters Kluwer; 2017.

Sinha R. Radiology assistants and radiology physician assistants. Published March 16, 2020. https://collaborativeimaging.com/2020/03/16/radiology-assistants-and-radiology-physician-assistants/

Study.com. Federal & State Regulation of Healthcare Organizations & Providers. Updated September 3, 2021. Accessed February 12, 2022. https://study.com/academy/lesson/federal-state-regulation-of-healthcare-organizations-providers.html

Study.com. How to become a radiation physicist: education and career roadmap. Accessed June 15, 2021. https://www.indeed.com/career-advice/finding-a-job/how-to-become-radiation-physicist

Sylter K. LVN vs. LPN: is there really a difference? Published December 17, 2018. Accessed December 23, 2021. www.rasmussen.edu/degrees/nursing/blog/lvn-vs-lpn

Wikipedia. Accessed February 14, 2022. https://en.wikipedia.org

CHAPTER 2

American Hospital Association. The patient care partnership. 2003. Accessed January 1, 2022. www.aha.org./other-resources/patient-care-partnership

American Society of Radiologic Technologists. Radiography practice standards. 2021. https://www.asrt.org

Kübler-Ross E. *On Death and Dying.* Macmillan; 1969.

Massat MB. Changes in reimbursement to propel digital radiography. *Appl Radiol.* 2016;45(7):24-27. doi:10.37549/ar2296

The Joint Commission. Mission statement. 2016. www.jointcommission.org

CHAPTER 3

Bell MD, Daniel J. Medical abbreviations and acronyms. Published July 2019. Accessed October 19, 2021. https://radiopaedia.org

HMP Global Learning Network. How generational factors impact patient engagement. Published May 2016. Accessed February 18, 2022. www.hmpgloballearningnetwork.com

Kourkouta L, Papathanasiou IV. Communication in nursing practice. *Mater Sociomed.* 2014;26(1):65-67.

Meola A. The aging US population. Published January 2021. Accessed September 30, 2021. www.businessinsider.com/aging-population-healthcare

National League for Nursing. Communicating with people with disabilities. Accessed October 11, 2021. https://www.nln.org/education/teaching-resources/professional-development-programsteaching-resourcesace-all/ace-d/additional-resources/communicating-with-people-with-disabilities-e030c45c-7836-6c70-9642-ff00005f0421

Patti Higgins RN. Developmental disability etiquette. Accessed February 18, 2022. https://www.slideserve.com/michalg/developmental-disability-etiquette-powerpoint-ppt-presentation

Traylor V. What are the 5 developmental disabilities? Published August 11, 2021. Accessed February 18, 2022. www.njddc.org/5-developmental-disabilities

University of California San Francisco. Communicating with people with hearing loss. Accessed October 4, 2021. https://www.ucsfhealth.org/education/communicating-with-people-with-hearing-loss

Wikipedia. Cultural competence in healthcare. Updated November 26, 2017. Accessed October 11, 2021. https://en .wikipedia.org/wiki/Cultural_competence_in_healthcare

World Atlas. Largest ethnic groups and nationalities in the United States. Valnet Inc. Updated June 2019. Accessed October 11, 2021. http://www.worldatlas.com/articles/largest-ethnic-groups-and-nationalities-in-the-united-states.html

CHAPTER 4

Akdeniz M, Yardimci B, Kavukcu E. Ethical considerations at the end-of-life care. *SAGE Open Med.* 2021;9.

American Hospital Association. The patient care partnership. Accessed February 25, 2020. www.aha.org/other-resources/ patient-care-partnership

American Public Health Association. What is public health. 2021. Accessed January 20, 2022. www.apha.org/ what-is-public-health

Bhandari P. Ethical considerations in research. Published October 18, 2021. Accessed January 19, 2022. www .scribbr.com/methodology/research-ethics/

Bhatt J, Bathija P. Ensuring access to quality health care in vulnerable communities. Acad Med. 2018;93(9):1271-1275.

Gledhill A. Professionalism, meeting the standards that matter. Published November 27, 2021. Accessed January 20, 2022. www.mindtools.com/av44li2/professionalism

Hajibabaee F, Joolaee S, Cheraghi MA, Salari P, Rodney P. Hospital/clinical ethics committees' notion: an overview. *J Med Ethics Hist Med.* 2016;9:17.

Human Rights Careers. Accessed January 17, 2022. www .humanrightscareers.com

Kapp MB. Ethical and legal issues in research involving human subjects. *J Clin Pathol.* 2006;59(4):335-339.

Lander V. Structural racism: what it is and how it works. Published June 30, 2021. Accessed January 20, 2022. www.theconversation .com/structural-racism-what-it-is-and-how-it-works-158822

Matthews EP, Matthews TM. Medical ethics and law in radiologic technology. *Radiol Technol.* 2015;87(2):163-184.

Oxford University Press. Incompetent patient. 2022. Accessed January 21, 2022. www.oxfordreference.com

Swanton D. FAQs for ethical rights. Published January 2, 2019. Accessed January 17, 2022. www.ethicalrights.com/about-ethical-rights/faqs

CHAPTER 5

ASRT. Essential education. In *Safety Essentials.* Module 4. 2014. https://www.asrt.org/

Drugs.com. How to transfer a person safely. Updated March 2, 2022. Accessed March 4, 2022. www.drugs.com/cg/ how-to-transfer-a-person-safely.html

Mercy Health System. *Rules for the Transfer of a Patient.* Mercy Health System; 2016.

National Institute of Health. Division of Occupational Health and Safety (DOHS). Safety Data Sheets. Accessed March 9, 2022. www.ors.od.nih.gov

OSHA. Sample Safety Data Sheet. Published June 2015. Accessed March 10, 2022. www.osha.gov

The Joint Commission. *Advancing Effective Communication and Cultural Competencies in Patient-Family Centered Care: A Roadmap for Hospitals.* The Joint Commission; 2016.

CHAPTER 6

Goldberg C. *A Practical Guide to Clinical Medicine; Vitals Signs.* University of California. Accessed February 12, 2022. https://meded.ucsd.edu/clinicalmed/vital.html

Goodwin M. About glomerular filtration rate (GFR) and diabetic kidney disease. Published October 26, 2021. Accessed February 12, 2022. https://www.healthline.com/health/ diabetes/glomerular-filtration-rate

Health Library. *Vital Signs (Body Temperature, Pulse Rate, Respiration Rate, Blood Pressure).* Johns Hopkins Medicine. Accessed February 12, 2022. www .hopkinsmedicine.org/health/conditions-and-disesases/ vital-signs-body-temperature-pulse-respiration-rate-blood-pressure

CHAPTER 7

ASRT. Patient-centered care for diverse populations. Modules 2, 3, 4 and 6. Essential Education Series. 2015. Available as an online continuing education series at https://www .asrt.org/

Centers for Disease Control and Prevention and the Alzheimer's Association. Alzheimer's disease and healthy aging. Accessed March 14, 2022. http://www.cdc.gov/ aging

Federal Interagency Forum on Aging-Related Statistics. *Older American 2020: Key Indicators of Well-Being.* U.S. Government Printing Office; 2020. Accessed March 14, 2022. http://www.agingstats.gov

Golden Beacon USA. Why is America called the melting pot? Published October 30, 2020. Accessed March 31, 2022. https://goldenbeaconusa.com/why-is-america-called-the-melting-pot/

Healthy Children. Child abuse and neglect: what parents should know. Updated March 16, 2022. Accessed March 23, 2022. https://www.healthychildren.org/English/safety-prevention/ at-home/Pages/What-to-Know-about-Child-Abuse. aspx?_gl=1*enq464*_ga*MTU4MTk5NDc3OS4xNjcw MDQzMTY3*_ga_FD9D3XZVQQ*MTY3MDA0MzE 2Ni4xLjAuMTY3MDA0MzE2Ny4wLjAuMA..&_ ga=2.63665641.773304117.1670043175-1581994779 .1670043167

Linn-Watson TA. *Radiographic Pathology.* 2nd ed. Wolters Kluwer; 2014.

Mayo Clinic. Child abuse. Published September 24, 2021. Accessed March 23, 2022. www.mayoclinic.org/ diseases-conditions/child-abuse

National Institute on Aging. http://www.nia.nih.gov

United States Census Bureau. Quick Facts. Published July 21, 2021. Accessed March 28, 2022. www.census.gov/ quickfacts/US

United States Census Bureau America Counts Staff. 2020 Census will help policymakers prepare for the incoming wave of aging boomers. Published December 10, 2019. Accessed March 14, 2022. https://www.census.gov/ library/stories/2019/12/by-2030-all-baby-boomers-will-be-age-65-or-older.html

CHAPTER 8

Ainsworth CR. Head trauma treatment & management. *Medscape.* Updated June 2, 2021. Accessed April 5, 2022. https://emedicine.medscape.com/article/433855-treatment

American Society of Radiologic Technologists. Patient-centered care for diverse populations. Module 4. Essential education Series. 2015. Available as an online continuing education series at https://www.asrt.org/

Centers for Disease Control and Prevention. Traumatic brain injury and concussion, Get the Facts. Accessed April 4, 2022. www.cdc.gov/traumaticbraininjury

Khalek A. Keep it simple: acute GCS score as a binary decision. *George Washington School of Medicine and Health Sciences.* Published March 6, 2017. Accessed April 5, 2022. https://smhs.gwu.edu/urgentmatters/news/keep-it-simple-acute-gcs-score-binary-decision

Lafferty K. Smoke inhalation injury workup. October 15, 2021. Accessed April 7, 2022. https://emedicine.medscape.com/article/771194-workup

Perez E, Foley M, Karlin R. What are the classifications of burns? Published November 1, 2019. Accessed April 11, 2022. www.nationwidechildrens.org/conditions/health-library/classification-of-burns

Lee S, Rahul, Ye H, Chittajallu D, et al. Real-time burn classification using ultrasound imaging, *Scientific Reports.* Published April 2, 2020. Accessed April 7, 2022. www.nature.com/articles/s41598-020-62674-9

Pew A, Shapiro D, National Center for Health Research. Football and brain injuries: What you need to know. 2022. Accessed April 4, 2022. www.center4research.org/football-brain-injuries-need-know

CHAPTER 9

American Diabetes Association. Accessed June 22, 2015. www.diabetes.org

American Heart Association. 2020 American Heart Association guidelines for Cardiopulmonary Resuscitation and Emergency Cardiovascular Care. Published October 21, 2020. Accessed February 12, 2022. https://professional.heart.org

Centers for Disease Control and Prevention. Living with diabetes. Accessed February 12, 2017. www.cdc.gov/diabetes

Centers for Disease Control and Prevention. National Diabetes Statistics Report 2020. https://www.cdc.gov/diabetes/data/statistics-report/index.html

Kalil A. Septic shock. *Medscape.* Updated October 7, 2020. https://emedicine.medscape.com/article/168402-overview

Kumar A, Sharma S. Complex partial seizure. *StatPearls [Internet].* Updated June 27, 2022. https://www.ncbi.nlm.nih.gov/books/NBK519030/

Mayo Clinic. Asthma. Accessed February 12, 2022. https://www.mayoclinic.org/diseases-conditions/asthma/symptoms-causes/syc-20369653

National Institutes of Neurological Disorders and Stroke. https://www.ninds.nih.gov/health-information/disorders/stroke

Williamson L. After years of decline, death rate from lung clots on the rise. Published August 17, 2020. https://www.heart.org/en/news/2020/08/17/after-years-of-decline-death-rate-from-lung-clots-on-the-rise

CHAPTER 10

Ahmed R, Boyer TJ. Endotracheal tube. *National Library of Medicine.* Published November 9, 2021. Accessed April 20, 2022. www.ncbi.nlm.nih.gov/books/NBK539747/

American Heart Association. Implantable cardioverter defibrillator. Published September 30, 2016. Accessed on April 26, 2022. https://www.heart.org/en/health-topics/arrhythmia/prevention--treatment-of-arrhythmia/implantable-cardioverter-defibrillator-icd

Knott L. Surgical drains: indications, management, and removal. *Patient.* Updated October 20, 2021. Accessed April 25, 2022. www.patient.info/doctor/surgical-drains-indications-management-and-removal

McGill RL, Ruthazer R, Meyer KB, Miskulin DC, Weiner DE. Peripherally inserted central catheters and hemodialysis outcomes. *Clin J Am Soc Nephrol.* 2016;11(8):1434-1440. doi:10.2215/cjn.01980216

Robinson J. What are central venous catheters. *WebMD.* Updated December 16, 2020. Accessed April 25, 2022. www.webmd.com/heart-disease/what-are-central-venous-catheter

Say S. Suctioning 101: special considerations for assessing the pediatric patient. Published July 10, 2017. Accessed April 21, 2022. https://blog.sscor.com/suctioning-101-special-considerations-for-assessing-the-pediatric-patient

CHAPTER 11

Bernstein S. Prion diseases. Published July 15, 2020. Accessed April 1, 2022. www.webmed.com/brain/prion-diseases

Centers for Disease Control and Prevention. Mission, role and pledge. Published April 29, 2022. Accessed May 5, 2022. www.cdc.gov/about/organization/mission.htm

Centers for Disease Control and Prevention. Standard precautions for all patient care. Published January 26, 2016. Accessed May 9, 2022. https://www.cdc.gov/infectioncontrol/basics/standard-precautions.html

Centers for Disease Control and Prevention. Hand hygiene in healthcare settings. Published April 29, 2019. Accessed May 5, 2022. https://www.cdc.gov/handhygiene/index.html

Centers for Disease Control and Prevention. Linen and laundry management. Published March 27, 2020. Accessed May 16, 2022. www.cdc.gov/hai/prevent/resource-limited/laundry.html

Cliffs Notes. Growth requirements for microorganisms. Accessed May 13, 2022. www.cliffsnotes.com/study-guides/biology/microbiology

Connecticut State Department of Public Health. Multidrug-resistant organisms (MDROs): what are they? Accessed May 6, 2022. https://portal.ct.gov/DPH/HAI/MultidrugResistant-Organisms-MDROs-What-Are-They

Kandola A. Everything you need to know about communicable diseases. Published June 16, 2020. *Medical News Today.* Accessed May 6, 2022. www.medicalnewstoday.com/articles/communicable-diseases

Mayo Clinic. Polio. Accessed May 6, 2022. https://www.mayoclinic.org/diseases-conditions/polio/symptoms-causes/syc-20376512

McLay C. Infection control oversee cleaning of linens and protect from contamination. *Environment of Care Leader.* Published May 26, 2014. Accessed May 16, 2022. https://apic.org/Resource_/TinyMceFileManager/Environment_of_Care_Leader_May_26_Carol_McLay_linen_storage.pdf

Med Law Advisory Partners. Universal precautions vs. standard precautions. Published February 18, 2021. Accessed May 9, 2022. https://medlawadvisory.com/universal-vs-standard-precautions/

World Health Organization. Ebola. N'Zerekore, Guinea, February-June 2021. Accessed May 6, 2022. https://www.who.int/emergencies/situations/ebola-2021-nzerekore-guinea

CHAPTER 12

ACR Committee on Drugs and Contrast Media. *ACR Manual on Contrast Media.* American College of Radiology; 2021. Accessed June 18, 2022. www.acr.org/-/media/ACR/files/clinical-resources/contrast_media.pdf

American Addiction Centers. How are drugs classified. Published March 22, 2022. Accessed June 10, 2022. www.rehabs.com/blog/classification-of-drugs/

American College of Radiology. ACR appropriateness criteria. Published 2022. Accessed June 26, 2022. www.acr.org/Clinical-Resources/ACR-Appropriateness-Criteria

Bell D. Iodinated contrast media. Published May 17, 2022. Accessed June 22, 2022. www.radiopaedia.org/articles/iodinated-contrast-media..

Iyanam Y, Nakaura T, Kidoh M, et al. Relationships between patient characteristics and contrast agent dose for successful computed tomography with a body-weight-tailored contrast protocol. *Medicine.* 2018;97(14):e0231. doi:10.1097/md.0000000000010231

Kim J, De Jesus O. Medication routes of administration. Published February 17, 2022. Accessed June 22, 2022. www.ncbi.nlm.nih.gov/books/NBK568677/

Linn-Watson T. *Radiographic Pathology.* 2nd ed. Lippincott Williams &Wilkins; 2014.

Muhammad Farooq R, Pham C. Intra-articular drug delivery systems for joint diseases. *Curr Opin Pharmacol.* 2018;40: 67-73. doi:10.1016/j.coph.2018.03.013

National Cancer Institute. Complementary and alternative medicine. Published March 21, 2022. Accessed June 10, 2022. https://www.cancer.gov/about-cancer/treatment/cam

RadiologyInfo. Contrast materials. Published June 15, 2020. Accessed June 28, 2022. https://www.radiologyinfo.org/en/info/safety-contrast

Wikipedia. Mechanism of action. Accessed June 22, 2022. https://en.wikipedia.org/wiki/Mechanism_of_action

CHAPTER 13

ACR Manual on Contrast Media. *ACR Committee on Drugs and Contrast Media.* American College of Radiology; 2022.

American Society of Radiologic Technologists. *ASRT Practice Standards for Medical Imaging and Radiation Therapy.* ASRT; 2019. https://www.asrt.org/main/standards-and-regulations/professional-practice/practice-standards

Dirckx JH, ed. *Stedman's Medical Dictionary for the Health Professions and Nursing.* 6th ed. Wolters Kluwer/Lippincott Williams & Wilkins; 2008.

Dix M. What you need to know about phlebitis. Published December 14, 2021. Accessed July 7, 2022. www.healthline.com/health/phlebitis

Indrajit I, Sivasankar R, D'Souza J, et. al. Pressure injectors for radiologists: a review and what is new. *Indian J Radiol Imaging.* 2015;25(1):2-10. Accessed July 6, 2022. www.ncbi.nlm.nih.gov/pmc/articles/PMC4329682/

IV infiltrations and extravasations: causes, signs, side effects, and treatment. Published May, 2020. Accessed July 7, 2022. www.ivwatch.com/2020/05/27/iv-infiltrations-and-extravasation.

LibreTexts Medicine. *Clinical Procedures for Safer Patient Care (Doyle and McCutcheon).* Last updated August 14, 2020. Accessed July 6, 2022. https://med.libretexts.org/Bookshelves/Nursing/Book%3A_Clinical_Procedures_for_Safer_Patient_Care_(Doyle_and_McCutcheon)

Merriam-Webster. Dose-response. Accessed July 24, 2022. https://www.merriam-webster.com/medical/dose-response

Phillips LD. *Manual of IV Therapeutics.* 5th ed. F.A. Davis Company; 2011.

Romans L. *Computed Tomography for Technologists Exam Review.* Wolters Kluwer/Lippincott William & Wilkins; 2011.

CHAPTER 14

American Cancer Society. *Guidelines for the Early Detection of Cancer.* American Cancer Society. Accessed August 4, 2022. https://www.cancer.org

American Registry for Diagnostic Medical Sonography. 2017. Accessed August 13, 2022. https://www.ardms.org

American Registry of Radiologic Technologists. *Post Primary Pathway.* ARRT; 2022a. Accessed July 30, 2022. http://www.arrt.org

American Registry of Radiologic Technologists. *Cardiac Interventional Radiography.* ARRT; 2022b. Accessed August 4, 2022. http://www.arrt.org

American Society of Radiologic Technology. *Vascular-Interventional Essentials.* Accessed August 4, 2022. www.asrt.mycrowdwisdom.com

Black BP. *Professional Nursing: Concepts & Challenges.* 8th ed. Elsevier; 2017.

Conant EF, Zuckerman SP, McDonald ES. et al. Five consecutive years of screening with digital breast tomosynthesis: Outcomes by screening year and round. *Radiology.* 2020;295(2):285-293.

Craig M. *Essentials of Sonography and Patient Care.* 3rd ed. Elsevier; 2013.

Eastern Radiology Associates. *Dexascan.* ERA. Accessed August 4, 2022. www.erabillings.com/services/dexa/

Linn-Watson, T. *Radiographic Pathology.* 2nd ed. Lippincott Williams & Wilkins; 2014

Long BW, Rollins, JH, Smith BJ. *Merrill's Atlas of Radiographic Positioning and Procedures.* 13th ed., Vols 1-3. Mosby/Elsevier; 2016.

Medline Plus. *Pulmonary Ventilation/Perfusion Scan.* MedlinePlus; August 3, 2020. Accessed August 8, 2022. www.medlineplus.gov

National Association of Proton Therapy. *Find a Center Near You.* NAPT. Accessed August 13, 2022. www.proton-therapy.org

Nuclear Medicine Technology Certification Board. Accessed August 13, 2022. http://www.nmtcb.org.

Patel D, Weinberg BD, Hoch MJ. CT myelography: clinical indications and imaging findings. *RadioGraphics.* 2020;40(2):470-484. doi:10.1148/rg.2020190135

RadiologyInfo.org. *Bone Density Scan (DEXA or DXA).* April 15, 2022. Accessed August 4, 2022. www.radiologyinfo.org

RadiologyInfo.org. *Body CT.* June 15, 2020. Accessed August 8, 2022. www.radiologyinfo.org

Urology Care Foundation. *What is a Kidney (Renal) Nuclear Medicine Scan?* 2022. Accessed August 8, 2022. www.urologyhealth.org/urology-a-z

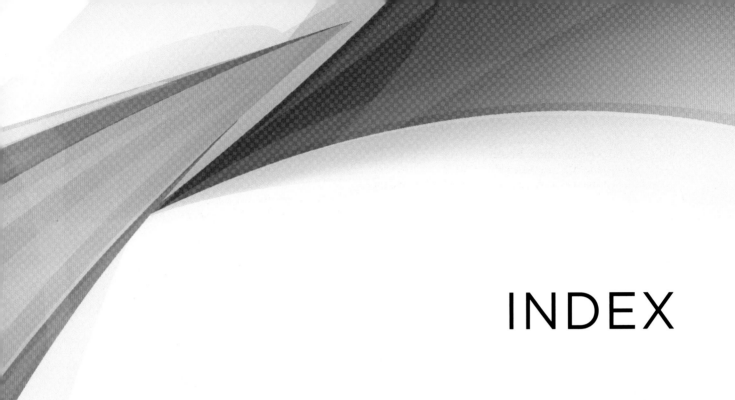

INDEX

Note: Locators followed by the letter '*f*' and '*t*' refers to figure and table respectively.